HEALTH AND WEALTH
ON THE BOSNIAN MARKET

HEALTH AND WEALTH

ON THE BOSNIAN MARKET

Intimate Debt

LARISA JAŠAREVIĆ

INDIANA UNIVERSITY PRESS

Bloomington & Indianapolis

Publication of this book was made possible, in part, by a grant from the First Book Subvention Program of the Association for Slavic, East European, and Eurasian Studies.

This book is a publication of

Indiana University Press
Office of Scholarly Publishing
Herman B Wells Library 350
1320 East 10th Street
Bloomington, Indiana 47405 USA

iupress.indiana.edu

The paper used in this publication meets the minimum requirements of the American National Standard for Information Sciences—Permanence of Paper for Printed Library Materials, ANSI Z39.48–1992.

Manufactured in the
United States of America

Library of Congress
Cataloging-in-Publication Data

Names: Jasarevic, Larisa, author.
Title: Health and wealth on the Bosnian market : intimate debt / Larisa Jasarevic.
Description: Bloomington : Indiana University Press, [2017] | Includes bibliographical references and index.
Identifiers: LCCN 2016038362 (print) | LCCN 2016051562 (ebook) (print) | LCCN 2016051562 (ebook) | ISBN 9780253023728 (cl : alk. paper) | ISBN 9780253023827 (pb : alk. paper) | ISBN 9780253023858 (eb)
Subjects: LCSH: Medical anthropology—Bosnia and Herzegovina. | Traditional medicine—Bosnia and Herzegovina. | Bosnians—Health and hygiene. | Bosnians—Social conditions—21st century. | Bosnians—Economic conditions—21st century.
Classification: LCC GN296.5.B54 J37 2017 (print) | LCC GN296.5.B54 (ebook) | DDC 306.4/610949742—dc23
LC record available at https://lccn.loc.gov/2016038362

1 2 3 4 5   22 21 20 19 18 17

CONTENTS

CONTENTS

ACKNOWLEDGMENTS

THANKING WILL NOT DO. THIS BOOK IS NOT A DONE DEAL, ALL packed and buttoned up for a final departure, so that I can thank so and so for helping me push it out the door. It is stuffed full of unsettled scores, open accounts, still sustaining or consequential encounters. To thank, I feel, would be to hasten the accounting of past transactions with hopes of squaring and closing them, or discounting them as definitive "gifts." Instead, I would rather take stock and acknowledge ("admit the existence or truth of; make notice of; express gratitude or appreciation," according to the Oxford English Dictionary) the vital, critical, nurturing, indebting, some daunting, contributions to the venture that became this text.

Judith Farquhar has always been my first reader. Inspiring, tactful, and conceptually unpredictable—hers were oracular interventions. Her own work on materialities, medicine, and salience of traditional metaphysics set an example for just how tightly the ethnographic can embrace the philosophical. Sue Gal, John Kelly, and Moishe Postone at the University of Chicago profoundly shaped this project in its initial years.

Friends were variously involved with the making of this text and the undoing of the author that such process entails. Larisa Kurtović, who restored the sense of the writing task too many times to count, and who also delivered vital staples at critical moments. George Meiu, who made us laugh, seriously. Caryn O'Connell, who kept me on a rich diet of words, words I could savor in my mouth, forever unstable in English, even when the meaning was flat.

Many colleagues, readers, and listeners—kind beyond measure— literally granted vital attention to what was too raw, too tentative, too awkward to have been thought of as text. I shall only list a few of them who lent ears at critical points: Tatiana Chudakova, Andrew Gilbert, Andy Graan, Chris Hann, Keith Hart, Jim Hevia, Azra Hromadžić, Stacey Kent, Owen Kohl, Aleks Prigozhin, Matt Rich, and Marko Živković.

Students who took part in the classes I taught over the years at the University of Chicago have no idea how substantially they changed what I had to say in the *Health and Wealth on the Bosnian Market.* I want to acknowledge the collective marvel that is the UoC undergraduate thinking body, though I can only list a handful of names: Yandy Alcala, Jennifer Cohen, Harry Backlund, Deniz Inal, Meltem Kaso, Sarah Mendelsohn, Michael Pierson, Myra Su, Laura Tong, Melisa Unver, and Treva Welsh.

Indiana University Press gave the manuscript a chance—who would have thought!—as did the anonymous reviewers, whose given time show how alive and well is the present, smack in the middle of the academic traffic. The field research was generously funded by the Advanced Research Fellowship of the American Councils Southeast European Research Scholar Program, and the Individual Research Opportunity Grant (IARO) of the International Research and Exchange Board (IREX), and the writing was comfortable thanks to a Mellon Dissertation Year Fellowship at the University of Chicago.

In Bosnia, people who shared their experiences; who let me into their market stalls, shops, cars, clinics, pharmacies; who invited me to their homes and gardens; fed me or worried that I did not eat; intervened in my health and wealth are the first to acknowledge. They were the many interlocutors, acquaintances, contacts, friends, thinkers, experimenters, medical practitioners, experts in the kitchen or in the field. Among them, some knew me before I wore an ethnographer's hat—we knew each other forever—while others and I were brought through the contingencies or logistics of fieldwork. Sandra, Melika, and Šejla made sure that returns were always, somehow, homecomings. My parents were mostly eager for this writing to end. Still, they have been most patient and most present (at a distance). They are as grounding to my being as all the many trees are to the orchard in which they live. My aunt, among the brightest spirits I know in Tuzla, was sometimes also a field guide or a buddy, especially on issues of domaće foods and medicine. My nieces are my trusted source of common sense and fashion advice. (And how do they laugh!) My brother-in-law has been kind and resourceful beyond belief—tending to save the day when obscure paperwork was missing, obtaining critical medicine seemingly nowhere to be found, and such. My sisters . . . if I were stranded on a desert island, I would bring nothing but the two of them, and this is sort of how it felt over the years of writing: stranded, insular, but, thank Goodness, with the two of them.

Acknowledging is a form of renewed indebting, and certain debts in Bosnia call for forgiving as often as settling. This I learned firsthand from my grandmother (*rahmet joj duši*) who overwhelmed me with offerings, and from whom I now regret not taking more, each and every gift ventured at our annual parting that I, stupidly, refused by pointing to my overfull suitcases. At a doorstep, seeing her guests out, she always asked to be forgiven (*halali*[1]): the unintended wrongs or too indulgent hosting. I too would ask all those acknowledged—and those unmentioned and unnamed—to forgive my slights if not my debts.

---

1. Unless otherwise noted, all translations are my own.

HEALTH AND WEALTH
ON THE BOSNIAN MARKET

Introduction

Oddly Bodily Lives in the Market

🌿 Waiting rooms of a home medical practice in a village of northeastern Bosnia fill up with patients every day except Tuesdays and Saturdays. Seventy to one hundred people hang about waiting—forgivingly—until they hear their names called out by the assistants. Some are obviously unwell, held up by their companions or propped up by the wall, slumping on the chairs, eyes shut, wearing bandages, gripping crutches, visibly tense, growing silent. There is nothing obviously the matter with others: a motley crowd of young and old, women, men, and children. Dressing styles, dialects, postures, and hairstyles are social clues, avidly read in a casual manner of resident experts who can hear, pick up, and tell apart salient differences in lifestyles and habits: provincial, regional, professional, urban, rural, refugee, or diasporic. Far less obvious are ethnic or national affiliations among patients who seek out this powerful woman's help from across ethnic and religious distinctions, and entity and state borders. Her patients call her the queen, a vernacular honorific that signals greatness and a streetwise "coolness," a mastery of some craft. From 2006 to 2007, this anthropologist was among the patients: waiting, observing, asking questions when allowed, taking notes, feeling painfully awkward at first, precariously admitted, challenged, tolerated, and mistrusted. Things changed over the years, as I kept visiting over the summers and felt more welcomed. I first heard of the queen at a flea market in the nearby town of Lukavac, economically depressed since the socialist, heavy-industry complex had shrunk to a few foreign-owned metallurgical coke and by-products factories that employ a fraction of the former labor force, export profits, and massively pollute the air.

Many of my regional ethnographic itineraries led from or to various market sites, where people trafficked in health complaints and medical recommendations as often as in produce, commodities, and second-life, second-hand goods. It was the only way to learn about the queen. She rarely appears in public. She will not speak to journalists. There are no commercial advertisements of her practice in the sorts of media that conveniently lead patients to the well-established or the emerging practitioners of alternative and traditional medicine in the region but that also, inevitably, make the readers suspicious: genuine healers and real doctors, it is commonly said, need no commercial advertising. Rather, they are found by word of mouth through support networks that spring up spontaneously in response to someone's medical problem or are actively mobilized through family and friends for the sake of someone ill. Reputation of medical practitioners is thus established through narratives of past encounters, told and rehearsed in evidence of their therapeutic efficacy or incompetence, with reference to personal narratives and health histories or with vaguer precision about what exactly happened to so-and-so. Real healers and genuine doctors are expected to practice an inherent gift, a curative talent that obliges them to lifelong, selfless service, without a price. They can, or rather, they ought to, be given gifts, however.

In the eventful space of the queen's practice, a corner of her desk attracts regular traffic in money and envelopes that patients drop off before leaving, and solicits the polite inattention of other patients and the queen's indifference even as she occasionally collects the bills into her wallet.

This book starts with one hugely popular, yet publicly invisible, home-based medical practice to unfold a number of ethnographic itineraries across places of exchange and bodily experience in post-socialist, post-conflict Bosnia. My writing gesture throughout is thus both itinerant and looping, as I investigate dispersed, quotidian ways in which the economic and bodily intersect but keep returning to recurrently significant or regularly visited places, such as the queen's, where money is missing or changes hands and where care, or the lack of, profoundly or minutely transforms visceral affairs, generates incomes, crashes hopes, renews appetites, restores vitality, and patches up or tears apart intimacies. It will soon become obvious that this is not a portrait of Bosnia usually found in scholarly, popular, or professional writings, although the writing climate is changing, new research projects are brewing, and excitingly different manuscripts have been recently published (Hromadzic 2015; Kurtovic 2012; Jansen, Brković, and Čelebčić 2016). At the risk of annoying at least the fellow scholars of the region who are rightly weary of many writerly promises to uncover the hidden, and hence more authentic Bosnian experience, so characteristic of texts and films in the wake of the Bosnian war, I suggest that *Health and Wealth on the Bosnian Market* traces connections that are not obvious, between places that have been simply overlooked, and speaks of issues that are shared across formal differences. Popular health, gifts and informal debts, medical and market experience may seem like themes irrelevant to the harsh realities of ethnonational identities and divisions, of traumatic memory, and yet, I will propose, they are woven into quotidian practices that are practically significant and, in a certain way, politically salient in their own right.

However, my project in this book is more ambitious still as I hope to start from Bosnia but venture propositions about bodies elsewhere, everywhere. In many ways, this book concerns this body of ours, supposedly so familiar and common, upon which everything hangs—including this writing and your reading—and whose nature is nothing if not uncertain, constantly undone and vigorously remade through so many practices and accidents involved in the oddly bodily lives we live. In order to speak of Bosnia I must estrange the notion of the human body as enclosed within its proper carnal interiority, a sovereign individuality set apart from others by the skin and, for as long as all is well, uncompromised by viral, microbial, toxic, technological, or too insistently intimate incursions. This ontological fantasy, so central to Western political and biomedical practice, does not materialize in Bosnia any more than it does in North America or anywhere else. I want to join the many productive interrogations of bodily materiality by emphasizing the oddly bodily ways in which contemporary economy is experienced and registered in Bosnia to the point where visceral and monetary, affective and promissory, abdominal and extensive, but intangible, are stirred up together. Anxiolytics, herbal remedies, or therapists' skillful hands are expected to meddle in and mend both domains while acts of generosity may amend both fiscal and visceral affairs. To make my point, I will start by parsing apart the therapeutic insights from exchange encounters only to return to their insistent intersections.

DRAWING PRECISION

The queen works on her patients with her hands, without touching, sometimes with her eyes alone, without meeting their gaze. She intervenes powerfully while preserving a distance. She examines them just as remotely and rather than ask about their symptoms or health histories, she gives them diagnoses and tells them whether or not she can help, what the treatments will entail, how often must they visit. Her diagnostic rubrics bundle together rather than neatly order symptoms, causes, and effects. Her responses hybridize biomedical and folk categories, personal dispositions and psychological disorders, environmental conditions and variously toxic materials, relational dynamics, and economic circumstances. Sometimes she issues a biomedical label or at least a working translation and with such a rubric sends them to health centers, laboratories, and clinics to request specific tests, biomedical images, or surgical procedures. Whatever her knowledge technologies, the queen's readings zoom in on an organ or a gland, an inflammation or a fracture; she estimates hormonal, cellular, and chemical imbalances; evaluates arterial blockages; sees malignant growths; takes heart rates; and estimates levels of blood pressure. But just as often she will excavate a detail from her patients' history or an object in their domestic inventory and invest it with etiological relevance. The accuracy of her readings tends to impress her visitors and anticipates the lab and clinical tests. Nonetheless, for all her references to the biomedical diagnostic lexicon, the connections that she draws between bodily points and pathological causes are not likely to be found in formally medical claims. The queen does not mimic biomedical science so much as develop several working translations between what she sees and knows and what may be formally discernible or technologically measurable.

Patient records in the queen's office are full of photographs and diagnostic images, which she doodles, especially on the first visit. One sketches a medical case from 2010 that the queen described as a treatment of an adrenal gland cyst. On a page of her archived patient record, a pen portrait of a right kidney sits next to the photo of a child in eye-catching, raspberry-red shoes, striking a boisterous pose sometime before hospitalization. "I saved her from bacteria in nine days," the queen says. The gland looks as if it has been ladled onto the organ, more voluminous and dripping a mass than in conventional anatomical representations, but is otherwise a true copy. Bacteria, not pictured in either representation, is the hidden actant working out a causal dissonance between buoyancy, health emergency, and exuberant innards, but it is the queen herself who is working out viscous, efficacious connections between and via the images and the two absent bodies—bacterial and human. Distance, detour, and deferral are necessary means to administer these intimate, therapeutic interventions effectively, whether the patients are in the office, stretched beneath her air-gliding hands and arms, or very far but within the grasp of her eyes, which see before the phenomenal and thus remotely present, across time zones and transnational spaces traversed by her patients from across Bosnia and ex-Yugoslavia, or by refugees, emigrants, and transnational labor migrants from Europe to America to Afghanistan to Australia. She is the medium for a sympathetic bond between copies and the objects copied, between her own, perceptual elasticity, and the internal organs' tissues, the girl's bodily being, and invisible bacteria. What she treats is not simply the pathological condition, caused by a generic encounter of some bacterial and anatomical forms, under who knows what circumstances that spell out the odds of someone developing an adrenal cyst. She treats this particular girl named Emina, her irreducible singularity reiterated with biographical detail—a date of birth and the parents' names.

Once, fondling a page with an illustration of a central nervous system in an anatomy atlas, the queen asked me: "Can you imagine, I see all of that? Except that I see it alive, and these are pictures of dead [organs]." A fantastic vision. Unlike the cadaverous stillness that founds biomedical anatomy, what the queen grasps are living organs, flows and currents, rising pressures, discharges and depletions, distensions and contractions, ongoing or obstructed exchanges—neurological, viral, bacterial, mineral—movements of heart, heart pumping, heart desirous, sometimes a pining heart, obsessive thoughts, excesses and lacks of everyday habits, tantrums, privations: in short, the inexhaustible repertoire of constantly particular, more widely familiar, because shared, states of what underlies being alive. Because it is the vital animacy, if not life itself, that the queen grasps, it is only appropriate that she grasps it remotely: life being no obvious object, but an intensity, a regenerative, disseminating force that is never by itself but corporeally elaborated, biographically complicated, socially implicated, and materially extended into the world, and, inevitably, overextended. Hence, neither disorders nor bodies can be fixed to a manageable number of references. The embodied animacy, I think, adds flourishes to anatomical depictions that the queen produces upon examining her patients. Images sometimes sprout rhizomic growths and leafy constellations rather than recognizable body parts. A tassel of squiggly threads depicted the torn-tissue state of one basketball player's leg; he complained of nagging and traveling pains, and the queen decided that his knees were as worn out as a soccer player's, his left meniscus was damaged, his pelvis imbalanced, and something was the matter with the 5th and 6th cervical vertebrae. But sports injuries in this clinic were not unrelated to the ways the basketball player otherwise played and lived: the queen interrogated about his fall as well as about his current intimate relationship and noncommittal habits (which he denied). One's passions and dispositions, everyday habits and recurrent frustrations, one's living arrangements and familial relations, have everything to do with health and illness. The queen tends to put it very bluntly, to the patient's face, provoking them to contemplate, to change. She is particularly harsh on women who, as she puts it, "neglect themselves": they dress carelessly, age prematurely, and are otherwise excessively generous, selflessly caring for everyone else's well-being but their own. In Bosnia more generally, one's appearances are scrutinized for clues about how well one is doing and these are freely commented on. You need not complain about feeling under the weather: your messy hairdo, wrinkled shirt, careless outfits, unshaven or pale face, sunken cheeks or a new weight-gain, or finally something about your eyes and gazes, will raise concerns, inspire inquiries, and prompt much advice as to what to do for the symptoms, how to handle the problems, should you care to share them, and more generally, how "to take care of yourself" (*pozabavi se sobom, čuvaj se*) or how "to order yourself" (*sredi se*). A long-term patient of the queen's, treated for cancer and recurrent malignant growths, reported among her health improvements an apparently curious development: she no longer cleans the house obsessively, she said, nor does she starch the decorative embroidery. Along these lines, the queen has little patience for overly anxious parents who meddle into their children's lives or spouses and lovers who are too jealous, controlling, nitpicking, emotionally or sexually stingy—all of these excesses and dispositions are within the realm of her therapeutic practice. She treats illnesses that are literally physical and affective manifestations of relational dynamics. Both illness and its treatment emerge in an always unique constellation of a specific physical composition and the subject's dispositions, these existential circumstances or that accident, some random or medicinal ingredient. This is why the queen repeats that no two women are alike, no two illnesses ever the same. She resists all of her patients' (or the anthropologist's) attempts to solicit generic advice on how to live or care for health.

LIVELY EXTENSIONS

The queen worked on the girl I call Emina, grasping an image of Emina's right kidney adrenal gland long before meeting her, at the frantic request of her parents whose little girl was hospitalized. Between the queen and the patient there were, first of all, anxious kin and the child's photo, which were the material resources—photographic as much as familial—from which the queen drew the anatomical image. The queen's body is not the only one elastic in this etiology; rather, everyone's flesh is radically unstable, distended onto and accessible via people, objects, and substances to which it is related. Emina's images were at once diagnostic and therapeutic: they made palpable the difference between a copy and the organic original, between a child's trace and parental presence, and rendered effectively traversable the distance between the queen's body and the girl's. Images, situated within the biographical details of birth dates, names of parents, children, and spouses, initiate access to present extensions of the absent patients. It often happens that people approach the queen with requests on behalf of their intimates who are too sick or too far away to visit. The remote contact works better still when mediated with another technology of remote contact: on the phone, the queen picks up people's voice timbre, the fleshly rhythm of their breathing-speaking, the sense of their mouthed event of being at once here with her and elsewhere, neither properly here nor there, and she works through and beyond the speaker-receiver, claiming, moreover, a synesthetic grasp: working on the phone she sees blotches of what her interlocutors see on the other end of the phone line. Similarly, Skyping with a patient, she plugs in, VoIP, voice over Internet, into their digitalized vocal and visual vitality, putting a different spin onto the classic Skype advertisement about "a whole new world of staying in touch." Finally, photos and posts of her Facebook friends serve both as medical and social media: messages, questions, and updates issue alarms, as often as greetings or gratitude—"Help, sweet queen, I am unwell!" or "Hello, beautiful. Am I having a reaction to your treatment or what is the matter with me?" And reassurances, diagnoses, and dietary and medicinal instructions travel back to them, in a two-way traffic of Facebook messages behind the public busyness of the wallpaper, posts, and announcements. The queen and her friends keep her Facebook page fresh: some post poetry devoted to the queen, with heart signs and pixelated flower bouquets, someone once crocheted her photoshopped portraits onto elaborate backgrounds, floral and dense, with swirling stars and bursting rainbows. They "like" her looks and posts, praise her powers and generosity, and wish her all the world's goodness.

Whatever it is that the queen does with some sense attuned to a telephonic or Skyped voice, to the sonic, digital, virtual index of a breathing, singular being on the other side, and however it is that she works through the visually stuffed Internet domain of being social, she affects a workable tactile extensity and dilated relation. She also stretches our commonsense of being in touch and being together. Thus flexed, we are in the good company of Jean-Luc Nancy, a devoted thinker of touching at a distance, and Jacques Derrida who reads closely, rather tenderly, Nancy's corpus on touching (Nancy 2000, 2008a, 2008b; Derrida 2005). Nancy blows our mind, for as long as we are fantasizing about intimate closeness and some uncomplicated familial or communal belonging, he shows again and again that touching always presumes and preserves distance. Take hold of a skin, for instance, and all you have within your grasp is the surface of a flesh, your own or another's, and the more you press, the more reassuring the sensuous feel of a skin against a skin, the more voluptuous is the hollow your hand claps, sensing as it does the promising yet receding, elusive more or rest of you. Groping, I never get a hold of wherever you are disseminated beyond these points that I am hurriedly nipping, frustrated and doomed, unless I come to terms with the proposition that one is most intimately here in departures (Nancy 2008a:37). And I am just as untenable: feeling myself on the outside, darting the skin, while intuiting that I am no more there than someplace deep within. Touching always touches the surface, but superficiality is not an envelope of some primary interiority wherein lies the buried subject. Rather, the subject is extended, point by point, each a limit to appropriation, preserving the singularity against the ambitions of subsuming one into another, into the identity of one and the same. Moreover, touching is an encounter between the tangible, fleshly medium, the untouchable sense that gets prodded, and the least locatable of all, the sensibility that picks up the other senses sensing, and which Nancy will not shut in, within a mind, a gut, or an inward psyche. The intangible extensity of sensing, thinking, and affecting spreads the body far out into the open: bodies are open spaces of existence, each specific and placed (15). Put simply, by thinking through the impossibilities of grasping, once and for all, and by thinking through layering of subjective presence and its dissemination along the embodied surfaces and beyond, Nancy is venturing a theory of bodies without essence—unbound by skin, unfixed in place—and of subjects that exist only through extensions and, inevitably, relations that never subsume them.

At a shorter distance, Derrida attends to the visual tactility of eyes and gazes. Interlocking eyes focus on what is visible and watching, the organic, retinal, phenomenal, while ever on the alert for the invisible gazes, pre-phenomenal but perceptible, though imprecise, and consequential. Similarly with reading, Derrida suggests, there is the *aporia* between a visible word and the intangible but discernible sense it evokes. In between the untouchable and touchable is "the very heart of the flesh," Derrida adds, where the "originary intrusion" of technics takes place: visible, audible word (2005:113). Voice, like eyes, touches at a distance. Breath to mouth to air, dispersing, to ear, collecting, a mouth to receiver, to wire or cordless network, converting and routing. What Derrida calls "telephonic caresses" between those separated but connected, depend on ears that listen for but do not alone sense the other. Rather, he writes, a communication hinges on the "telephonic memory of a touch" (112). For Derrida, this is a phantasm without which conversation might convey information but would not effectively put in touch, if touch is on the order of striking or ecstatic, smacking of sensuous pleasure whose possibility a phone conversation excites, and except for the invocation—and the specters that respond—misses. What is delivered "across the cordless cord of these entwined voices" is the "ecotechnics of other bodies" (112–113). To Nancy and Derrida, contact takes place between inviolable singularities that are, nevertheless, thoroughly interrupted and inextricably related to each other and to each other's technics.

However, the queen's bodies require us to flex the philosophical imagination beyond what may be comfortable to the post-foundational, post-structuralist thought on the body that, ultimately, leads to political hopes for some particularly resilient collectives that always preserve singularity and intense connection that never compromise with lasting, demanding commitments. On the phone or over Skype, the queen makes out, part to the whole, the real-time singularity of the other: not only a particular bodily being, tangible-intangible, but the state of its current disorder, which changes constantly and variously, including under her influences. She is asked to intervene, and when she does there ensue vital exchanges between bodies, affects, capacities, and thoughts that are unpredictable, often unpleasant, and substantially alter all parties in contact.

The queen's working worlds might be Nancy nightmares, or what he calls the *immunditia* or the underworld: messy, "clogged," wanton, where space between the bodies gets abolished, where bodies as spaces-places are pressed to each other too closely to bear, causing pain, inflammation, itchy outbreaks, discharges, "in a promiscuity thick with microbes, pollutions, defective serums, excessive fat, and grinding nerves" (2008a:105). The queen's working worlds are of contagious contiguity, of contact that, invited, tactlessly crosses the limits, disrupts, makes substantial, experiential difference and lasting carnal or lifestyle changes and all precisely on the account of bodily superficiality and extensions. Nancy's writing on immundita starts ominously: "Touchings are infected, places are just so many spasms, rubbings, viral and bacterial swirls, gasolating bodies" and spirals down to an image of a disaster: "an overpopulation of acidic, ionized psyches, bristling with the blind signals of a world of bodies in which bodies, identically, decompose the world" (ibid.). The viscous proximity, contagious intimacy, and operative tactility are too alarming ("bristling"), distasteful perhaps ("gasolating"), and politically pernicious ("blind signals," "decompose the world") for the philosopher of the *Corpus*. In Bosnia, close proximities are the most immediate routes to securing health and wealth: life-saving, emotionally sustaining, and yet often also pressing in ways that are neither benign nor salvific.

Derrida's reading, however, already takes Nancy's thought in some other directions, where bodily extensity is promiscuous and indeterminately consequential. Ecotechnics speaks to the entwining of human and technology that are originary. This is a starting point for many contemporary voices committed to including all kinds of things, technical devices, and actants in the constitution of a human that is also always more than human (Braun and Whatmore 2010). For some, a scholarly lingering on the issues of the human body is theoretically and politically nostalgic, since biotechnologies, cyborgian accessories, sped-up temporalities, and virtual spaces, pop cultures, and queer subcultures have already moved us post-human (Halberstam and Livingston 1995). To my ethnographic eyes, the post-human move seems too hasty given how much wellness and illness preoccupies people, not only in Bosnia. Post-humanism is also ethically untenable for a book that is concerned with the shared object of bodily suffering, which is the post-socialist market. Moreover, the Bosnian history of genocidal violence and the ongoing exhumation of the war missing will not allow us to denounce the human and not least because, usually, debunking the human first of all presumes stripping down all the differences (biographical, cultural, ethnic, religious) to get to the bottom line of the universal humanity. The stripping down is unnervingly similar across these gestures—genocidal, militant and post-human, theoretical. Rather, I find allies among theorists who rework our sense of a human by pluralizing imaginable bodily ontologies as well as our political and medical epistemologies.

Lock and Farquhar, for instance, invite us to consider lived and historical worlds of material bodies that undermine classic scholarly tendencies to distinguish between subject and object, textual and real, cultural and natural. They emphasize an interlocking of four terms that are also key to this project: materiality, embodiment, experience, and practice. None of these elements is fixed nor found prior to the situated encounter that stirs up the vital dynamic of being a body in relation to the world, exercising historical appetites and new skills, encountering the material surroundings that substantially make up what and how one feels. If embodiment is contingent and experience effectively trans/formative and if the world is populated by multiple bodies that biomedical reference to the normative universal ("the body proper") cannot accurately anticipate let alone claim to define or treat authoritatively, then it follows that we ought to similarly pluralize our range of medical knowledges and diversify what effectively constitutes a therapeutic practice.

This is a point that Stacey Alaimo (2010) also makes, concerned as she is with bodily natures and illness experiences that demand "more capacious epistemologies" and that allow ethical and political positions more responsive to the realities of the twenty-first century. Alaimo writes about environmental illnesses and multiple chemical sensitivities, disorders that not only challenge the biomedical reason but also radically question the common sense by which we live within the industrialized environments of convenience technologies whose basic ingredients—dryer sheets, processed foods, emulsifiers, pesticides, heavy metals—require scrutiny for unintended animacy of xenobiotics and toxins, traces that wreak havoc on some bodies. The embrace of bodies and toxic environments suggests that the human is thoroughly enmeshed in the material world and that, as Mel Chen puts it, the question becomes how any bodies can sustain "the fiction of independence and uninterruptability" (2012:199). Alaimo proposes the concept of trans-corporeality to register the contiguity between material natures, be they human or not, and the exchange of influences across surfaces whose traffic is often uncomfortable, unpredictable, and unwanted (2, 14–15).

Thinking through oddly bodily lives draws attention to the ordinarily strange materiality, extensity, and animacy of the bodies, the kind of vitality that is uncontained, worked up irresistibly through bodies' contact with so much else, potentially everyone and everything else; caught up, indecently, inconveniently, in the wider social environment with rippling implications for subjective and collective experience; for visceral, medical, and economic matters. Oddly bodily also gives room to some extraordinary experiences that are had not by the virtue of a retreat from the everyday but, on the contrary, are in the midst of concrete dwellings of post-socialist urban and provincial landscapes: around a kitchen table, in the waiting rooms, in a supermarket, in fleshly readings of death notices posted on town squares, at a hairdresser's, outside one's window on the seventeenth floor of a crumbling apartment block. It gives room to considering medical interventions and rituals that require impressive, occult skills of experts, be they medical professionals, families' designated cooks, or unlicensed practitioners of healing arts, as well as relying on responsiveness of bodies whose imaginative and visceral potentials are infinitely varied and unanticipated. Oddly bodily gives room to the generativity of shared experience and thinks it by moving from ethnographic situations and propositions to philosophical speculations, and to Nancy's in particular. Finally, or first of all, oddly bodily rehearses, descriptively and analytically, a sense picked up while in the field, that bodies and illnesses have changed since the war and the peace and have been unstable ever since, becoming ever more vulnerable, more responsive, and insistently threatened: by some strange new illnesses, by some old maladies that once were safely relegated to folk superstitions, by premature deaths and evidence of generally poor health, by the pervasive spread of the new market as much as by the explosion of commercial magic. What I picked up is a vernacular sense of bodies' historical metamorphism, a sense that also practically orients therapeutic treatments, be they traditional, revamped, alternative, or domestic. Because bodies are historically metamorphing, the authority of clinical medicine is compromised not only by suspicions of professionals' corruption and negligence but also more profoundly, by evidence that medical science and its diagnostic and treatment technologies cannot effectively keep up with shifts in medical objects—patients bodies, signs and conditions of illness and wellness.

MEDICAL ITINERARIES

The queen is a powerful figure in the new medical milieu whose influence has been silently growing for almost two decades across Bosnia and the greater post-Yugoslav sphere, including across transnational, diasporic networks. People usually arrive at the queen's at the recommendation of someone they trust or someone who, upon hearing them complain of a medical problem, has persuaded them with sufficient evidence—whom has she treated for what, how she cured them and how fast, is she for real, and what does she charge—that they should give the treatment a try. It takes a complicated health complaint to send someone traveling widely in pursuit of care and beyond the first, obvious consultations with the local pharmacy, health centers, private practices, and regional clinics, or with those among friends and family who are properly versed in herbal medicine and medicinal meals. It takes a complaint that is urgent or desperate, that describes a condition which is persistent or stubbornly resistant to various therapeutic interventions. Such complaints are regularly and fervently rehearsed for the sake of concerned intimates and strangers one meets at the typical points of public convergence—in the markets and shops, in pharmacies and health offices, on public transportation—and yet their airing, as well as the advice they earn, hinges on subtle cues that solicit speaking of matters that strike some ears as incredible or that risk to portray the speaker as gullible or superstitious. Some such complaints turn into exemplary narratives of persuasion, used by all those familiar with the medical case—the family, friends, colleagues, and neighbors familiar with the medical case—for one's health in Bosnia is rarely a private affair.

Socialist Yugoslav medicine effectively spread general health-care coverage through a network of public health facilities, pharmacies, village outposts, and regional clinics and taught values of scientific materialism and secular modernity through lessons about hygiene, public health, and dietary tastes (not least for industrial and convenient foods).

Nonetheless, forms of healing and magic-making have also been practiced on the margins of scientific socialism, just as herbal medicine and homemade (*domaće*) remedies referenced a long folk tradition, collected in volumes of venerable folk herbalists (Sadiković 1988; Mijatović 1982; Pelagić [1888] 2008), while cosmopolitan practices of self-care and holistic medicine have entertained urban imaginations since at least the 1980s. Multiplication of imaginable medical directions and indirections is both rather new and different. Privatization of medical and pharmaceutical care and the impoverishment of the public health system, which in Bosnia remains large and supported by comprehensive health coverage, have not only brought about a crisis of trust and access, as in so many post-socialist contexts, but have also submitted biomedical, pharmaceutical, clinical, and professional authority to new scrutiny on the basis of criteria used to evaluate all therapeutic claims: efficacy and price. Health in Bosnia is less than ever an exclusive domain of licensed professionals. In a reversal of the very logic that Isabelle Stengers (2003) proposes foundationally differentiates modern medicine from various medical traditions and charlatans (that have historically stalked it with competing claims to efficacy), the question relevant to health seekers in contemporary Bosnia is whether a remedy is "curing" rather than whether it is backed by clinical trials (see chapter 4). In other words, the new medical milieu is inseparable from epistemological and ontological shifts in the ways of being a body, knowing a body, and feeling with and through the body (see Pedersen 2011).

It is a fabulously dense new medical field, expansive and expensive, treacherous, teeming with invitations, solemn recommendations, with traditions, sometimes strangely revamped or repurposed, and with never-before-heard-of treatment technologies. Everyone is weary of cheats, many are suspicious of advertisements that circulate on television and radio and in the mainstream newspapers and specialized magazines dedicated to health, folk and herbal medicine, and alternative lifestyles, though these ads often seem the best place to start (see chapter 4). This field calls for pedestrian strategies of traveling, trying, asking, listening, wondering, doubting, complaining, and, most of all, waiting and detouring. At each stop of the popular medical itineraries, one arrives at a new constellation of possibilities.

Seeking medical attention in public health facilities, and seeking specialist consultations in particular, entails collecting precious paperwork at multiple, confusing sites of primary care and family medicine, including referrals to clinical departments, to diagnostic units, and to laboratories. For those fortunate enough to have them, intimate connections (*veze*) work behind doors to facilitate appointments and sidestep the waiting process. Others are left waiting, frustrated, exhausted, hurting, dejected, impatient, in pain, scared, slumping, pacing, going out for a smoke, joking at each other's expense, hushing up children, shadowing or comforting the injured and the elderly, and occupying various nodes in the time and space ordered by the logistics of bodies and health cards and by the more opaque arrangements made by administrators, nurses, doctors, and other patients, including those better connected with the staff or more familiar with the system. A man whose veze used to spread effectively across Tuzla health centers and clinics and who was thus asked to manage health appointments and itineraries of his extended family, friends, and friends' family and friends, and whom I saw breeze through health centers and clinical units in 2006, told me: "That's how it's done. Everyone has someone." "What about those people waiting?" I asked. "Well, they are waiting for the order" (*oni čekaju red*), Mrki responded, leaning on the plural meaning of the word *red* as a waiting line, a procedural order, and, more generally, a social and moral sort of order. Waiting is formally organized through prior appointments, submission of health cards and referral forms at the reception window, and preferred access granted to emergency cases, families of war martyrs, war veterans, and veteran blood donors. In fact, waiting translates to joining a mass of well over a hundred people at some clinical units and health center laboratories, without knowing exactly where to submit your health card, where to expect your name to be called, whether it will be audible, how to signal your presence or flag someone's attention to your appointment time, to your special-access privileges, or to circumstances that make your case an exception. You learn how to know if you are waiting at the right unit, are assigned a doctor, and whether he is on duty or elsewhere, and what seems to work in a given context: waiting patiently on the fringes or right by the doctor's door, appealing to a nurse, or staying on guard for other people's attempts to cut into the line. Everyone suspects that presents to the health staff circulate secretly, as envelopes stuffed with bills or as more openly concealed gifts in decorative gift bags that one sees moving in and out of doctors' and nurses' offices. Tagging at different strings of the Bosnian cultural habit of generosity, alms-seekers who tend to be children, often Roma, or adults with exposed disabilities or injuries stalk clinical corridors regularly, asking for *sadaka* (Turkism, from Arabic *sadaqa*, translates to mercy, alms, and merit), an exercise of monetary gift giving that is always prospectively charged but especially so by the context and the seekers' wishful words: "may sadaka save you, and save all your dear ones." People respond with change, perhaps more eagerly then elsewhere, more forgiving of the vocational begging, prompted by the request of a gift, which is presumed to engender non-monetary surpluses that can redistribute fortunes and reorder health.

Gifts to the professionals, however, are also complicated and productive of generosities and surpluses, despite the extortionary circumstances of their being given and taken within the public health-care institutions. Money is not the principle currency here[1] and it is rarely a matter that settles the accounts between the parties, since a medical encounter is not so much a transaction as a moment brought through a contingently composed web of differently concerned and variously related, sometimes through intermediaries unknown to each other, characters (see Rivkin-Fish 2005). One can be left with no one obvious to pay or extend a gift, but might feel obliged and indebted in a convoluted way that leaves one with no means of responding graciously.

Waiting in the public health facilities calls for suspended subjects with no other options, nothing left to do, no pressing claims, confident in the workings of the system or compliant with its temporalities, procedures, and ambiguities. In fact, it generates an agitated mass, bodies on the edge, breaking up the lines, asking obvious questions, pushing and clustering, smelling, itching, shouting, insisting, going with the flow, hoping for a diagnosis, solution, an end or an exit, exploding, issuing protest and insults. "You horse!" one woman blurted, closing behind her a door to a doctor's office in the regional clinical center. Such waiting affects are anticipated in a sign posted on a door of a cardiovascular unit:

WARNING NOTICE!!!
Patients and their company are not allowed to:
Disrupt order by quarreling, shouting, or behaving rudely;
Maltreat or physically attack others, provoke a fight or behave in any other
manner that is threatening or causes disquiet [*uznemirenost*].

This biopolitical regime has clearly come to terms with the unspooling of its subtle powers to arrange the logistics by means of spatial clues and bureaucratic records or to anticipate compliance with prior lessons on respectful conduct. The sign is not a pedagogical device so much as a stern warning, published in the wake of past transgressions, a sole paperweight against the structural conditions of possibility, brewing discontent.

Waiting in the public health facilities, however, also mobilizes people more quietly around practical issues: What to do, under the circumstances? Patients and their company bond and swap histories of illness; interpret each other's symptoms, diagnoses, and tests; jointly complain or recommend patience—someone whispers to the woman who departed the doctor's office calling him a horse, to be sensible, for her own sake—evaluate particular practitioners and medicines, and generally rely on each other to negotiate the given order. Sometimes, these are sources of good advice, as they indicate which paperwork is essential and where to get it; other times these conversations are practically useless to a particular listener as they rehearse strategies that have already been tried or that recommend treatments that one suspects will fail or that show clearly a speaker's limited knowledge. For those who care to engage, the waiting encounter becomes a give-and-take of leads on treatment strategies, on private practitioners and alternatives to clinical and pharmaceutical medicine, and on home treatments with herbal medicine, homemade recipes, and folk and dietary remedies.

Formal medical facilities variously inspire onward journeys, most obviously to pharmacies. Pharmacies, especially in small towns, are similarly not grounds of brief and straightforward transactions but provide intensely social occasions to make other people's health issues one's own business, while waiting your turn, to learn about illnesses and remedies and about professional mishaps and therapeutic miracles. From across the counter of one provincial town pharmacy, I observed time and again how most prosaically physical details and inconvenient bodily flaws are laid out for the pharmacists and others to hear and ponder. Since prescriptions are often filled on behalf of others—grandparents, spouses, children, neighbors—distant bodies, not just one's own, are exposed in collective examination. Circumstantial intimacy rather than privacy marks these therapeutic settings. Pharmacists' advice is collectively heard and open to commentary and questions by the general public: Could they repeat what that medicine was good for? Do they know of an herbal substitute? How to match diuretics and blood pressure medicine? The intimacies here can be tender, as in the informal address between pharmacists and patients (grandma, doll, sister, friend) or the kind that push uncomfortably close, elbows into ribs.

A trip to a pharmacy or a market may swing you by some treatment opportunities. Say, Dr. A.'s. He parks his mobile pharmacy on the grounds or just outside the open-air weekly markets across Tuzla region. Speakers blast a crackling advertisement of "traditional Tibetan medicine," drawing attention to the display of tonics, tea mixtures, and creams. Most intriguing, however, is the tentacled, button-laden device that promises a hassle-free, comprehensive diagnosis, which Dr. A. uses with a playfulness and a vaguely stated authority of his alleged apprenticeship in Tibet. He is a charming cheat, ready to cure for a bargain, willing to negotiate further discounts. It would take more concerted efforts at seeking help to find another Dr. Ahmed, working in a smart clinic on the outskirts of a provincial town. This one cannot be caught fumbling for explanations of his training, expertise, or equipment. Elegant, eloquent, and effortlessly charismatic, he runs a rare establishment, not least because it is taxable, state-registered, with neat patient histories collected and kept by professional nurses. Dr. Ahmed's "natural and spiritual medicine" calmly translates across the idioms of Islamic medicine and psychiatry, technologically savvy energy medicine and remote healing by hands and gazes, without touching. His handsome image travels widely and frequently on pages of *Aura*, a hybrid genre for alternative medicine and newsworthy curiosities from divergent registers, from occult interferences to skin issues, and he is known to offer a reasonable price, discounts for seniors, and free treatment for children.

Other routes turn you up at much different therapeutic settings. The expectations for a genuine practice—genuinely generous and gifted—

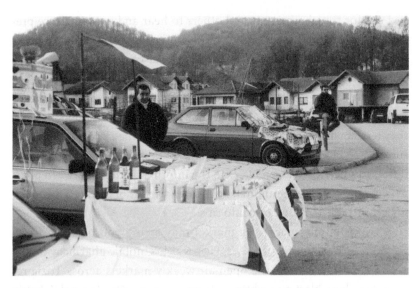

Figure 0.1. Dr. A.'s mobile pharmacy. *Photograph by the author*

are especially high in the case of *strava*, as this is traditionally the domain of wise, elderly women in the neighborhood, whose hands are endowed with remarkable powers but are, nonetheless, primarily occupied with kneading the proverbial bread and nurturing a family, keeping a home, and working the land. Moreover, strava manipulates lead and water and with suras of the Koran and with *dove* (supplications; see chapters 5 and 7) whose potency very much depends on the women's receptivity/near-ness to the ultimate source of Mercy, which requires rootedness in the Islamic practice of praying, remembrance (*zikr*), and proper conduct. As I show in chapter 5, finding a genuine strava practitioner, however, can be equally difficult and confounding.

By traveling, this book approaches medicine sideways. It affords a wandering perspective that comes at the heels of the health travelers, following their movement across medical establishments, asking where itineraries begin, whether they ever end, and how people get ideas of where to go and what to do, especially given the conflicting advice, the repeated failures, and the prohibitive prices of therapeutic remedies and trials. Medicine emerges as a broad domain, daunting and shift-ing, always navigated with the concerned, sometimes unsolicited, help of others who share their own well-trodden, convoluted, resourceful, and exasperating cure-seeking routes. Looking sideways affords insight into how economies that underwrite medical encounters intertwine, as well as how expectations and values are extended from other, seemingly unrelated sites of exchange of money, commodities, or gifts. Following the itinerant logics of practice, I do not privilege the sites of professional medicine, public and private health offices and clinics, as the proper reference point against which all other therapeutic repertoires emerge as "alternatives," global fads or folk practices the resurgence of which has to be somehow explained by means of a cultural logic of sorts. Rather, multiple therapeutic repertoires are not explicable solely by post-social-ist, post-conflict, or global traumas or dis/enchantments but, I propose, have also to take into account the convergence of experiential evidence: of changing bodies and of shifting limits and possibilities of variously medical claims. Finally, this lateral move seeks and stumbles upon un-expected vantage points to foreground the questions of bodily material-ity and medical efficacy, thus allowing the pathways of popular health pursuits to redefine what health and illness mean, what makes a medical practice relevant, where and how a body is implicated in the world, and how it works and ails.

BODILY ECONOMIES

I went to the field in 2006 to study the pervasive spread of informal lend-ing and borrowing and stumbled upon evidence that the economic and bodily were contiguous domains. When, for instance, I asked people how their work was going, they often presented me with the contents of their purses or pockets, stuffed with pharmaceuticals or herbal or di-etary supplements. When traders took stock of daily losses or when my interlocutors openly fretted over looming loan repayments, they would predictably cap their accounting of negative numbers with a seemingly unrelated comment, sounding anxious, obligatory, heartfelt or half-hearted: "but [all is well] as long as there is health," or "but [never mind] so far as one's healthy" (*ma dok je zdravlja . . . , ma nek je samo zdravlja, ma nek se zdravo*). Does health hinge on sales or debts? I eventually won-dered, and if so, how? Where do economic forms end and bodily points begin? How are their various intersections—monthly repayments rubbing against one's embodied rhythms, budgetary contractions sharpening appetites and tightening the possibilities, employment prospects brightening, or retirement checks stalling or slimming—felt and handled, and with what consequences?

Critical thought has long worried about the snug embrace of life and capital, sensuous experience and mass commodities, about co-productions of subjectivities and historical realities. Divergent theories of mediation, alienation, or overdetermination are the staple of cultural and political economies, be they concerned with classic sites of production, circulation, and advertisement or places of cutting-edge technological innovation and financial speculation (Mazzarella 2003; Miyazaki 2009; Rajan 2006, 2012). Grateful for the politically salient inquiries that these texts are sustaining but attuned to some local lives for whose etiologies and ontologies critical theories did not prepare me, I profess different interests, interests that are somewhat literal-minded. I wonder how might we think of bodies as extended with the new market? And if so consequentially and contiguously extended, what kinds of things, then, are bodies? What are the economic matters if they are effectively managed with therapeutic regiments, if they are evaluated by the looks of one's skin or anticipated and prodded by techniques that seem principally to stir guts, cleanse embodied fears, soothe psyche or soul, anticipate affairs of the heart, and reorient dispositions toward sharing or giving or forgiving? What is such a bodily being in the market?

To raise an ontological question about the nature of being, Nancy argues, "does not mean we have to leave the realm of economics and sickness, any more than we have to abandon the order of *praxis*. On the contrary . . . this question is simply that of what is called 'capital,' and even the question of 'history,' and 'politics.' 'Ontology' does not occur at the level reserved for principles, a level that is withdrawn, speculative, and altogether abstract. Its name means the thinking of existence" (2000:46–47). Nancy's argument is worded defensively, and although anthropology as of late is enjoying an "ontological turn" (see Langwick 2011; Pedersen 2011; Kohn 2015), I join Nancy's tone as much as his argument, trained as I am in cosmopolitan lessons of critical theory and in the Yugoslav pedagogies of historical materialism, which underpinned my education through the mid-1990s. I anticipate objections that my points are divorced from the realities of global capital, its systemic temporalities and historical dynamics that render Bosnia, as a matter of course, open to violent dispossession and evacuations of productive capital, and that my interests are irrelevant to the political questions of what would be a just, more proper alternative to the transitional policies, neoliberal solutions, and the regional entrepreneurial alliances of politics, crime, and business. Perhaps it's true; I can do no more than perform an academic exercise of saying something counterintuitive and add in a tried anthropological trick of staying close to some situated commonsense while suggesting that the critiques of global capitalism cannot be radical enough if our imagination of its efficacies is kept on the strict diet of a disenchanted, scientific, bodily materialism. Hence, I proceed to think existence by reading Nancy as a found, strangely coincident theoretical complement to my interlocutors' cues and propositions about riotous corporeality underskirting market and medicine, health and wealth.

In an economy marked by mass unemployment or informal and intermittent income opportunities, where salaried employment and state pensions were regularly lower than the cited estimates of monthly expenditures on subsistence, nothing can be taken for granted: neither food nor clothing needs, neither essential medical supplies nor a settlement of heating bills. Bosnia, next to Kosovo, has been consistently ranked among the poorest countries in southeast Europe. As elsewhere in the formerly socialist East, economic uncertainties have been folded into the structural logic of "transition" by means of hasty privatization and "primitive accumulation," by fervent neoliberalization of the markets and deregulation of foreign investment. The usual stories of postsocialist crony capitalism regularly fill the newspapers in the Bosnian-Serbian-Croatian language with exposés that, time and again, trace genealogies of new capital to the bloody grounds of frontlines and war crimes, humanitarian corridors and arms traffic. Contemporary scandals also make obvious that the ongoing plunder of public resources in the public eye, whether perfectly legal or legally fuzzy, more or less hides shady promiscuities of bureaucratic and brute power that cushion the electorally secured posts of elite alliances. The sheer weight of the new Bosnian state's administration, whose massive troops have much to do with the constitutional safeguarding of the three ethno-national communities' interests, is inflating public taxation, exhausting the bloated budget, and, steadily generating budgetary deficits. Put simply, in the Muslim-Croat Federation of the Bosnian two-entity state that was the geographical focus of my ethnographic travels, not even those dependent on the federal budget could count on their salaries and pensions being regularly paid.

On the other hand, the felt textures of the rough economic reality, which people were "merely surviving" (*jedva preživljavamo; samo preživljavanje, baš preživljavanje*), are met with historically minded sensibilities whose benchmark is no "bare life" but, rather, a "better life" (*bolji život*): life as remembered through the iconic events of splendid consumption, as recorded in the archives of family accounting books, promised and aspired to, always almost tenable during Yugoslav socialism. As I show in chapter 1, quotidian complaints about mere surviving register not so much the wartime surviving as the "better life" that was commonly expected to materialize after the end of the Bosnian war. The 1992–1995 war is often conceived of as a historical exception that suspended the telos of socialist biographies between two proper horizons of possibility. While the year of 1995 has come to mark both the end of the war with the signing of the Dayton Peace Agreement and the beginning of a routinized, peacetime struggle for existence under the conditions of post-socialist, post-conflict uncertainty, bodily habits of consuming, computing, spending, and giving are involuntarily or self-consciously rehearsing older lessons of what makes a life good, beautiful, and worth living. The economic instrument of "minimal consumer basket" (*minimalna potrošačka korpa*) used across the region to statistically grasp household consumption against the index of changing consumer prices, essential caloric values, and basic human needs does not capture the contents of purchases made or omitted any more than it appreciates the historical adornment of the essential expenditures on people's shopping lists: not just food but a rich birthday cake, baked on borrowed funds; not just clothing but monthly sewing classes for a teenage daughter with a fine sense of fashion and worrisome tendencies toward depression; not just meeting winter heating bills but affording summer vacations by the seaside, which the socialist history of leisure hailed as restorative (see chapters 1 and 2).

Ever since the war ended, the quotidian is regularly interrupted by monetary emergencies and intersected by things, and these contacts are fleshly. Skin-deep, at times, as when a trader is fondling displayed goods absentmindedly, unsticking the urban dust and smog that are attracted more duly to the plastic, shimmering, faux-furred surfaces than are the eyes of the passers-by whose wallets and debt-ledgers are scraping the bottom of the "high date" (*visok datum*), which is the second half of the month, when people are overstretched between the next and the last incomes. Superficial, in the deeply compromising ways with which people tend to practice their skills at reading your faces, outfits, hairstyles, your tolerance for cold, the volume of your appetites for the signs of a financial emergency. Abdominal to the extent that digestive faculties, intestinal lesions, and bile secretions are said to be highly sensitive to the tension between resources and expenditures, to the blocked flows of capital. Abdominal also in the sense that folk herbalists and vernacular experts treat the stomach with special reverence and foreground it as the principle site of encounters between a subject and a world. Visceral, in a sense that one common disorder, *struna*, with a long history in folk medicine (*narodna medicina*), registers causal links between excessive worry (*sikirancija*) and a stomach organ unhinged (*strunila se*) within a belly mass distending and hurting, which some skilled hands can massage back to its place, just beneath the bellybutton (see chapter 4). My point here is that the economy is an object of health experience and that such visceral affairs are variously informing and forming the monetary and commodity traffic. But the ethnographic phenomenology leads further still: from the question of experience to the variously practical postulates about the curious matter of bodily objects to be known and protected, altered and tended.

Being literal-minded about the extensity of bodily matter does not necessarily evacuate the more subtle stuff that has been traditionally stuffed within an enclosed interiority of the subject but rather, finds a biographical, thinking-feeling-knowing subjectivity, psyche—or soul, even—similarly spatialized: surface upon surface (Nancy 2000, 2008a). Take, for instance, the folk medical therapy strava. Strava is increasingly popular and repurposed to treat common anxieties, insomnia or obsessive fretting, uncanny or traumatic events, as well as affective dullness and loss of purpose that the emergent rubric of "depression" was just beginning to catch in the clinical and pharmaceutical lexicons as well as in the street. Strava is a therapeutic ritual whose implements work at the closest distance from the patient's physical frame, all on the outside, barely and rarely touching the skin, to flush out viscerally enfolded, stressful deposits and influences. In the process, what the therapist reveals is the biographical-circumstantial bundle of the patient whose ailment is inseparable from disastrous business relations, marital disputes, tempers and dispositions, hemorrhoids (see chapter 5). Just as there is no hierarchical ordering of causes at play in case of a disorder that would, for instance, grant more sway to the historical conditions of capital flows than to digestive processes when it comes to vital imbalances, the object of strava's diagnostic and prognostic attention at once relates to health and wealth (*nafaka*). The ties between owing, having, earning, spending, gifting, and being are ornately intertwined in the market as often as in therapy, so much so that generosity is often recommended, not least by a strava therapist, as both a business and health improvement strategy. The queen, too, is in the habit of saying that what most of her patients suffer is the lack of money while, in the course of the treatment, she shows that monetary shortages exercise circuitous effects, involving commodities obtained, renounced, or gifted and quickening through the ties that expect settlements or allow deferrals to interrupt or shift embodied rhythms. Indebtedness summarized the most prevalent complaint about the economic condition and the most viable, if discomfiting, strategy for surviving, whether this entailed provisioning for subsistence or running a business.

INTIMATE DEBT

Remember the detail I quickly described in the queen's office: a corner of her desk attracts a pile of money that people leave on their way out, without her asking for it. Hands dropping gifts, however, fail to attract the queen's attention whether the bills are dressed in envelopes, crisply stretched euros, handsomely round numbers of 50 or 100 (KM) konvertibilna marka, or, more often, crumpled and folded modest figures of 10 or 20 KM. Some patients hand her bags with gifts of clothing or accessories, while others give nothing. I have also seen the queen refuse money offered to her and give money to the children among her patients. The queen's practice has no set price even if the queen has no other source of income, sustains an extended family, hires salaried assistants, and admits to be barely surviving. No matter how much money a patient gives, his or her giving fails to approximate the queen's original gift of her own embodied, extended, restorative potency; of her caring intervention; of her radical generosity that is the condition of her healing: "It is myself that I give." Whether one gives or not, one remains indebted, repeatedly, hopelessly, irreversibly with each subsequent return visit, with each sign of recovery. Whether one gives much or little, one receives a surplus that spoils an attempt to give adequately, which in terms familiar to many Bosnians means to give more than minimally expected, to give lavishly, to give what is beautiful or very necessary so as to be of help (*pomoć*) or to give joy (*obradovat*). And yet, at least outside her practice, the queen, too, owes money. To the audience of her patients she would often tell: "I too am human. I too am indebted, like everyone else." The queen's reputation for curative potencies and for efficacies, super-extended across great distance, makes her rather extraordinary. And yet, by means of debt she establishes her commonality with everyone else in contemporary Bosnia and beyond, for she often points out that the entire world is likewise indebted. The queen tentatively defines the human not by means of an essence but a commonality: what human beings have in common is being indebted. What are the theoretical implications of this proposition? What would a theory of an economy sound like if we started with the being-in-common of being indebted?

Debt has been the prime financial instrument of the global neoliberal economy since the late 1970s. Critiques of political economy have convincingly made this point while placing different emphasis on the key historical dynamics, from financialization of the crisis tendencies of capitalism and the problem of over-accumulation (Harvey 2010), to the exercise of US imperial powers (Strange 1986), to the emergence of most interesting co-productions of biotechnological and speculative imagination (Cooper 2008; Rajan 2006). Ethnographers, by contrast, have shown how people live with indebtedness while handling peculiarly local notions of credit and debt, which in popular economies often entails generating value and cycling wealth through practices of care, ritual or indulgent expenditure, and generosity toward kin, neighbors, gods, or the nation (Chu 2008; Williams 2004; Han 2012; Klima 2002).

In Bosnia, too, discretely economic forms were rare as informal loans sustained everyday economies of all scales. Investment capital could only come through the networks of fellow traders, suppliers, distributers, and intermediaries who, in turn, counted on others for funds to procure their supplies and meet repayment deadlines. Incomes and profits hinged on one's willingness to lend money to others, to extend goods and services on credit, to wait for payment, and to secure alternate sources of money if the clients' deferrals of debt settlement upset one's own schedule of loan installments and investments. Since 1995, money and capital were mostly cycling through the trade and consumption. Markets of all kinds presented the initial entrepreneurial opportunities when peacetime opened the roads to an unregulated, untaxed flow of goods that were greedily welcomed after three years of war-rationing and were afforded by the influx of capital in remittances as well as in humanitarian and reconstruction investments. The sphere of the market vigorously spatialized in the familiar forms of open-air marketplaces, flea markets, door-to-door and sidewalk sales, as well as in numerous small shops, pharmacies, and supermarkets. In the Yugoslav visions of socialist modernity, such traditional forms of trade appeared hopelessly backward. Marketplaces were sources of peasant produce and products that were promisingly "natural" and "homemade" (*prirodno, domaće*) and increasingly precious in the world of industrial agriculture and processed foods; in the late 1980s, they were attractive sources of bootleg commodities and counterfeit brands that were at once desirable and disappointing, given their inauthentic labels and provenance. Presently, masses of Bosnians who would prefer shopping in the appealingly modern spaces of supermarkets, boutiques, and department stores turn instead to the suspiciously "peasant-looking" (*seljački*) street markets or to the cluttered neighborhood stores to negotiate advances of bare necessities as well as of luxuries. In the cash-based market where money is missing, promises of later payment keep the informal economy afloat and entirely invisible to the macroeconomic eye except as a surplus of money in circulation unaccounted for by the records in the formal banking (see Pugh 2005). Debt ledgers keep track of borrowing and lending out of view, in plain notebooks with bent spines, their pages softened and gently looped around the edges by the hands handling, leafing, and inscribing. Promises were sometimes committed to paper furtively and only after the transactions, so as to avoid embarrassing the borrowing party with a show of indebtedness or to avoid the signs of doubt about either parties' given word. Traders "worked on debt" (*na dug*) while their clients said they lived on "[debt] ledgers" (*na teku*) or "on pencil marks" (*na olovku*).

Working "on debt" entails cashing in, piecemeal, the outstanding promises, borrowing short-term and small sums from multiple sources, from one's work companions to friends and family. Living "on pencil marks" includes relying on familiar vendors and on borrowed funds, including at times from those who are worse off, struggling, and whom the lender typically supports, say an elderly parent living on a minimal state pension. Making money from the promissory potential of a social network is a busy, optimistic, and anxious affair. People worry that money will not materialize, complain of a looming financial disaster to all who might care or might help, gently nudge their debtors to help out by giving back however small amounts, think creatively and perform accounting against the odds, while counting on other people's generosity, sheer chance, and good fortune that saved them in the past. Remarkably often people do collect, in the nick of time, just enough funds to meet the nonnegotiable monthly credit installment with a micro-lending agency or a bank, to settle a debt with a supplier or with a department store, to invest in the procurement of equipment or stocks, to pay for a health intervention, a wedding, a funeral.

What coordinated work and life in promissory extensions was not simply trust, as so much scholarship on debt stresses while emphasizing contractual encounters between lenders and borrowers who evaluate, anticipate, and mitigate risks with appeals to the wider social, moral, or legal background. Rather, what plays out in informal debt practice is less instrumental and more tacit, more thoroughly embodied, and thus a more comprehensive bundle of principles, constitutive of a habitus— to recover Pierre Bourdieu's (1990) fine analytic, now somewhat out of vogue. Habitus *foregrounds* embodied dispositions and felt obligations that diffusely coordinate lending–borrowing, owing–owning, practices within an economy where debts are most efficient routes to cash and capital, though routes that are neither entirely predictable nor quite avoidable. In other words, the practiced play of inclinations and calculations registers the political–economic conditions of possibility while also—departing from Bourdieu—working despite or against them, referencing compelling values and expectations of what is proper or what constitutes wealth.

Attention to popular practice in the contemporary Bosnian economy foregrounds the noneconomic expectations that involve the market squarely with values of other forms of exchanges. Generosity and discretion that otherwise guides gifting sensibilities are implicitly expected under the circumstances of informal borrowing and lending. Loans are negotiated free of interest and with flexible return timelines. Shopkeepers would record advances of commodities only after the customer left, making sure that no one else was there, ethnographer excepted, so as not to embarrass the indebted fellow neighbor. People were commonly uncomfortable requesting loans of money or advances of commodities but, also, when approached for loans, found it difficult to deny them even when lending would strain their resources or when a would-be lender seemed financially irresponsible or unreliable (see chapter 2). However, preferring one trader over so many others running adjacent shops or market stalls entailed considerations that made loyal debtors generous patrons. I learned of lenders' reluctance to inquire about their debtors' outstanding debts. "How could I ever?" a tombstone maker in a provincial town responded to my wondering why he did not call the people whom, he complained, have been long owing him money. Deferrals were expected. Many such considerations were more akin to gifting circumstances than to professional lending as modeled by the banks and micro-credit lenders, whose steep interest rates and nonnegotiable installment plans made them less accessible and never solely adequate to run a business. More often than not, people relied on informal loans to meet institutional repayment deadlines and, in turn, used formally loaned capital to patch the yawning gaps between incomes generated, payments still pending, and expenditures due. Underwriting the distinctions between informal and formal lending was also the constant, buoyant traffic of ordinary gifts and caring gestures between people involved. Traders would give little gifts to their clients or their children or would invite them to have coffee or sweets. Traders would also receive jars of homemade preserves or fresh produce and flowers from their frequent shoppers' gardens. Whether or not a sale was made, people offered each other health advice over a market stand, exchanged recipes for restorative meals, or, if a need or opportunity arose, presented a remedy at hand, or else a pill, and tranquilizers in particular. Gifts laced encounters that were persistently and readily converted into more complicated transactions while debt relations only furthered the flow of gifts. In one town pharmacy that still worked "on debt" in 2007 as well as issued medicine in advance of the prescriptions eligible for subsidized drugs and where pharmacists were particularly helpful, their patients would bring them fruits or a homemade meal just in time for their lunch break while the pharmacist found ways or collected funds to give, in turn, something more than their professional service (see chapter 5).

Gift is a notoriously ambivalent thing whose possibility has exercised anthropologists' imagination ever since Marcel Mauss's classic essay on *The Gift* ([1954] 1990). The gift's career in critical thought has taken many turns; early generations of anthropologists wielded it as a powerful critique of the universalizing discourses on *Homo economicus* (Mauss [1954] 1990; Malinowski [1921]; Sahlins 1972) while those writing in the wake of Bourdieu's (1990) skepticism of the economic innocence of "the gift islands" treated it as a market instrument, though of a different kind. Derrida's critique of gift's impossibility uncoupled Maussian vision of the gift as a hybrid of self-interestedness and genuine generosity, and anthropologists have since been hesitant, though a number of voices, not only anthropological, have explicitly called for another look at the gifts that are possible, and that can or ought to be such (see Schrift 1997). In extended ethnographic meditations on funeral exchanges and public acts of generosity in Thailand, Alan Klima (2000, 2008) suggests that Western and (neo)liberal sensibilities get in the way of appreciating the unruly mixing of market and nonmarket in the domains of popular practice and thus shortchange the gift's critical potential. There is no economy outside a gift economy, Klima suggest, since gift stresses the enduring responsibilities, relationships, and obligations that the formal market logic would discount and that post–Cold War historical narratives would absolve.[2] Gift has too often been premised on a stark distinction from obligations and debts. On the contrary, Bosnian informal economy suggests that we attend to relations where generosity underlies both lending and borrowing and gifting irrevocably indebts in ways that are effective because they are acutely felt, stimulating someone to give well, to give better, to give constantly. Far from undoing a gift, debt affirms it, but to the extent that debt is about lingering responsibilities that make no one being entirely sovereign, but one commonly indebted, "like everyone else," debts precede any event or a lived memory of giving or taking (see chapter 5). This is not to say that gifts and debts are not suffered at times, felt as the pressure of close relationships and commitments unresolved, unforgotten, left dangling and cluttering one's affective space. Gifts to the queen are the extreme examples of impossibility to give properly or to give, finally, and yet futility cannot prevent one from trying.

Nancy's corpus does not have a rigorous theory of capital, but pursuing his proposition that ontological questions inquire about existence under the conditions of capital, across a terrain of popular economy that Nancy did not have in mind, I suggest that informal relations of debt enable circumstances, experiential as much as material and monetary, that alter the formidable power of the Capital, with its particular dynamics and tendencies, and generate relational opportunities and limits to circulation and appreciation. The ontological implications of shared indebtedness cannot be appreciated solely within the encounters of the two parties involved in an exchange. Rather, with the sense of a general debt crisis and with expectations that others ought to know how it feels, the meantime of overextended investments, overdue promises, life-saving loans, and multiple income and repayment schedules becomes the place of existence held in common.

CARNAL COMMONALITIES

Moving beyond the body proper—biochemical, anatomical, universal, and discrete—I tour some curious, fantastically responsive, and fleshly economic domains, to arrive to the conditions of existence held in common and formative of collective possibilities across mundane spaces of Bosnia. I described economic conditions that are intimately and collectively shared while having already proposed, from within the queen's office, that a bodily domain is no private property but is extended, far into the world. Moreover, I want to take the implications of sharing beyond Bosnia, as the ground from which to address a "we" and imagine an "us." Imagination that queers bodiliness tends to whistle a mischievous tone, out of tune with the political sensibilities that invest in individual rights and votes, choices and immunological defenses. Critical readings of biomedicine have already made this point rather obvious (Lock and Nguyan 2010; Good 1990; Lock 1993, 2008), as when, for instance, Ed Cohen (2011) reads against the grain the public health policies of viral containment to suggest that we already contain viruses, parasites, and microbes. These life forms are more than hostile invaders but are also actants in the shared cellular ecology, coopting, managing, collaborating with the cells we might call our own. Except that the idea of body, our own and owned as "proper and proprietary given, a natural fact" becomes a different thing in the light of viral incorporation (26). This may be becoming more widely obvious and legible in the speculations readily found in popular-science writing on human microbiomes and in Do-It-Yourself activisms of fermented and raw foods in North America. Michael Pollan, whose public voice carries far and takes issues of health and food into the messy mix of nature-culture and politics, opened up his 2013 article in the *New York Times Magazine* with a metaphysical musing prompted by a lab test. Hundreds of species of resident bacteria found in his skin and gut made him think of himself "in the first person plural," as a "superorganism, that is, rather than a plain, old individual human being" (1). The "superorganism" sounds like a buoyant curiosity[3] rather than an existential crisis at the evidence that sums up the human precisely as the remainder in the microbial stock: "to the extent that we are bearers of genetic information, 99% of it is microbial" (2). In a nutshell, Pollan and the microbiologists he cites write up a cellular communism when they describe human health as a collective property and a "function of the community, not the individual" (3). My writing takes the proposition about being singular plural elsewhere, in two directions: one opened up by Nancy's philosophical meditations on being premised on sharing and the other anticipated by Lock and Farquhar (2007) when they write about contingent forms of embodiment that are "refusing all biological reductions and proposing a new politics that seeks solidarity among bodies" (4). What would such political and bodily solidarities look like? What could they ever achieve for our understanding of Bosnia? And how far would Nancy's idea of being as always singular and plural get in thinking Bosnia?

For as long as it may seem obvious what bodies are, properly speaking, the temptation is to speak of Bosnia in terms of genocidal and identity politics. After all, the country has become the figure of intimate ethno-national violence among former companions, neighbors, friends, and kin. Regional communitarian ideologies foregrounded bodily matters while violence operationalized ethno-national ideals, putting to work the assumption that flesh is the medium of ethnic essence that binds an individual to the communal and allows the identification of the self-same and separation from essentialized others. Regional politics since the 1995 peace declaration are similarly preoccupied with ethnically marked voters, refugees, and returnees, with heroes and civilian casualties, with the missing dead whose remains are exhumed by joint efforts of forensic and legal experts and are reburied in media spectacles of commemoration. I do not mean to be irreverent; I have no heart to take lightly the grave local history. I am, however, compelled to trouble the reduction of the matter and meaning of the bodies to the bodies made formally relevant by the war and the peace that institutionalized many of the wartime ambitions for policing the difference. Politically relevant bodies are indexed by flesh, blood, bones, and by circumstances of birth and death. Murderous and discursive attentions fixate on torture, bloodshed, skeletal remains of the martyrs and the missing. Or else, bodies are treated as mediums of connection that presuppose degrees of proximity and milieus of mixing: countless debates over Bosnia's age-old pluralism evolve around the vicinity of neighbors, promiscuity of markets, and, iconically, on sexual intimacy and procreative work of ethnically mixed couples. "Cleansing" is the striking gesture of a knife, a pen, a keyboard writing out a decisive distinction between a Serb, a Croat, or a Muslim. Even when the object is molecular—a DNA strand or traces of mortal remains—the molar to which they are made to relate is the body, reassembled to the point where its identity is reconstructed (see Wagner 2008). It is customary to point to Bosnia as an example of bodily politics even when the authors themselves venture more complicated ways of thinking about subjects and bodies (e.g., Csordas 1994). Scholars of Bosnia, even when skeptical, take up a study of the very rubrics that politics of essence have opened up. Scholarship has, understandably, turned the history into an object of inquiry, but it has also been inadvertently obliged by the normative description of what the body is, what sensible ways there are to relate to body, and what bodies make sense. Oddly bodily imagination is no fit replacement for the preoccupations of identity politics, but it offers a supplement that points to other carnal matters and experiences that are not only otherwise consequential in Bosnia since the peace but are formative of unexpected, fleeting, but effective collectives. Let us think back to the queen's therapy.

The queen draws close to the others in a visceral adjacency that rearranges them, affecting multiple changes that patients feel, that others notice, or make legible by means of clinical or lab technologies. Further still, immediate relatives, or sometimes dearest friends removed by time zones of two continents, reportedly sympathetically resonate with the queen's treatment: the queen works on a woman's stomach while the woman's friend, mother, or sister gets nauseated. Imagine a flesh so unstable that the queen could slide between the lower ribs to the glandular tips, and from there shower throughout with their secretory potential. Imagine, further, that your nearness to others is sympathetically charged and tactually amplified with the technology whose convenience and frustrations you take for granted. The queen too, though, is a vulnerable subject. I heard her say: "I feel what you feel, I go through it, for how else could I treat?" After a day of working in the clinic, she regularly points to her bloated stomach that stomached hours of her connectedness with the ill. Or sometime in the summer of 2012, she rolled up a sleeve to show me hives she developed from an hour-long session with a ten-year-old girl who suffered head-to-toe skin rashes that a medical doctor diagnosed as a "psoriasis." The queen orders that patients abstain from pharmaceuticals twenty-four hours before they visit lest they somehow contaminate her. Similarly contagious are traces of inhaled or ingested transcriptions of Koranic suras, solicited from imams who could be either in the business of healing or harming (*sihire*, see below). "I feel what you feel" is an admission of a curious therapeutic potency and vulnerability, one inseparable from the other. Thinking viral, microbial incorporations, Ed Cohen almost anticipates her words when he says that "our vitality and our vulnerability coexist," (29) but not quite. Both presume a remarkable bodily responsiveness, but the queen also speaks of radical empathy, which she puts to curative uses—at the thought our cool head spins or shakes doubtfully—but which is also more generally in evidence, outside her office.

Not only is the economy an object of shared experience, where people expect each other to know how debt feels, but the bodily economies I encountered were more closely attuned to misfortunes of others than may be expected. News of death, grave illness, or financial ruin, sometimes of perfect strangers, affected listeners to the point where they reached for tranquilizers and grew anxious about surviving the world gone wrong. Empathetic sharing, people admitted, was unwise, unhealthy but unavoidable—just as impossible as keeping one's calm in the face of quotidian economic disasters. As I describe in chapter 3, my hairdresser consumed anxiolytics one day after she learned of her colleague's son's premature death; she could imagine how the mother must have felt, she said. These are radical examples of "solidarity among the bodies," most manifest in the collective readings of publicly posted obituaries. People paused to read and worried in groups that would assemble, disseminate, and reassemble, suspending briefly every body in the act of collective, affective reading. They read together and in the flesh, and they took the story and the readings' traces onward, on their quotidian journeys, re-telling, remembering, reliving. Upsetting events and quotidian disasters in turn provoked concerned interventions, advice given and taken not to "burden yourself" (*nemoj se opterećivat*), not to worry oneself sick, to gain some perspective, some distance. Similarly, market and medical sites were ever opportunities to sympathize and strategize together, in waiting rooms, waiting lines, or at prescription windows. From public readings of obituaries to exchanging health complaints and advice to figuring out treatment tactics, I saw intermittent, intense, practically minded collectives gather and disseminate, again and again across the fields of mundane practices.

Significantly, streets, marketplaces, and clinics that occasioned the assemblies around common concerns with health and wealth did not hinge on ethno-national distinctions and casually made formal politics beside the point. Reading the implications of these spontaneous gatherings with Nancy, I would call these communities "political," acknowledging their associational potential around the matters of good life, communication, and sharing—which is one definition of political objectives—as well as marking their inherent distinction from the sphere of formal, institutional politics, within which they take place by default.[4] Nancy's rethinking of the political away from electoral parties or formal mobilization is motivated by a desire to capture the critical potential of gathering, experience, and sharing that cannot be formally recruited, routinized, or rhetorically corrupted. In other words, he is interested in the political as it pertains to disposition, inclination, and experience that take place spontaneously and energetically and disappear as quickly from one occasion of being social to another. Nancy's investment in the promise of "the political" travels with a rather compelling argument. In his words, there is an urgency to thinking the possibilities of something that we all may have in common and that cannot be lost despite all the disappointments in socialist, communist, and welfare-state experiments, and that cannot be perverted nor recruited for nationalist and fascist identity projects (which played out in the Bosnian war with a genocidal bluntness). This political thought, first of all, evolves around a community without a corporate life or identifiable body, with nothing of substance (historical, ethnic, national, institutional, symbolic, or corporeal) to precede or succeed gatherings of singular humans drawn to each other. A community that is neither imagined nor represented, neither named nor fixed onto a political platform, neither organized nor called for. Such a finite community could only take place in the space with and between others because it is always already at the very heart of every singular being, not as an identity that one has or must affirm but as an irresistible attraction of one being toward another.

Secondly, the promise of the political in Nancy's writing requires rethinking the singular being and bodily experience. Each body is contiguous with others but is also singular, unlike any other, while, at the same time, it is "plural to begin with." He suggests that a relation with others is a minimal ontological condition, a condition of possibility for each "I" (2000:27). Self-knowledge is already a relationship with an outside. The possibility of thinking and conversing with the self is premised on relationships with others, on the position of self as an other, as well as on social forms—of addressing, touching, sharing, and exchange. It is the originary plurality of singular being that engenders the political potential, right at the place where an experiential community comes into play. The political for Nancy rests in the very "outlines of each being"; it registers not institutional power relations but concerns a social life, which Nancy defines as a life of sharing.

But what kind of a community can be formed in quotidian activities of gathering and dispersing? What can ever become of superficial bodies without proper essence, except as a togetherness lost-and-found in evasion and deferral? This book picks up these questions but with a light hand, without privileging the political or blanketing all other practical and vital energies into a single notion of (political) effort. Chapter 3 attends closely to the sites and objects of collective sharing, but ethnographic detours in chapter 4 move us away, by default, from formal politics and identity concerns. In stepping into conventional, alternative, and traditional therapies we find people from all walks of life seeking health care regardless of their backgrounds, spiritual practices, and ideological convictions. As is the case in anxiety therapy (strava), practiced in the local Muslim tradition, the common rule is that "strava is for everyone" (see chapter 5).

BETWEEN MAGICAL AND METAPHYSICAL

No one knows how the queen works, nor what "it" is that she practices, for she disassociates herself from the medical categories in regional circulation: from conventional medicine and traditional healing, from bio-energy and Islamic medicine. The uncertainty is unnerving but the promissory potency it advertises is hard to resist. People say that she has a "power" (*moć*) and report how they feel it acting, what changes it affects. The anthropologist has not cracked the queen's secret nor do I intend to dodge the challenge it poses to my observations and narration by shifting attention entirely to the issues that are more conveniently graspable because they concern social and historical contexts of this home-medical practice rather than its oddly corporeal matters. The queen too claims ignorance: "I don't know how I work. If I were making a pie, I could tell you, 'here, this is how you do it.' As is, I don't know."

Magic is a more marked word for potencies and phenomena that, in Margaret Wiener's words, "Euro-Americans would ascribe to chance, coincidence, luck, or charisma—words whose English definitions are essentially confessions of ignorance" (1995:58). Magic is at once a generous and a compromising word for what escapes comprehension or appears as the outer side of reason, *logos*. Because for Jean-Luc Nancy the outsides, edge surfaces of contact are where the significant events of being and being together, of thinking and gathering, take place, *alogon* is not an underbelly or an unconscious so much as "the extreme, the excessive, and necessary dimension of the *logos*: the moment we speak of serious things (death, the world, being together, being-oneself, the truth), it has never seriously been a question of anything other than this dimension. It is the *alogon* that reason introduces with itself" (Nancy 2008c:8). Nancy is writing about the concerted exclusion and persistent creeping in of (Christian) metaphysics into Western scientific, philosophical, and secular thought, while Wiener attends to how magic was excluded from the historical records of key events of Balinese and Dutch colonial encounters. *Health and Wealth on the Bosnian Market* attends to efficacies, promises, and potencies that trail both the magical and the metaphysical, but sits comfortable in neither rubric: because medical practitioners and their patients rather insist on inarticulations of therapeutic powers, efficacies, and objects; because they do not interrogate ultimate causes nearly as often as they worry about the secondary and intermediate ones; and because they indignantly, often anxiously dissociate therapies from conventional magic that has proliferated in the postwar professional service market.

Suspicions and complaints about sihire (plural, from Arabic *sihr*, which translates to sorcery, spell, or magic), "magic" or "black magic" (*magija, crna magija*), "bad" or "low" energies, and all kinds of spirit or jinn interferences were part and parcel of the popular medical journeys I followed. Except that broaching the subject of magija or sihir entailed more circuitous conversation between casual interlocutors that first established confidence or made the topic unavoidable for the sake of advising those who might be seeking or needing a cure (see chapter 4). Talk of magija, sihire, and intangible agents made people self-conscious and embarrassed in anticipation of secular, modern, skeptical ears over-hearing them and judging them as uneducated, gullible, superstitious, backward, peasant. Moreover, those complaining were often caught by surprise, caught in the illness rubrics, experiences, and treatments that they themselves found beyond belief. Many have also learned what a splotchy, treacherous terrain is the magical market where false promises sound no less ambitious than the claims that made a difference, where genuine cheats are hard to tell from those who do real magic, and from those who can undo it. Ameliorative and self-help practices are many. Is-lamic healing manuals are especially popular, selling across northeastern Bosnian bookstores next to texts on folk and herbal medicine, medicinal diets, bio-energy, meditation, and dream interpretation. The manuals speak in a practical, try-it-at-home language. A complicated world flies off their pages, the world of human passions, wills, and relentless striv-ing, intersected with nonhuman agents, from jinn to talismans to potent objects, and leafing through the manuals recommends recruitment of a specialist. In case of sihir or jinni-related affliction, one looks for an imam, a dervish, or, less often, a Wahabi community willing to help.[5] Is-lamic medical manuals and experts and many other remedies, medicinal objects, texts, and practitioners are also advertised on television and in special periodicals, such as *Aura. Aura* advertises an open market where all kinds of claims, proofs, articles, and testimonials compete in narrat-ing strange new affliction, marvelous new cures, and nervous journeys between them.[6]

Magic and healing comprise a busy field of popular practice in Bosnia whose disappearance was taken for granted since at least early twentieth-century Austrian-Hungarian imperial efforts at modernization, educa-tion, and urbanization. Late nineteenth-century collectors of folklore rushed to capture the curious repertoire of magical concerns and inter-ventions, from accidental encounters with spirits to resourceful tricks of low-key love-magic, from sorcery attacks to the ever popular talis-mans and biblical or Koranic inscriptions for the protection of health and wealth.[7] A few scholarly texts on magic during Yugoslav socialism site it similarly in the charming Slavic past, while a recent study of the National Museum's collection of inscriptions and talismans places their earliest mention to the 1400s while confidently dating their disappearance to the twentieth century.[8]

Proliferation of strange new medical practices in the region has been officially noted with amusement and embarrassment, when not with downright alarm. This is especially so when strangeness, otherwise held in its proper place—below the radar, circulating in hushed, intimate conversations or advertised in marginal venues—bursts out into the open: say, at the scale of tens of thousands of people, who queued for two seasons in 2010 and 2011 at the Olympic Sports Hall of Sarajevo, the capital, to see Moroccan healer Mekki Torabi who healed at distance, free of charge, charged water bottles with medicinal energy, and was himself powered by disputed sources (see Jašarević 2014b). Amid accusations of charlatanism and millennial entrepreneurialism, critics indignantly contrasted mass pilgrim enthusiasm with gross voting apathy, linking mass enchantments and ethno-national passions, magical frauds and the sham electoral democracy. The public scandal of mass healing and credulity was, inevitably, made political, packed into formal electoral and ethno-national politics, leaving the inconvenient questions of Torabi's knowledge claims or imputed efficacies out of public debate.

Magic, in short, causes discomfort, which is turned into a joke, into a properly political issue, or else into an embarrassing question of who could afford to believe it or be openly mixed-up with it. Such play of public affect must be considered in the wider, ex-Yugoslav perspective, since socialist modern sensibilities and the uncanny returns of the peasant, folk, the Balkan, or the neighborhood Oriental are shared and remain entangled. Prior to his Bosnian tours, Torabi was a returning guest in nearby Croatia. Moreover, curious and largely invisible flows of magicomedical tourism bring clients from as far as Slovenia to famous Bosnian healers, imams, or magic-makers or hook them, at a distance, via eco-technic and communication technologies (see chapter 2; Jašarević 2014b).[9]

Magically inflected health practices have been described across wider post-socialist medical markets, attracting patients in numbers—and not only the usual suspects, the peasants and the superstitious—while soliciting varied scholarly analytics. Some observers rely on analytically lean concepts of "New Ageism" and "cosmologies" to grasp the "post-communist epistemological multiplicity" and, often, rescue symbolic anthropology's search for veiled native meanings and worldviews (Lūse and Lázár 2007; Portata 2007). On the other hand, Gallina Lindquist (2006) speaks of magic as a technology of hope in times of the pervasive uncertainty of the new Russia; Frances Pine and João de Pina-Cabral (2008) introduce a shift in perspective from the grand theory of magic (and religion) to the scripts of popular pragmatics in the fuzzy margins of religions. In post-Mao China, Judith Farquhar (1996) speaks of magic as an embodiment of local powers and claims to efficacy that appeal to nonscientific desires of patients in the entrepreneurial medical landscape and more recently. Pedersen (2011) shifts the terms of analysis significantly when he insists that the resurgence of spirits and the improvisational, fast-learning, half-remembering responses of not-quite-shamans raise more generally ontological questions about the post-socialist present.

Magic is the conceptual milieu that anthropologist have largely exited—guilted by the imperial projects that their universal object of interest, "the magic," corroborated; a little embarrassed by the calls for symmetrical anthropology; not a little awed by the comparative edginess of Science and Technology Studies; and often disheartened by crude misunderstandings that the mention of things magical earned them or their communities of affiliation. Nonetheless, magic and a looser fit of speculative and promissory potential of a magical quality—magicality—seem too relevant to retire, too potent to surrender to a reductive framing: it is repeatedly suspected in the ethnographic fields; too appealing to lay publics everywhere; too casually invoked and dismissed by natural scientists and philosophers alike, even those brandishing speculative thought.[10] Perhaps it takes a lobbying by an unlikely party, such as Isabelle Stengers, to nudge us into revisiting magic, as she puts it, precisely because it creates discomfort that is conceptually productive, not least of a hesitation before hasting to claim "to know better" (2012:6–9).

With eyes on Bosnia, rather than revisiting magic, I wish to repurpose the domain of inquiry and intervention, from pragmatic to fantastic, from preposterous to metamorphic, that sits between the conceptual realms explored by the classic and contemporary anthropologies of magics and the newly open lanes of speculative thought. Taking a cue from local lexical discomforts I join the travels across this tricky zone overfull with indices of practically wild imagination, with critical world-making and -breaking implications, and with suggestive or unlikely but palpable connections and consequences that butt against cosmopolitan, scientific epistemologies. As I show in the subsequent chapters, the ethnographic journeying, at the heel of the people concerned about health and wealth, helps me rehearse a recurrent point: popular economic and broadly medical practices flesh out lived bodily possibilities that may seem odd, or at least unanticipated by the formal economic or biomedical logic, and that are decidedly unanticipated by the politics of ethno-national identity. Patients enter strava regardless of their national identify or their religious convictions, entrusting themselves to wise old women (*nene*, sg. *nena*) who whisper Koranic suras over their bodies and wash them gently in a manner of Islamic ritual ablutions (*abdest*). Devout Catholics sometimes make a sign of the cross as the nena initiates the treatment, in the name of God, *Bismillah*. The queen sees patients from all corners of Bosnia, claims to belong to all three faiths and not to any of the ethno-national categories, which identity markers she boldly, inventively reshuffles to the point at which there are no criteria left to any listening patients to ethno-nationally easily identify with (see chapter 6). *Health and Wealth on the Bosnian Market* presents an ongoing inquiry into the efficacies of contact and consequences of close connections and these therapeutic encounters are only the most excessive manifestations of alogon, folded in all the talk of "serious things," as Nancy puts it. Contact, of course, has always been an especially magical concern. Attentive ethnographers showed it to be not obviously contagious; its sticky or rippling ultimacies are achieved, courted, and cultivated. Contact relies on finicky connections and fortuities attractions as much as on skillful managing of aversions, deferrals, and defenses. All along, however, a prior sympathy, a possibility of affective coinciding and irritation is presumed: it is the underlying, fermenting actuality of the originarily plural being whose configurations and consequences are mostly below the threshold of experience but can be manifested concretely and sensuously in close encounters and coincidences, and can be mobilized, synthesized, and exercised to a point.

The trouble with effective contact is precisely that it connects, often whether or not we like it and long after we would like to cut short, push back, exercise, or at least fantasize about having some control. This text cannot enjoy a claim to an authorial immunity, if ever there is one, afforded by a distance between the ethnographic ground that variously attracts, compromises, and sustains us, the gleaners of other peoples' eventful lives, and the zones of academic production where we can reflect, not least on problems of voice and representations. Reflexivity has been our professional inclination for a while, only made more acute by the growing likelihood that we will be read by those we write about. I worried about this book while trying to write it responsively, not only responsibly: following my interlocutors' cues and taking leads from the circumstances that shaped my being in the field, not always nor primarily as an ethnographer.

During the fieldwork, I was never immune from the queen's power, her influence, or her charm. Over the years, I only grew more attached and more compromised, visiting her year after year, persisting with questions, annoyingly curious, slow to understand. "How will you describe me?" she challenged me, initially. Her loyal patients, too, rallied around the question, some suspicious, others sympathetic, not envying my task. Eventually, the queen relaxed, encouraged me even, and prodded onward when words failed and when my writing life caved in under the pressures of illness and mundane troubles of a life lived under the privilege of a cosmopolitan displacement. The distance between us was not stable; it compressed, softened, and grated uncomfortably. Via Facebook, phone, and otherwise, we kneaded the connections, she in ways that are more skilled in the ecotechnics of being remotely social. She read some of my texts and drafts—sometimes with the aid of Google Translate, which I protested—and while she was rarely pleasantly surprised she grew more patient and indulgent, but never conclusively so. In the process of writing the final version of this text, I omitted all the biographical details, including her name, as the prospects of earning her dismay seemed ever greater than the chances of finding adequate language to avoid it. I too grew hopelessly indebted. Responsiveness does not simply resolve issues with a compromise; it acknowledges failures, it faces limits.

Writing responsively goes beyond the queen's office. Responsiveness is neither collaboration nor engagement, two admirable visions for the discipline of anthropology (Low and Merry 2010; for an admirable example of a collaborative work see Farquhar and Zhang 2012). It is a writing in reaction to the dawning awareness that the academic genre regularly edits the conditions under which ethnographic objects arise, conditions under which doing and writing ethnography, and just being alongside, coincide. Debts, and the suffering they caused, the generosity they enabled, the arguments they inspired, and the lives they torqued, were never far from home. The field was home, although I have lived displaced for a long time. Deaths, misfortunes, cravings, and habits of closest kin, dearest friends, and many others with whom I grew close over the years presented me with "ethnographic material," not always by design, which I rarely hesitated to take but whose particulars remained nonconsumable, indigestible, acting as remainders—like a fishbone stuck in the throat—and reminders of what is being manipulated into scholarly material. However, writing responsively remembers all the ways in which I was being manipulated in the field, while doing research, revisiting places, or writing about it all. Healers, herbalists, and so many other vernacular experts on health and wealth scrutinized me and advised me on terms that, outside Bosnia, could be embarrassing or at least easier to avoid. Being vulnerable in the field is the condition of being responsive and, perhaps, the condition of doing certain kinds of ethnography: of embodied life, of common experience.

BOOK ITINERARY

Chapter 1 begins in one woman's apartment, after an ordinary argument over the family's overextended budget and after her stumbling upon an exquisite item, at a bargain price, in the local supermarket. Taking stock of the family's furnishings, closets, prized acquisitions, and traces of prior living arrangements, the chapter begins to tie the quotidian, biographical micro-circumstances with greater historical events and longer trends while describing what it might look like or mean to be "just surviving," as Bosnians tend to put it. Just surviving, as I show, entails selective remembering of the better life passed and of resourceful, wartime strategies, but it also presumes ardent striving to live well at all costs under the present conditions. The chapter gathers a bundle of surviving practices while asking how tastes and tactics work through the quotidian shifts between sources of pleasure and comfort, acts that feel natural or aspire to the beautiful, and sources of greatest discomfort. Market, broadly speaking, is the primary site where unease and possibility mix up even if the spread of the market seems disorderly, evidently misplacing goods and people and obscuring sound qualities by preferred temporalities of all things inexpensive and "most-modern." The chapter describes the shared existential conditions and experiences of surviving that underwrite medical and market interventions in the subsequent chapters.

Chapter 2 starts with a curious medical diagnosis of manic generosity that one man earned in a regional mental health clinic. Since the clinic figures widely in the popular imagination as the site where the border between the common and the pathological is made unclear by the historical events of the recent war and the post-socialist present and since generosity seems to be more generally and recklessly practiced, the chapter evolves around the puzzle of excess and gifting under the conditions of precarity. I attend to gifting expectations and dispositions that frame the informal, interest-free lending–borrowing that underwrite local markets and inquire into the implications of the local ideas of intimate debt. Rereading the classic controversies surrounding the gift's improbability or impossibility, I object by showing how in the Bosnian context, gift is not canceled by but rather conditioned on debt; I ask "What kind of wealth is made out of debts?" The proposition of this chapter is that one cannot understand Bosnian popular economy without attending to the effective, practiced, pleasurable, discomfiting, in short, material and embodied implications of everyday gifts. In addition, the intimate relationship between gifts, debts, wealth, and bodies outlined in this chapter is further explored, entangled, or sidetracked in each of the book's chapters.

Chapter 3 takes up a challenge that one trader shoved in this ethnographer's face when I asked her how her work was going in the market. In response, the woman reached into her bag and pulled out a fistful of medicine, saying, "Here is how it is. Write as you will." Translating her gesture into a broader question, the chapter first of all asks what it might mean to say that market is an object of health experience. Reviewing the problem that experience has always posed to the social thought, I collect ethnographic evidence for the lives that are lived on the edge: compromised, every day, by market trends, general indebtedness, and ample evidence that people are falling ill and dying unnatural deaths. Moreover, since concerns over poor health and premature death tend to drift back and forth between one's own circumstances and the misfortunes of others, I am most interested in thinking how experience is so readily shared or, perhaps, plural and shared to begin with. From some sites of intensive sharing—of health complaints and accidents, news of illness, deaths or suicides, around obituary postings and readings—I explore and play up the resonance between vernacular and philosophical imagination and, specifically, Nancy's thought on experiential communities and the political promise of their spontaneous inclinations.

Chapter 4 takes off from the corner of a grandma's kitchen table to pick up questions that issue so readily from the mushroom jar if one attends closely, with voracious curiosity, to some seemingly simple matters or simply amusing domestic and dietary habits. Such attention prods questions concerning materiality of medicinal objects, from remedies to technologies to the bodies, whether or not human, intervening or intervened upon. What interests me here are various things that enter and exit popular health-care practices as well as the circumstances that promote their therapeutic relevance, that discern potencies, that make remedies available, promising, potent, or mute, and that shape treatment regimes while nurturing, relating, and recomposing bodies. Contemporary health matters in Bosnia may be plural or etiologically and epistemologically muddled to the extreme, but my point is that they also speak more generally of the extent to which biomedicine, anywhere, is the domain of supreme uncertainty. The chapter follows in the footsteps of people nervously traveling, seeking genuine healers and real cures, to tell stories collected on the go, while traveling by train, eavesdropping on a bus, shopping at the market, visiting a few home practices, waiting in the pharmacy, or hanging by an herbalist's stand.

Chapter 5 arrives at the grounds of a traditional but presently tremendously popular therapy for everyday stress and exceptional worries.

I examine the terms and objects of the therapeutic encounter, postulates for the medical efficacy, and the practical knowledge of what are bodies and psyches. Strava advances three claims (it is for everyone, regardless of their beliefs or affiliations; it cures everything; and it has no price) and illustrates a tactile economy that can only be appreciated, I propose, with an analysis oriented toward both ontology and phenomenology. Particular treatments that I describe show what little difference strava makes between affective, digestive, and accounting habits, between skin and relational inclinations, while it engrosses a singular, biographical person and a psyche in consequential relations to the point where each bodily person is potentially and inconveniently extended into the space of collective affairs. To grasp such tangible–intangible extensions and the distance across which the therapist's hands, objects, and the ailing bodies meet, the chapter finally suggests, we need to turn to more metaphysical propositions. And we may just as well run out of arguments, especially having found a healer for real, finally.

Chapter 6 is composed of two parts that are intricately but never explicitly related, not least because doing so would greatly displease the sources from which I am drawing. The most obvious connection between the two parts is the profound, more or less ongoing speculation on whether a healer is for real, and if not real, but still efficacious, what or who is he or she? The first part returns to the queen's clinic where she works, with her hands, without touching, and draws daily crowds of new and returning patients. She has no fees, runs no advertisements, and keeps a low public profile (but an active Facebook page). Observing the encounters between the queen and the people she assembles, this part of the chapter continues the book's overall project of troubling the phenomenological and conventional notions about proximity and suggesting that it is a certain form of "superficiality" that matters and renders the therapeutic and collective experience around the queen effective. The second part of the chapter takes up the problem of the source of medical efficacy while reading three practical guides to healing by the Koran; a kind of medical practice that the queen finds most irritating. Selected readings belong to the genre of recently prolific medical texts and, in their own terms, elaborating, in plain language, basics of Islamic metaphysics of body and health; they further destabilize the sense of what counts as bodily matter and what is real. This book has intermittently wondered about the ways in which the magical and the metaphysical seep into the most mundane sites and practices of post-socialist medicine and market; these two parts explore the space between the magical and the metaphysical, under the auspices of mysterious medical efficacy and practical advice.

One last note: most chapters end with a rubric that I call "open items." I borrow a term from a business dictionary, which defined *open item* as: "A record found in an accounting ledger that keeps track of a particular type of financial activity over a given period of time."[11] What I find so wonderfully suggestive about the idea of open-item accounting is the tracking of unpaid balances over time, which I repurpose for the particular ethnographic gesture of being at once loyal to my notes and archives—painfully aware of how much I betray them by the economizing conventions of telling a printable story—and forgetful of all the gifts given or received and of the many surpluses that find no room in any vital ledger. Items entered here are bits of unfinished stories, sometimes merely lists, or else full accounts that were missing from but invoked by the preceding chapter's pages. Many of them take into account time that passed or flowed variously between field collecting, revisiting, writing, and rewriting, providing not so much an update on the ethnographic materials as adding veneers to their historical and circumstantial density.

NOTES

1. I mentioned Mrki breezing through the health centers. One morning he did so on my behalf. As I tagged behind, he led me to one Dr. Gogo, who phoned to schedule an appointment with a certain Dr. A., at the regional clinic, five minutes before 8 AM the following day. If Dr. A. were to ask, I was to say that it was nurse H. who sent me, since Dr. A. knew neither Dr. Gogo nor Mrki. I was also instructed to call the nurse, if there were issues. The reception desk was not yet open when I arrived, yet the hall was full of patients already waiting, their health cards stacked on the closed counter. I was lost as to what to do—to wait or to walk into a room—and I phoned nurse H., who was still in bed, who instructed me to find nurse R. or nurse D. and introduce myself as H.'s friend or a cousin with an appointment with Dr. A. Soon after, I had a referral and abdominal scan finished, but the doctor could not tell me how I should pay. He advised me to ask nurse D. who ignored my question. Mrki did not know either and asked me to ask H. who had me ask D. again, which is what I did, some hours later, while collecting the X-ray images. Nurse D. simply smiled and moved onto other patients. "She did not want to charge you," nurse H.

explained on the phone, "for my sake. If you ever need anything else, just tell me." In the telephoned voice of H., the woman I never met, I thought I heard notes of care as she proceeded to inquire about my scan results and my health complaints. I felt indebted, in a complicated way, without anyone able to tell me whom I could or should pay.

2. His examples include surpluses and afterlives of gifts and commodities alike, from American Cold War military alliances with Thailand, whose history of military dictatorship and civilian massacres recycled the value of military knowledge and technology, to public acts of ritualized, Buddhist generosity that collected funds for the National Treasury, which emptied out after the currency crash of the 1990s.

3. Pollan's optimism has much to do with the therapeutic promises of the human-microbial "interior wilderness" that can be tended and whose micro-climate changes urge us to reverse the learned, modern habits of eradicating bacteria and viruses with harsh chemicals and pharmaceuticals.

4. Oliver Marchart (2007) explores the implications of the emerging distinction between the political and politics, while he gathers the sense of "post-foundational political thought" in the works of Nancy and several other French thinkers (Badiou, Lefort, and Laclau). Some of the complexity and nuances of society versus community in Nancy's corpus gets lost in Marchart's attempt to read for commonalities across different authors. Nevertheless, the idea of post-foundational political difference captures nicely the project that might be otherwise confused with other alternatives to foundational politics: politics of affect (see Panagia [2009]), political ethnography (see Schatz [2009]), and Foucauldian politics of subject formation, or the politics of deconstruction in general. Marchart historically situates these post-foundational investigations within a certain retreat of the political brought about by proliferation of genres of "politics": from Michel Foucault's idea of capillary exercise of power, to Deleuze's everyone's everyday fascism, to feminist claims that personal is political. The expansion of the "political" makes politics at the same time everywhere and nowhere to be found. Marchart also speaks to the crisis of political theory that fails to grasp contingency adequately with positivist forms, from identity to ideology. Furthermore, Marchart proposes that the difference between the political and politics is unbridgeable and akin to a distinction between analytical levels: ontic, material, empirical, the domain of political science on the one hand and ontological and philosophical, on the other. It is the impossibility of grounding society, in any final instance, that grants the political import to the moment when the social appears in its potential and disappears in the act of its actualization in any one modality of conventional politics that aims to arrest the community with definitions of essence: class, ethnic, or national.

5. Two popular Koranic healing manuals, first published in the 1990s, forward the impression that healing is a sanctioned Islamic practice, while also offering quite different reflections on its place in the broader historical context. Muharem Štulanović references the Islamization of Bosnia and affiliates itself with lessons of the more authentic Islam (2007). Vehid Pekarić, by contrast, acknowledges a long local history of healing among imams whose practice was outlawed but informally continued throughout communism (1998).

6. Often advertised in *Aura* is an impressive set of CDs and DVDs of a Sufi sheikh's *Protection from and Healing of Sihir, Black Magic, Jinn and Sheitan's Evil*. See also a volume

published by students of Islamic studies: *Zaštita od Džina i Šejtana u Svjetlu Kur'ana i Sunneta, Hamajlije, Talismani i Ruk'je u Svjetlu Kur'ana i Sunneta"* (Tuzla, 2006).

7. See, for instance, Leopold Glück's 1980 account. A practicing physician, Glück was intrigued by his patients' talismans, published a comparative survey of these curiosities made and worn by all confessional communities, suggesting that "Mohammedan" talismans were most complex and custom-made, Eastern Orthodox and Catholic ones were ready-made for a host of uses, and Sephardic Jewish ones, *kameje*, came from Jerusalem at a significant price (48).

8. Reading the collection with the help of several regional histories, Fabijanić (2004) suggests that talismans were the "common good" (*opšte dobro*): Catholic priests used them to treat Muslims, Catholics sought imams or Eastern Orthodox priests. A mention of 1866 Shariat court license granted to a Catholic priest to treat an Eastern Orthodox patient suggests that the traffic in religious medicine was somewhat regulated.

9. The regional status of magic is well expressed in the figure of Milan Tarot, a regional celebrity who made magic into show business, on television and online networks from Serbia to Croatia to Bosnia. His media is tarot, which he explains as a navigational tool for resolving issues related to health, love, or business that are hindered by negative influences and black magic. His problem-solving paints a world congested with agencies, human and nonhuman, a world that could make one panic. He reads the cards to suggest the most impossible array of remedial actions or else makes magical implements for his clients. There is no making sense of Tarot (I capitalize Tarot when I refer to Milan for this is his artistic surname) since he so fabulously, so outrageously, so industriously produces nonsense: from call-in television, radio, and internet shows to reality shows and, since 2013, to the private consultations behind the closed doors in his new "tarot salon" in northern Serbia. Milan Tarot compresses the negative dialectic of faith and skepticism (Taussig 2003), masking the magical trick with unbelievable disguises that unmask cheating throughout the real act of making money, making fun, and claiming efficacy. And making magic obviously political: in 2012, Tarot's website ran a dead-serious mock electoral campaign. Posing as an independent delegate in the Serbian National Assembly, he appealed to those who would otherwise not vote, promising to end "the joke" that is the current state of Serbian politics. Against meditative musical backdrop, a gentle, bashful Tarot in a lemon-yellow blazer foresees being "the only wizard in the Assembly" and spells out a series of untenable and unrelated electoral promises of plenty: 6000-euros salaries for all and three meals a day, which he itemizes in detail as if reading a menu.

10. In his *Prince of Networks*, Graham Harman invokes "magic" and "magical" with an unreflexive tenacity that can only be described as a verbal tick—and always to designate what is improbable, presumed, unreal, preposterous. And this from a prince of wild philosophical speculation! Similarly, in the introduction to the *Political Matter: Technoscience, Democracy, and Public Life*, Bruce Braun and Sarah J. Whatmore ask that we seriously consider the political potential of objects—how they compose the world and recruit their publics—but offer an anxious disclaimer: "The idea that "things" might condition political life is seen to return us to a primitive state, attributing magical qualities to inanimate objects" (xiv). The hasty gesture of distancing is telling: social scientists and political philosophers concerned with science and technology seem not to be aware of contemporary studies on magic, which show that 1) energies, technologies,

and objects have a long and active political career, everywhere; and 2) magic or fetishism has never been a thing of the past, but has been actively produced within the projects of modernity, science, and disenchantment (see Stacey Langwick, *Bodies, Politics, and African Healing: The Matter of Maladies in Tanzania* [2011]; Brigit Meyer and Peter Pels, *Magic and Modernity: Interfaces of Revelation and Concealment* [2003]; Bruno Latour, *On the Modern Cult of the Factish Gods* [2010]; Isabelle Stengers, "The Doctor and the Charlatan" [2003]; Lawrence Principe, *The Secrets of Alchemy* [2013]; Katherine Park and Lorraine Daston, *Wonders and the Order of Nature: 1150–1750* [2001]).

11. My source is an online Business Dictionary, http://www.businessdictionary.com /definition/open-item.html.

ONE

Just Surviving

Living Well since the Better Life

🖋 Back from a supermarket, the woman was beaming. It was late autumn 2006. She had gone out on a morning mission to spend, wisely, no more than 2 konvertible marks (KM, about 1.25 USD) on essentials: fruit, sweet cream (*kajmak*), and milk. The family of four has nearly run out of money for the month—2 KM is a third of their usual daily funds. Her excursion was preceded by a heated domestic argument about managing the budget better and resolving, once more, to do things differently next time, so as to truly make the two pensions, hers and her husband's, last. The woman oversaw the family accounting and ran out of steam and money by the twentieth of each month: her expense log regularly registers minuses, over expenditures, and loans for making do until the pensions arrive. She is a retired economist applying her professional skills to minute accounting of household expenditures; the smallest item at the time: "1KM to the beggar," reads one budget entry. Here are a select few entries, which do not do justice to the care with which expenses are catalogued under each household member's name, under the utilities for the flat and for the house in the country, or under the rubric of the "miscellaneous," placed right next to an unnamed column that seems to be opened from month to month to capture the unexpected (house and car repairs, medicines, education costs, etc.). From June 2007: "electricity 28,30 KM; laundry detergent 9,35 KM; hairstyling 26 KM, medicine 9 KM, magazine 3 KM, rattles × 2 for the neighbor's (newborn) twins."

That autumn morning she had walked out feeling the mood that sinks in when repetitions of a failure make us suspect that it's our fault, or still render us so hopeless even though we are not entirely to blame, but she came back from the store buoyant, impatient to tell what she found: on sale for just 10 KM—imagine, a bargain!—was a pair of beautiful green gloves, made of "genuine leather," perfectly matching the hue of her older daughter's new boots. She buried the pair at the bottom of the heap, hoping somehow to come up with the money. Had the gloves been in any one of the seven small stores clustered in her neighborhood, she could have promised the trader a later payment. But no such arrangements were possible with the supermarket staff. Still, the gloves were not lost, just out of reach and not impossibly so: the price was right, irresistible, the gloves well hidden for later retrieval—a surplus or a secret stash of money just might turn up. It had happened before.

I've known her for a long time. I care for her anxiously and fiercely, though I cannot presume to know her well: she keeps her secrets, like her poetry and her diaries, to herself, although she opened her budget logs, her drawers and closets, and her family door to the ethnographer, whom she sometimes calls "a child" (*dijete*). How can I turn her into an ethnographic character without enacting a fantasy of authorial power that, clearly, I could not have in a relationship where the woman's age, wisdom, and life experience urged her to confidently address me as "my dear child"? And not least when she itched to give me advice or when she got me out of awkward situations into which my research curiosity sometimes misguided me. Besides, who knows how her diaries describe me, in the privacy of handwritten Bosnian–Croatian–Serbian, free from the pressure (or the pleasure) of an address to a wider, English-reading audience? In response to her secrets and to her own representations of what I call "our ethnographic encounters" and to account for the too many known and unknown fine details that bind us in a relationship, I will speak of her briefly, leaving her unnamed. She is my guide to the quotidian, sensuously historical experience of "just surviving" (*samo preživljavanje, baš preživljavanje*).

Her home is a comfort zone furnished with clues about lives that were deliberately cultivated and ornamented in the last decades of Yugoslav socialism, interrupted by the 1990s' war ("I feel that the best years of my mature life have been stolen," she often says, reflecting on the war and the years right after, when the couple was getting back on their feet), and lived beautifully, though the family was merely surviving, ever since the 1995 peace. The war upturned routines, habits, and expectations, and repurposed the objects in the domestic inventory, making room for emergency responses: a wooden stove in a corner of a high-rise apartment; duct tape over the windows, anticipating a shell blast; plastic water barrels; and volatile gas lamps. From her home I step out onto the streets of Tuzla, and when she is willing, I gladly join in on her routes. Otherwise, I go on my own, trekking further than she wants to, getting into the crowded spaces of marketplaces, waiting rooms of health centers, and pharmacies, lingering around shops and market stands long after the customers have left or before anyone has appeared, gathering a sense of what was so strange about the present (*čudno neko vrijeme, čudna vremena*) that people generally complained they've been weathering, enduring.

The two-bedroom apartment was furnished in the early 1980s with solid wooden pieces meant to last—shelves, cupboards, a dining-room set—and hastier purchases of cheaper plywood that were still bitterly regretted since they did not age so well and their flimsy joints and surfaces needed propping, gluing, nailing, painting, disguising, and upholstering to retain a functional and decent shape. The dark wooden shelves in the living room host a home library whose many titles, it seems, were on the essential reading list of their worldly-minded generation: de Maupassant and Zola, Marquez, Dostoyevsky, Selimović, Sartre, complete works of Marx and Engels, a few of Kardelj's, splendid volumes of *Arabian Nights*, *Health and Beauty* and *You and Your Child*, two hardcover, instructive reference books, and *Tito*, a glossy biography. New titles have been acquired since the 1990s, in particular the Koran, the Bible, and texts on Islamic practice and philosophy. However, the book collecting seems to have stopped. Prohibitive prices and small pensions orient the family toward the public library.

The honey-hued dining room furniture lends itself to joint meals, coffee rituals, important meetings, like this morning's dispute, and display souvenirs from earlier travels—a vase from Greece, a tea set from Germany, Sienna pottery, Czech crystal bowls. High above anyone's reach, on the corner of a cupboard, sits propped, a fat, sumptuously illustrated volume of a *Svjetski Kuhar* (*Worldly Chef*). It was never more frequently consulted nor ever so closely read than during the war years, when the family—like so many others—cooked creative meals out of the basic staples of humanitarian aid packages, out of foods found or gifted from the war black market, and with whatever produce and weeds urbanites managed to cultivate or glean on the town fringes or in the nearby forests, villages, and fields. Stacking an ottoman onto a chair, the youngest child would reach the *Worldly Chef* and pour over it. Other household members joined in, decoding the unknown culinary words while feasting vicariously on picture-perfect dishes between the inadequate and repetitive meals they were grateful to have.

The family closets attracted me most. To my ethnographic-voyeuristic eyes, they afforded peeks into a history of consuming habits, a collection of tastes, a display of desires: a color-coded history of sorts, finely threaded with smells of moth-repelling herb sachets, trailing perfumes, and trace odors of bodies and their brushings with the outside world: a whiff of cigarette smoke, city smog, or a bakery. What closets no longer contain, the photo albums and coffee-prodded tales invoke in a full contextual and textual richness: a yellow mid-1970s coat, perfectly cut, wool tweed that proved elusive during a cold month of one late autumn, which the determined woman spent searching the stores of Frankfurt until, so the story goes, she ended up in a hospital with pneumonia. Her husband showed up with the yellow coat on his arm, on his first visit, and it was just right, just as she wanted it. Or the smart, green evening dress, gently bell-shaped on the bottom, which matched her husband's moss-green, rich velvet suit, in which they danced into a New Year's Eve sometimes in the 1970s, and many years since. Silk blouses. Clever blazers. Yellow, green, brown, shy pinks: a small history lesson could be had around these colors, from primary to more ambivalent hues, and around the fabrics and cuts: the clothing items were carefully collected, registering splurges and savings, and from the mid-1980s to the last years of socialism, purchases above one's means courtesy of a mass speculative shopping scheme known as *na čekove* (on checks) and more accurately *na čekove bez pokrića* (checks without the collateral), issued confidently in advance of a salary in agreement with some friendly sales staff about a delayed release of a check. The closets present clothing as collections, composed with a particular sense of ownership as a relation between self, the milieu, and things, guided with a stated preference for a few items only but of finest quality (*jedno al' vrijedno*), tailored in ways to outlast finicky fashion trends while dressing up the person as sharp and "classy" or "most modern" (*klasika, najmodernije*). Clothing collections hang together memories of items' provenance, memorable shopping events, and special occasions, as well as the sedimented but constantly stirred traces of familiar moods and past occupations.

Since the woman retired from a career in now abolished socialist enterprises in the city of Tuzla, the capital of Bosnia's northeastern region, and had attempted jobs in small, private, trade-oriented businesses that failed, her dressing habits included new, inexpensive, functional pieces. Much of her wardrobe was second-hand, handed down to her or purchased at the market. The elegant everyday clothes needed special occasions for wearing—an outing downtown, a doctor's visit, a celebration. This fall she had been managing some ordinary misfortunes, including a death in the family, with tranquilizers, which she consumed only when her other techniques, Islamic daily prayers (*namaz*—Bosnian Turkism) and a yogic breathing practice, brought no relief. There was no medicine, however, for the chronic money troubles, which dressed her domestic quarters like an oppressive wallpaper periodically before the war and constantly, ever since, erupting at times, like water stains or wall cracks that furrow bumpy, busy patterns but remain contained within the taut fabric of the everyday. The rhythm of her monthly accounting, beginning with optimistic expenditures and diligent payment of bills (from utilities to her daughter's fashion-design classes and French lessons) and slowing down to negative numbers, borrowed funds, and disciplined appetites, exemplifies the more general struggle to live on average incomes or state pensions (from around 400 KM or 250 USD in 2007 and up to 800 KM in 2015. The minimal incomes and pension remain below 400 KM, though). Let alone to live beautifully, *lijepo živjet*. What else was there to do but to keep trying?

<h2 style="text-align:center">SINCE THE GOOD LIFE PAST</h2>

This chapter is interested in the shared existential circumstances and experiences of surviving, as well as in the mundane modes of pursuing a good life. It attends to spaces, objects, and practiced habits in present-day Bosnia—from dressing to eating, from caring to craving, from valuing to accounting—that regularly enact a sort of historical unforgiving of the stark difference between the presently precarious life and a better life (*bolji život*) of the past. This is no simple nostalgic memory but a comparative disposition that is at once critical and indulgent, stubbornly committed to the values that seem out of step with the objective conditions of possibility, but often sympathetic to the logics of yearnings. I often heard such ambivalence articulated in the field, sometimes decidedly resolved into a harsh critique, as when a nurse on a lunch break at an herbalist's street stand remarked with dismay: "See? Everyone walks about beautifully dressed but with empty pockets." This was a serious young person speaking out for sensible consumption and from the position of an employed, single man devoted to cultivating his *iman*, the inward aspect of Islam, and *ihsan*, beautiful conduct, as opposed to fashionable appearances. I will describe others who are more hesitant to judge, more entangled in outstanding obligations, more easily swayed by the attractive commodity callings even when it means hammering with determination into the interior fixtures of bathroom walls to redecorate—not because anyone else will ever see the results, but because one learned to live in nice dwellings. By the end of this chapter, I will show how this particular costly resolve proceeded while generating debts, bodily aches, and serious doubts about one's own plans, making substantial yet only privately noticeable differences to the flat in an apartment unit that was seriously close to crumbling as a whole. In other words, investments in better life, bolji život, are often not simply about keeping up appearances, self-consciously tending to the skin of things, but are more complicated and more ambitious aspirations for goodness that inheres in a comprehensive, enveloping sense of being and having, that saturates life thoroughly, with quality.

Besides being historically minded, modes of surviving beautifully are also oriented toward the present where better life may be impossible but where pursuits of the good life are enthusiastic or quietly insistent, inventive and resourceful, disappointing and nourishing. Surviving in style entails selective remembering and learning fast and anew what makes life good, worth living, even if it makes little economic sense, strictly speaking, or precisely because it downplays the strictly economic priorities and economizing tactics.

Scholars of post-socialist Europe and the former Soviet Union have already noted how common the complaint about "surviving" is across the region. Studies have turned the rubric of popular grievance into a repository of local experiences and perspectives that critically diverge from macroeconomic portrayals of the necessary pains and inevitable gains of the transitioning economies. I pick up the task of listening for the local experience and take it further with a curiosity that is insatiably interested in the sensuousness that surviving presumes and invigorates. I am also intrigued by the possibility of following the experiential arc that involves an embodied sense of a good life with a memory of senses, retrained tactilities with familiar and brand new market objects, and finally, with wider historical materiality. Furthermore, surviving sounds and works differently here: not only was the end of socialism in Bosnia and ex-Yugoslavia obviously embroiled in the wars of the 1990s and post-conflict circumstances, but also the Yugoslav exceptional socialism, professing a humanist commitment to the better life in the future and a good life in the meantime, left in its wake particular expectations and disappointments. Thus, several historical reference points loosely orient present efforts to survive stylishly in Bosnia. One is the Yugoslav socialist and cultural economy, which formal records describe as going through four distinct phases, with the peak of its economic growth and life standard in the 1960s and the economic unraveling in the 1980s. Depending on the pace and context of storytelling, biographical memory may compress this history around key moments of economic plenty and of a more diffused range of possibilities that were taken for granted even in the moments of private privation and financial crises. The war of the 1990s is another reference point, although it figures in ways that are perhaps unexpected: less as stories of trauma, bleak despair, or mortal danger and more as offering witty tales of resourcefulness and simple pleasures that people managed to secure under extraordinary circumstances. The 1990s war is also tacitly operative in the complaint about present survival: it is a poorly hidden, grating note, dubbing the story of peace, which was long in the making and barely negotiated, and so, otherwise, a very much welcomed event; it is a grinding of teeth at the tales of peace as the end to all suffering. Insofar as the war conditions kept open the possibility that after the war life would carry on as before, or become better yet, complaint about surviving in the time of peace is an ironic comment on what was supposed to be a much more comfortable existence.

Because I'm mostly preoccupied with the present bundle of surviving practices, I attend to how new spaces and persistent habits toss up historical references and subject them to reliable old and newly acquired evaluative tastes.

MARKET SPREAD

Once, in a small flower shop while we were buying a gift for someone, I caught her looking at a pretty pair of sheer stockings, on display among flower seeds, gardening tools, and a number of random items that the florist was trying to sell on the side, since one could not count on flowers to keep one's business afloat, not these days anyhow. Thinking she liked them, I drew near only to hear her say in a low voice: "I have no desire for stockings, pretty or not, if I see them in a grocery store." Goods were neither mere utilities nor discrete items whose aesthetic qualities alone ought to compel or repel; their affective value, insofar as it registers a capacity to appeal, was contingent on their provenance. The stockings were out of place. It took an ideal context of a shopping experience for things' value to emerge. This kind of value is not inherent—though it concerns things' substances and qualities and invites pinching and rubbing the fabrics to discern their composition (an experienced tailor in Tuzla, giving classes to all generations of women within a small, local NGO-scheme, is quoted to me as saying "it is the classy people whose cloths are wrinkled," *gospoda je uvijek izgužvana*, because they wear the prized, natural fabrics: cotton, silk, and linen). Nor are the evaluation standards entirely consistent, as shopping preferences shift with needs, cravings, and opportunities. Remember, this woman seriously coveted a pair of green gloves found in a supermarket, when it was a question of composing, just perfectly, her daughter's outfit on a shoestring budget. Without such pressure she could afford to hesitate, to tune in to the affective value of a commodity that may arise or may not move her. Indulging children is an act more open to compromise.

The most obvious trend of the new economy ushered in by the 1995 peace, a trend that persisted at least through the first decade of the new millennium, has been the uncontained spread of the market. Trading venues that were familiar enough became too many—like corner grocery stores strung, side-by-side, along each neighborhood block. Some relatively new enterprises, such as private pharmacies, started proliferating, while others were old, traditional even, but reinvigorated beyond all expectations, as was the case with the open-air marketplaces. The new market has regularly, irreverently enacted a sort of misplacement of goods—like stockings in a flower shop—and people: involving "everyone" with the new business of trading and with new shopping venues and habits. Moreover, the new marketplace repurposed the social and commercial space itself, directing the flow of money and promises, needs and desires, pretty things and possible pleasures out into the open of face-to-face exchange, whether on the street or withdrawn into small, stuffy quarters of a family-run corner store. This is a frank surface of the circulation sphere whose everyday machinations presume less visible and more painstakingly occluded flows, blockages, transformations, and occultation of values into capital and cash. Its counterpart is actually the robust hidden economy made into a public scandal and the staple of local media, loudly denouncing criminal–political business schemes and their extravagant speculations. Far more occluded are the energies and investments that lubricate the consumer economy since the withdrawal of significant industrial capital, the dismantling of public industries, and the absence of formal value-generating enterprises. It is within this space of quotidian mystery that people go about their business of selling and shopping in the new market economy that not only works, although money is said to be missing (*nema para*), but appears hyperactive, consumed by the market.

In socialist Bosnia, open-air markets remained fringe sources of prized local produce, products of domestic and peasant (*domaće; seljačko, seosko, sa sela*) economies that were cherished as minimally processed and free of synthetic fertilizers and pesticides, though regularly suspected as being less than authentic. Or else, provincial markets afforded weekly social events that were variously outward looking, connecting people beyond their immediate kin and neighborhood alliances (see the classic study by Lockwood 1975). Visionaries of Yugoslav socialist modernity counted on the eventual disappearance of marketplaces with all their lingering vestiges of the backward, peasant past that even the villages were expected to leave behind as they grew sophisticated and affluent and moved toward the future of shopping in department stores and shops (Štahan 1974:151). Thirty-odd years after such optimistic projections about the rising Yugoslav standard of living, from 2001 through 2007, I followed the northeastern regional rhythm of weekly markets that overtook provincial and urban centers, one day at a time. Markets seemed to burst out of the designated grounds, spilling into stalls and street sales, with moods grave or giddy with business and bargain possibilities.

A market day in the northern town of Srebrenik, for instance: crowds join in on a Tuesday, many arriving early from the surrounding villages and districts, to sell or to buy, to have a look and see kin and friends, to hear the latest news while on the way to municipal offices, health centers, or pharmacies. The plenty has to be negotiated whether you join in or resist the pull of the people whose density engages your arms and elbows in a defensive or offensive stance; you check and adjust your stride, while the sounds, sights, smells, and surfaces claim attention and distract. The collective pushing and compelling spills with the exchanges over a tight passage between buildings that is supposed to separate the market square from the street. Instead, every exit is an entrance and an extension of the market exchanges. Narrow thresholds are occupied by small traders, here selling socks, there, baby chicks—trembling in downy yellows—and chocolates: three bars for 1 K M. Stalls extend onto the streets, block sidewalks, stop car traffic, occupy parking lots, drape over vehicle bodies to display herbal medicine or music C D s, over human bodies to move easily an assortment of choices through the crowd, past the outstretched hands of beggars whose incomes largely depend on such weekly affairs, and onward into the town center, all the way to the doorsteps of pharmacies and public health centers. One fresh morning I find a pool of bright, red blood at the market threshold and find the hue as bold as many featured on the commodities for sale, dangling from stands, urging, striking, calling to eyes and noses, bellies, and hands: red perfume bottles, red lipsticks, red shoes, red purses and belts, red toys and cookie boxes. Red was in vogue that fashion season (*crveno je "in"*) and the traders cashed in hastily, ever watchful for when the market glut and popular whims shifted the color wheel toward different hues: small

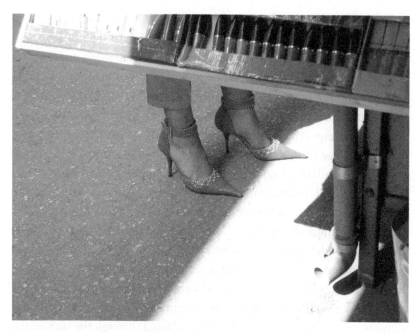

Figure 1.1. This market display of lipsticks featured all shades of red, which was the "in" color of the moment. The most eye-popping hue, however, was on the trader's feet. *Photograph by the author*

stocks could not afford outdated oversupplies. The street fashion sense keeps traders jittery and confident about their predictions: in just a bit, no one will be selling nor buying red for a while. The trace of someone's blood at the market will more permanently stain the pavement than the fluid commodity's flow will mark people's closets or memories: the new marketplace clothes being relatively inexpensive (but still barely afford-able), their cuts stylized to such perfectly current pitch—"the most mod-ern" (*najmodernije*) is the local term—their fabrics, hems, and threads flimsily sown, not meant to outlive by much the downward slide of the "it" or "in" color career.

The new market struggle could be hardly described as "bloody," al-though the iconic postwar markets have emerged literally from the for-mer frontlines and zones of separation between them. Arizona market, for instance. Situated along the northern stretch of a regional road, a meeting point between the Croat-Muslim Federation and the Serb

Republic, the two administrative entities of the Bosnian state, the town of Brčko, an independent district since 1999, close to the border crossing with Croatia, a former Yugoslav republic.[1] Trade was ongoing between the army trenches in the prized goods of war economies. Then, with the signing of the Dayton Peace Agreement and even before the NATO-implemented demilitarization, soldiers came out in the open, still in their respective uniforms, turning aside their weapons to trade, the very image of the classic anthropological idea of exchange as an act of forging alliances against odds, swapping hostilities for proverbial handshakes, and resuming reciprocity by other means. NATO found the image irresistible and invested in the mission of opening the market for peace, demining and patrolling the zone they code-named *Arizona* while advertising widely their patronage of interethnic reconciliations. Others soon joined in to try their luck in trade or to replenish the exhausted pantries, houses, drawers. "Everyone" went to Arizona regardless of their ethnic backgrounds, nationalist and wartime affiliations, religious convictions, or professional pasts. The boom lasted through the turn of the millennium, slowing down in 2006 partly due to the effective efforts to turn unregulated trade into a chain of strip malls and partly because the informal lending and borrowing slimmed down the available cash flows and the small traders from across the region gained access to Arizona's wholesale sources. The most enterprising traders took their business elsewhere or exited the trade to start small service shops or to enter transnational labor markets, especially in Germany, Austria, and Slovenia, or much further, as far as the recruiters for American defense contractors would take them, from Iraq to Afghanistan (see Jašarević 2014a). On our way to Arizona in autumn 2006, the driver of an unlicensed taxi told me confidently that sales were so low that "the traders, in debt up to their necks, will start hanging themselves."

Debt and death were frequently paired in quotidian stories of surviving (see chapter 3 of this book; Jašarević 2012b) but the ordinary economics of selling and shopping just as often register more nagging pains of persevering. Missing money provokes tedious, rhythmic fretting about the state of one's business or budget, especially around the "high dates" (*visok datum*) of mid-month when budgets are low, as well as a nurtured discomfort about being in the market. Many people feel misplaced at this new market and join the surplus labor in circulating the excess of commodities for the lack of better opportunities. A shoe vendor at a southern provincial market of Živinice, puts it like this: "It's hard to work at the market, the competition is fierce. Anyone who stayed without work came here, just to survive [*preživi*]." Džemila was an accountant with a branch office of Energoinvest, a successful Bosnian-based Yugoslav conglomerate with transnational contracts, doing business from Libya to Kuwait (or "from Mexico to Malaysia," as its webpage narrated its history) until the war broke out and she fled eastern Bosnia. She made do with humanitarian aid and odd jobs here and there, raising her two sons with the help of her extended family. In 2006 she supported her sons through their university studies and provided for their household of three, with this truly small business scheme: her stand features inexpensive slippers, shoes, and handbags, ranging in price from two to no more than 30 KM. Džemila's market incomes were very limited as she only kept the stand on market days and stuck to small stocks of items that were less "most modern" than indispensible and hence more reliably, though more slowly, sold.

Others pursued the new market currents more enthusiastically, taking risks and finding opportunities outside most people's comfort zones. Dragana, a woman of a sunny disposition, traded in luxury commodities, which she had been bringing over from Turkey since 1995. Initially, she supplied various sensuous commodities to the intimate companions of UN peacekeepers and foreign military personnel while also smuggling gold jewelry and lingerie that, she tells me, are always in demand. Her turnover capital was around 5,000 KM and she deployed an impressive range of resources to recover her investments and profits, sometimes against the odds. By 2006, she was complaining that everyone was "trying to sell something, and only a few can afford to buy." At that point she advanced a total of 25,000 KM-worth of commodities in exchange for informal promises of later payment. When even her trusted clients began deferring payments indefinitely, she shifted to a safer form of speculative economy. Having convinced a local clothing line to hire her as a traveling salesperson, she toured private businesses, public health facilities, and government offices, offering their employees goods on installment credit, provided that the employers guaranteed monthly paycheck deductions. She figured that the informal trade would bring no profits as long as people were "trapped" into repaying increasingly popular and available microcredit agencies and bank loans. "These credits do nothing but imprison people; they keep them captive," Dragana explained; "interest rates are tremendously steep, these lenders earn mighty well. Not everyone will take these loans, only those who are most desperate, those who have to. People take money to buy coal for the winter or to go to the seaside." It is a peculiar kind of desperation that articulates needs in what may seem to be different registers of urgency: a more economizing language would prioritize the expenses for the heating season in Bosnia's harsh winters over the summer vacations, which might be pleasant but not life-saving.

CLASSY SOCIALIST PAST

Yet, such broad articulations of needs are common across contemporary Bosnia, and often explicitly reference the good life of the socialist past. A traditional *strava* therapist (see chapter 5), a woman in her mid-eighties running a busy home treatment for anxiety, precisely in reaction to rising complaints about the new historical times, drew out a long sigh, between quiet smokes, and a single, wistful line from her thoughts that occupied her during a brief break: "Ehhh. Back then, in Yugoslavia, we had everything a human needed to live." *Everything* is ambitiously comprehensive. A broad understanding of the essentials for a good life was an integral part of Yugoslav socialist humanism that framed, rhetorically and methodically, the many projects of building a new society after 1945. The party programs of the League of Communists of Yugoslavia (Savez Komunista Jugoslavije; SKJ) reiterated the message about care for human needs and commitment to the good life. Its statements enjoyed a vast citational spread across vernacular, research-oriented, and policy-related venues. A 1970s SKJ statement, cited in a study on the Yugoslav living standard, is typical: "The essence of socialist political economy is the care for human needs, for the continuous improvement of material and cultural conditions and the lives of working people" (cited in Štahan 1974:151). Yugoslavia, like the rest of postwar Europe, East and West, was bent on reconstruction as well as on rapid industrial development and urbanization, especially given its initially precarious but eventually strategic liminality: not quite belonging to either East or West, doing business with both, and nurturing alliances with the Non-Aligned Third World. The new Yugoslav state's liminality also had much to do with the sheer mass of rural economies and peasant populations that it incorporated in the new state-national body; this fact was self-consciously cited as both an apology for the blatant cases of socialist underdevelopment or internal inequalities and as an obvious cause for concern and intervention. In 1964, at the peak of what is known as the Yugoslav economy's "golden age," during which its rate of growth was among the highest in the world, Branko Horvat, an influential political economist of international reputation, wrote that the existing social inequalities were inevitable, but were no more than historical baggage packed into the historical leap that Yugoslavia made from a "Balkan, peasant" society into an "almost modern economy" (1969:12). Inevitable but temporary and surpassable, Horvat and many hoped, for as long as earnest work was invested (earnest but aspirational, as to the tune of the uplifting labor song, "long live work, among us," "da nam živi, živi rad") and development well-planned, but neither implemented at all costs nor entirely at the expense of a pleasant present. The envisioned dynamic of development was held in check by the bundle of "human needs" that were irreducibly "material and cultural" according to the SKJ school of praxis, and oriented by two intimately related temporalities of quality: of the good life in the present and the better life, still in the future, but glowing brightly on the horizon. In the contemporary memories of socialism, the good life of the past is both the forward-looking, better life of the socialist ideal that saturated the narratives of socialist privation and shortages during the mid-fifties, early sixties, and the economic crises of the eighties, and the good life of relative plenty, enjoyed with oblivion to the signs of impending disaster.

President Tito's speeches variously emphasized that present concerns toned socialist development ambitions. In a 1951 interview for the Communist Party newspaper *Borba* (Struggle), Tito is quoted as saying, "People! Among us [socialist Yugoslavs], the human [*čovjek*] is everything. Our principal goal is to create, as soon as possible and in the most humane manner, a better life for the people, for individuals and for the

entire community. Even under the most difficult circumstances, we are
trying, first of all, to take care of the human, the human for whom socialism is being realized" (cited in Matić, Stojanović, and Štrbac 1972:37).
The emphasis is on the good life in the meantime; the possible contradiction between it and the urgency of development, "as soon as possible,"
is mediated by the caveat on the "most humane manner," a subtle but
sufficient reference to the distinction from the Soviet and Chinese paths
but also, at the time, a commentary on Yugoslavia's own attempt at land
collectivization, which was hugely unpopular and quickly abandoned in
1951. The formal socialist ethics of care for the human variously legiti-
mated pursuits of pleasant life and impressed, or dismayed, the visitors
and onlookers of the so-called Yugoslav experiment. In his 1956 travel di-
ary, John Kenneth Galbraith, an American economist on a first academic
visit to the socialist East of the Iron Curtain, admits being pleasantly
surprised at the sight of "well-dressed crowds, good food, pleasant promenades" in Belgrade, the Yugoslav capital, and nearby Novi Sad, especially in comparison to his bleak impressions of Poland. Galbraith relates
his observations together with a saying by Tito, which his interlocutors
rehearsed for him: there is no reason why workers shouldn't enjoy today
while they are busy building a better tomorrow. Tito's heroic biography,
endlessly reprinted, illustrated, and retold across many media, including
elementary school textbooks, appropriately mixes stories of privation,
morals on self-sacrifice, and anecdotes of mischievous childhood indulgence, while his presidential figure of elegantly tailored corpulence was
rounded off by the signature tip of a Cuban cigar. By his side, his spouse
Jovanka Broz modeled socialist style smarts, evidently preferring local
designers, clothing lines, and textile factories over Parisian fashion labels
(see Velimirović 2006).

The ideal of a good life and of properly human needs was translated
into the quantifiable, manageable, practical terms of a "living standard,"
a yardstick of development. Josip Štahan's (1974) comprehensive overview of the rising standard of living in Yugoslavia captures the trend with
statistics on appliances per household as well as some revealing indica-
tors of good life, such as the frequency of visits to hair salons and medical
doctors. Štahan's work was optimistic about the near future, an age he
anticipated to be well-groomed, finally modern without a tradition to

embarrass it. Human needs also translated early on into numerous governmental strategies and pedagogies, from encouraging production and consumption of consumer goods to advertising health-care services, personal hygiene practices, and scientific diets to rural mothers. Moreover, not only the Communist Party but all sorts of work and residential communities (*mjesne, radne zajednice*), activity clubs, and service-oriented public voices worked to educate popular tastes and aesthetic judgments, to cultivate urban spaces for cultured leisure and sociability, to tap into the subsidized sector of national tourism, to organize vacations or trips abroad for school children, students, and workers, and to establish sport clubs and communal venues for hobbies, from photography to mountaineering, to poetry writing. By the early 1960s, the Communist Party's repertoire of cultural concerns expanded to include a more forgiving treatment of Western popular art, a move that also furthered a need for critical education on just how to read bourgeoisie entertainment (Bokovoy, Irvine, and Lilly 1997; Luthar and Pusnik 2010).

Browsing through the archives of a Tuzla town newspaper, *Front Slobode*, one picks up reverberations of the broader cultural and national rhythms on a scale of what was newsworthy for one relatively small urban center and a handful of surrounding municipalities. Issues from the 1960s speak of intense investments in developing civic spaces and particularly venues that would give people something cultured to do after school and work. We learn of growing enthusiasm for the cinema: not only were the three town theaters under pressure to introduce screening times conducive to workers in uncommon shifts, but cinema projectors also toured the countryside on the back of a movie truck, setting up shows in the village districts' "homes of culture" (*domovi kulture*). On tour were the latest Hollywood as well as Yugoslav feature films, and while film critics regularly reviewed movies on the pages of *Front Slobode*, cuing the viewers to aesthetic and ideological value judgments, film clubs across the provincial capitals organized workshops, discussions, and classes to raise the moviegoers' aesthetic tastes (see also Bokovoy, Irvine, and Lilly 1997).

Cultivation and display of tastes were not only the objectives of governmental pedagogies but were also on personal and household agendas, inspiring quieter tactics to pursue the good life, under the circumstances.

While Jovanka Broz, for instance, performed socialist classiness by mixing and matching foreign haute couture with Yugoslav design labels and public fashion factories, she did not need to model her other style strategy: to have clothes made by small tailor shops—among a number of enterprises in a small but vibrant private sector—which is what many Yugoslavs, women in particular, did. Having clothes custom made, or else sewing or knitting their own or employing mothers, siblings, and female relatives to do so was the surest way to look smart. Compared to the shopping trips abroad, these tactics were inconspicuous, inexpensive, and significant: they dressed fashion-savvy masses in creative or authentic copies of cosmopolitan or store styles while reorienting distinction from literacy in labels to discernment of quality, even if the goods were unmarked. A trader from Arizona showed me black-and-white photos of herself with friends from the 1960s: at a municipal fair that village girls attended she was the one best dressed. With a smart suit and a handbag, she thought she stood out in the crowd of people wearing a motley range of outfits. She saved her daily lunch money that her parents gave her, during the years she commuted by train from a district in Srebrenik to a vocational high school in Tuzla.

PROPERLY HUMAN: BEING VERSUS HAVING

Bosnia was among the economically poorest constituents of the Yugoslav federation, and from 1947 it was on and off the list of recipients of federal development aid. Development aid was discontinued a decade later due to massive investments in the defense infrastructure, strategically located in the Bosnian mountainous interior, and resumed again in 1965. The investments Bosnia received, however, continued to fall below its per capita share (Plestina 1992:100) and this was just one of many contested issues in the Yugoslav internal-development policies. The Federal Development Fund allocated aid for various projects and sent experts to help Bosnia catch up, while leaving aside the questions of structural underdevelopment whereby the underpricing of raw industrial materials from Bosnian mining, steel, and chemical enterprises provided the initial impetus and ongoing supplies to the secondary industries of the northern republics, particularly Croatia and Slovenia. The status of the poorest among the equals and of an internal Orient, where modernization efforts confronted not only stubbornly peasant ways but also ethnic or Muslim traditions, contributed particular urgency to the socialist development initiatives in Bosnia and fanned a particularly self-conscious hankering for modernity among some aspiring Bosnian socialists.

The pages of *Front Slobode* display earnest effort and exasperation at small, repeating failures. "Once Again, How to Organize Good Fun [*dobru zabavu*]?" is the heading of an article that revisits the perennial problem of where Tuzla's young people could go out. The journalist informs us that one dance hall has been converted into a public reading room, which is a fine idea but too small a facility for all the visitors; the facility also lacked "basic hygienic standards." Besides, young students or workers, laboring hard six days a week, long to go out *at night*. The article surveys other venues that are either too expensive or unattractive to youth. It issues a number of appeals and suggestions to the municipal committee and also places high hopes on the Home of Youth (*Omladinski dom*) whose construction was expected in the early 1960s (*Front Slobode*, January 18, 1960, p. 8). The article is squeezed next to a brief press report on the latest activities of literary groups: a gathering of young poets and fiction writers from among medical high school students; the quality of the literary works was mixed but the journalist begs readers not to judge these beginnings too harshly, capitalizing his ending with a cheer: just carry on with writing! Snapshots of fashion shows held in a packed local theater that also hosts amateur theater groups and ballet ensembles on tour are followed by a welcoming coverage of a brand new restaurant, Expres, serving 5,000 meals a day—no other food venue in Tuzla since can boast of such traffic—and daily news of progress and growing pains from surrounding districts, municipal towns, and villages.

Some socialists were ambivalent about the popular appeal of modern values, as these were synonymous with consumption of Western goods and trends. In an editorial titled "Modern Times," the author sides with "a great number of us, the nonmoderns" (*nas nemodernih*) who are sifting through the loud, entertainment-hungry, provincial (*malogradjanska*) trends to look for what might be valuable after all about modernity. A cautionary tale is spun around the narrated figure of the author's friend, initially a shy, humble peasant child, hungry for knowledge and, the author suspects, secretly dreaming of escaping the family fate of hard soil toil. Snubbed by a pretty, urban woman for preferring "our folk songs and domaći films" over rock-and-roll and suggesting a date in a theater rather than a dance hall, he embarks on a personal mission to "modernize rapidly." Soon enough he is up to date on all the current cues: Marlon Brando hairdo, baggy corduroy pants, and black, pointed-toe (*šimi*) shoes. Shoes are not just a colorful detail here but a crucial sign of quality around which the story line turned, signaling the before-and-after moments in the metamorphosis of a noble peasant to a modern provincial. Although it was on the dance floor that the story's protagonist was first discovered to be a peasant, when his date, the young urbanite, saw clearly that he did not know how to rock, the story tells us that she reportedly later blamed herself for being in denial about prior clues: "I should have known right away by the looks of your suit and shoes," she is said to have said. A final blow: "You haven't even had a sniff of modern life" (*Front slobode*, April 18, 1960).

The editorial ponders how to be properly socialist and modern while being caught up in or resisting the changing seasons and trends "from Tarzan to cigarette-pants [*sulunar pantalona*]" (ibid.). He prefers his friend to be "genuinely peasant," honest, "knowledge-hungry," employing callous hands with books during the school season, but he nonetheless fears his ambition ("beware," he reports telling his urban friends, "no one will match his work effort, for he knows real toil"), portending a substantial change, no matter what. The author does not reflect on the critique of the urban privilege written out in the peasant's voice ("while you are vacationing with friends on the coast this summer, I'm only now headed to real work. My father and land await my help") but, rather, he carves out a niche for a "large number" of critical onlookers, decidedly "nonmodern." Being on the outside of the trends, they were true to themselves, discerning the lasting values beneath appearances.

The story speaks to the larger problem besetting Yugoslavia in light of the patent differences in incomes and lifestyles as well as in the vigorous vernacular distinction between the northern and the southern republics, between urban and rural Yugoslavs, between intellectual and manual workers. Amplified to the scale of international discourse, the internal differentiations and the market-oriented socialism fueled ideological scrutiny among the COMITERM observers, who debated whether and how Yugoslavia was socialist, given its exceptional politics and economics. In one of his early texts, Branko Horvat (1969) aims to distinguish the Yugoslav style of socialist humanism from bourgeois consumer democracy. Increased consumption and better life, Horvat argues, were only the essential means of making a socialist human, whose ultimate goal was self-affirmation, realized through forms of "being" rather than "having." Marx's early philosophical manuscripts are behind Horvat's dialectics of socialist encounter, but the intersubjective constitution proceeds only on the condition of a proper prior schooling in the arts of "social consumption": consumption of essentially nonmaterial goods, from education, arts, and culture to health-care habits and self-care techniques. While bourgeois consumption is individualistic and leads to alienation, social consumption orients the individual outward, to collective needs and common resources that shape individual tastes and raise collective consciousness as a whole, "beyond the psychosis of a consumer society" (Horvat 1969; see also Štahan 1974 and Šefer 1965). Social consumption was a redistributive administrative rubric, funded through Common Consumption Funds (Fondovi Zajedničke Potrošnje) that spread access to resources and opportunities, including, indeed, anything from winter coal to summer vacations, with the practical goal of minimizing and eventually transcending social inequalities.[2]

Socialist consumption resolved the ideological tension between having and being with a working compromise: acquisition and consumption were meant as teleological means, fashioning future socialist being with comprehensive needs but well grounded in the present of redistributive and collectively minded goods. As such, social consumption did not discriminate between material and cultural needs, between basic necessities and leisure time.

HEAD TO HEEL

In contemporary Bosnia, social distinctions still pivot around shoes and clothing styles. The general economic impoverishment, however, the vigorous return of repressed traditional forms, and the proliferation of market venues that promise to lend indiscriminate salience to people, habits, and things, all under the currency of most-modern, have made it at once more urgent and more difficult to discern underlying, lasting quality. Many modes of figuring out the ways of being and having involve learning and teaching others as well as rehearsing norms on what is proper, wholesome, desirable, or tasty. Present is a history lesson on small and collective habits that includes selective and sensuous-minded memory, prodded by quotidian discomforts, lasting irritations, misalignments, and misplacements. All along, however, pleasure and goodness are earnestly sought.

A pretty young woman stopped by a clothing stand at a southern municipal market of Živinice, run by one savvy businesswoman, Sanela, and one of her daughters in her early twenties. Barely skimming the stock with a half-interested look, she thanked the traders and turned to leave. No sooner had she turned her beautiful, freshly styled head, than the two traders scanned her from head to heels. The trader's daughter announced defiantly: "It's better to sell nothing at all than to sell to just anyone." Her mother added: "And this is what we've been telling you about who is in the market: peasants' kids. Did you see her heels? These are kids who just took off their rubber boots. She's dressed up and wears her purse just so"—here Sanela caricatured the latest manners of carrying the oversized, "most-modern" handbags on a bent elbow, and the traders laughed at the humorous show of folk couture, which they meant as a lesson to an ethnographer: "And you'll see later just how a city child dresses: normally. They know what to wear for this occasion [a market outing] and what to wear otherwise." To detect a peasant, a suspicious gaze may have to search to the ends of well-dressed, carefully groomed appearances to find an ill-fitting detail: rough skin exposed in high-heel sandals, showing traces of a quotidian habit of wearing iconic rubber boots across the proverbial village mud and manure. Moreover, because anyone can master new items and postures, the finer art of dressing up or down requires attention to timing and contexts. The task of teaching the ethnographer about local distinctions was ungrateful because the ethnographer at once looks and speaks as a native urbanite but displays a privileged cluelessness about basic social facts; such teaching is rarely a straightforward lesson because the tutorial attention could turn back on itself: Selma next started fiddling with her daughter's shirt, attempting to tuck the straps of her daughter's bra beneath her tank top, before giving up, frustrated: "Why didn't you sew those together?" The trader's two daughters married right out of high school, disappointing her expectations that, unlike her, they would pursue university education, which she still offers to finance. Sanela built a successful trading business after the war, managing to accumulate capital at just the right moment before the economic slowdown, which she met with consolidated assets and reliable networks of suppliers and clients. She wished, however, that her daughters and their children would exit the market for good.

Many traders were reluctantly employed by the market. One couple, a husband and wife in their fifties, traveled with flea markets that revolved across the regional towns one day at a time. Years after, they still felt out of place. Their discomfort is regularly renewed, and not only by the usual risks related to running a business in a precarious economy. Theirs was a gendered division of goods, displayed side by side: Amra handled clothing, accessories, and catalogue-order makeup, while Idriz kept an excellent stock of tools and household appliances. Here is a snapshot of an exchange from their stand one morning in the town of Brčko, where the market takes up several kilometers of the city edge, including the compound of a defunct socialist trading giant. An elegant woman returned to buy a blazer that she had tried on earlier, taking up the advice of her friends who, over coffee in a nearby café, thought it fit her perfectly. Having paid, she was in no rush to leave before speaking her mind about the present-day market, trusting the anthropologist to take note:

> Nowadays, everyone buys at the market, from doctors to doormen. We, people from the cities, all of us, we shop here. Before the war we used to wear top brands [*markirano*] but now have no means to do so. This Monday market is a special day. My friends and I get together here to socialize; all of us are city folk [*gradska raja*]. One is a medical doctor, another a high school professor, and so on. There's a green market nearby where we go to find healthy food, stuff homegrown [*domaće*] by the peasants, who only come on market days, so we primarily come for the produce but then we also come out here [to the second-hand market] and look for things. . . . Then we sit down for coffee someplace. And everything can be found at the flea market, everything can be found here, if one is knowledgeable [*ko se razumije*]. Those who can

recognize good stuff, good quality, those who know how can find all the good things here. You see, while I was raising my children, we would go to Italy every spring and every fall, and would buy them everything there, everything from socks to undershirts, and everything was brand-name. And my children are now returning everything I've ever given them, they are helping me out [financially]; I'm a lucky mother. But this, this is just surviving, surviving indeed [*baš preživljavanje*].

Our elegant interlocutor delivered these lines after a longer mono-logue, building an emotional crescendo from the initial excitement over the found bargain treasure and the pleasures of a weekly social event, to distaste for the market, anxiety about being confused for belonging there, to the grievances over the circumstances that brought her and her city people to market, ending on a note that sounded typically exasper-ated. My fellow traders and I also learned that she had been dismissed as redundant from a public financial institute after thirty years of employ-ment and without a retirement plan;[3] she could not make do on her late husband's pension without her children's help. That she was not used to this kind of living—without an income and shopping at second-hand markets—needed not just emphasizing but contextualizing to drive in the point that her condition is the new norm: everyone, from doctors to doormen, shopped at the market. The city people might have lost the financial means but they can count on their fashion sense and skills of discernment in recognizing value even when it does not come from the most obvious places: Italian department stores or boutiques. Memories of shopping trips abroad, and most often to Italy, are cherished among many Bosnians of certain generations, cited and variously embellished as evidence of the cosmopolitan mobility they once enjoyed, courtesy of the socialist Yugoslav lifestyle. This woman, however, adds another cru-cial element to the popular narrative of past conspicuous consumption acts: it was her children whom she dressed lovingly, devotedly, season-ally in foreign fashion brands. Moreover, it is this excessive investment of an indulgent caretaker and the stark reversal of the familial roles that, perhaps, choked her up as she spoke, with gratitude, of her children's present support. What they give is not the expected filial duty but more than that: a return on the surplus, which is "everything" she ever gave. A lucky mother.

The woman was a snob, Amra decided once the customer left. Some such people were too caught up in the "city folk" distinction, Amra explained, telling me, in confidence, that she never brags about the fact that she is a native of Tuzla, the region's capital. Like so many of her fellow traders, Amra never imagined herself working at the marketplace. She shared the elegant shopper's expectations about figures who were traditionally at home in the market: "genuine," *real*, peasants, selling homestead produce and handicrafts, provincials known as *šverceri*, handling counterfeit and smuggled commodities (derived from the German *Schwarzhändler*, black marketeer), and "Gypsies" (*Cigani*).[4] These figures issue from a powerful place on the cultural peripheries, from which they exercise the regional popular imagination with a fine, sometimes blunt, regularly unnerving force of ambiguous valence. *Real* peasants are presumed to be closer to nature and to venerable culinary and herbal traditions. Elderly peasants in particular are tenderly included in the familial addresses for grandparents (*nena, baka; djed*, or *deda*), but are also profoundly suspected of polluting, diluting, or faking domestic, domaće, staples. In stories and jokes, peasants' clichéd naivete and ignorance are only matched by the cunning they are imputed to have, especially when it comes to tricking and outwitting the urbanites. Far more troubling, however, is the closely related figure that earns an especially mouthed intonation of the word *seljak* or its adjective *seljačko* to mark all sorts of transgressions of propriety regularly performed by those whose typically provincial provenance confuses the boundaries between urban and rural, cosmopolitan and local, between having high culture and showing off affluence with lowly means. It is this figure of seljak whose ambitions exceed village boundaries and peasant economies to pursue the business of *šverc*, accumulating conspicuous wealth and building powerful alliances, not least in the nationalist political parties, that troubles the most contemporary sensibilities across Bosnian spaces. Not surprisingly, the "peasant" figure is shape-shifting, to the point where it cannot be reliably picked up in accents or dress, let alone in the geographical markers of work and residence, given how much the latter were confused especially since the population displacements and resettlements of the 1990s. Almost anyone could be possibly confused for a peasant and a peasant could potentially slip by unnoticed: well-educated, urban and polished, dressed with classic or most-modern touches. Finally, Roma have been the regional scapegoats, romanticized in cinematographic and popular culture; objectified in various governmental projects of reform, development, public health, or education; regularly vilified, or admired, for being ungovernable subjects; and reputedly especially talented in handling šverc commerce and servicing the occult market for black magic, sorcery, and divination.

Much of this ongoing distinction takes place outside the market grounds, in spaces where knowledgeable consumption shapes mundane pedagogies and saturates perceptual encounters, priming the senses, from a tender age, to the various pitches of sweet, sour, rough, or finely scented. So trader Amra's young grandchildren, for instance, are learning fast the art of what Bourdieu (1984) described as "distinction": quotidian processes of tasting and sorting that exercise class differences and shared dispositions in the seemingly most unremarkable acts of being a body: wearing slippers, home decorating, stomaching foods. Amra's five-year-old grandson wanted Grandpa Frost (the regional counterpart of Santa Claus who has been distributing parcels with sweets and fruits since socialism, and often on behalf of socialist enterprises [see Kurtovic 2012]), to bring him a Bulgari perfume so he could give a New Year's present to his kindergarten sweetheart. Amra was amused and told other, similar stories. How she once disappointed him with a gift of cheap chocolates bought at the marketplace. Remembering the child's sour face, she laughed and impersonated his objection: "Ugh, Grandma! Don't you know any classier chocolate [*gotivniju*]?" Of course she knew, so she took him to a corner store and let him choose a flavor of the decidedly favorite brand of "German" chocolate, Milka. "His mother is like that too," Amra explained. "As an adolescent, she would wait forever, if need be, to get a new pair of jeans, but back then they had to be Levis."

WARTIME SURVIVING

It is the various ways of being a body in the world that people practice, remember, worry about, and reinvent while feeling misplaced in the strange times of the new economy. Habitus here is far more contingent than Bourdieu imagined, especially given dramatic shifts in the brief history since the mid-1990s; it is neither efficiently nor conveniently matching what's likable with what is, anyhow, possible nor is it so easily disoriented as to produce a lag between the practice and its shifting historical conditions (1990:78). Rather, old habits are cherished or repurposed, variously rehearsed or retrained as the historically minded values of a good life orient practices and encourage improvisations under unanticipated, unimaginable circumstances.

In the 1990s, people were displaced from cities to villages and from villages to cities and to Tuzla, in particular, given its vital position in the largest unoccupied contiguous territory under the Bosnian army with access to an international border. The roads to Tuzla were lifelines for wartime movement of things and people. The mobility of a disaster and relief aid may have much to do with Amra's elegant customer's investment in the difference that sets "us, the city folk" apart: many Bosnian Muslims and Croats fled Brčko after its occupation by the militant Serb nationalists (Četnici), and lived for years in the surrounding village districts. Life in displacement, or more generally in a war emergency, is better appreciated if one listens for the small, muffled complaints about routinization of foreign acts: urbanites learned to flex their bodies onto the outdoor squatting toilets, picked up hoeing, seed-saving, weeding, and gleaning produce from the wild or abandoned fields, and cooked on fires. Refugees in the city collective centers and private accommodations learned under which conditions their causes earned humanitarian attention from the UN and NGOs. Rural refugees also quickly learned about urban distastes for the doubly other, "refugee" and "peasant" ways of dressing, speaking, spitting, squatting, and settling in the cities.

Remembering the war past in the present, however, registers not only privations and discomforts but also small-time tactics of surviving that speak of resourcefulness and improvisations, recycling and repurposing of overused things, ornamenting and upturning of familiar tastes. Stories of the wartime quotidian play up a selective memory of the senses and are meant to make one laugh as well as teach a lesson about living well—how simple this can be—under extraordinary circumstances. A mention of a banal item solicits eventful inventories of practices, events, and experiences, as when a 2008 conversation on the popular online Forum Klix.ba started off with the question about whether anyone remembered a wartime recipe for Eurokrem, the favorite milk and hazelnut spread that flavored childhoods of generations of Yugoslavs.[5] Entitled "Wartime Eurokrem," the discussion invited posts with recipes as well as longer, biographical essays on eating, drinking, smoking, knitting, growing food, making clothes, making up games, during the war, in displacement, or on frontlines. Recipes for cigarettes include smoking clover, mint, fig, and blackberry leaves. Recollections of smoke and smells saturate the tales: cooking tripe made the house smell revolting; *pače*, bone-marrow gelatin, was cooked with salt and pepper and was "fatty, smelly,"; people recalled smelly, coarse blankets; black, heavy smoke of lamps was variously improvised by adding a few drops of oil into a jar of water, with a cloth wick; or oil lamps were made from chunks of cocoa butter (found in the stock of a nearby chocolate factory) or lard. On the menu list of war memories are substantial meals, meals that are indigestible or impossible to chew, smelly meals that make a "smiley face vomit."[6] Some remember sour fruit jams, made prematurely because hunger could not await the ripening season, but others speak of counterfeits that could not be told apart from the real things, "or so we used to tell ourselves," the post adds, doubtfully.[7] Or traditional sweets (*hormašice*) that, stripped to the basics, turned so "super" tasty that, one contributor admits, she no longer bakes the peacetime version.[8] Included are also clearly nonessential foods: "here is another recipe for a wartime lollipop," writes one post (20 dkg of sugar, 3 tablespoons of water and ½ spoon of juice from a [military] lunchbox. Mix it all up, cook for three minutes, grease a baking pan, arrange toothpicks, pour the hot syrup over ⅓ of each toothpick).[9] What stands out in the online sharing of recipes as well as in the hand-scribbled ones I leafed through in people's homes is the resolute naming of the dishes—pizza, marzipan, Eurokrem, *pâté*, mayonnaise, torte—a mimetic practice in its own right whereby faint similarities between wartime ingredients or their cooking procedures and peacetime culinary assemblages were played up in resonances, priming the tasting and dining experience. Titles that offered disclaimers poked fun at the whole affair—"Pizza with nothing"—but humor was only one of the flavors in what goes without saying: there are no potatoes in wartime "French fries" ["1 cup flour, 1 cup corn flour, 1 teaspoon baking soda stirred in some vinegar. Mix up a hard dough, spread out and cut into French Fries shapes. Fry"[10]], nor is there dairy in wartime "Cheese" or meat in the item named a "Bread Steak." Contributions signal different ages, responsibilities, and gendered orientations toward the wartime supplies and appetites: some remember what cooking or providing supplies entailed, while younger respondents have "no idea how my mother and father's brother's wife [*strina*] made Eurokrem nor what did they ever put in it, but I know this was the best thing I ate." Then there are memorable acquisitions—gifts, purchases, handicrafts. Someone remembers "to this day" a green comb she received as a refugee in an aid package. Another voice speaks of a gorgeous sweater in "1,000 colors" ("ah, that was so very modern then") that her mother and cousin, more skilled knitters, made for her. Having fled homes with no change of clothing, she writes, they used to look for old sweaters to unspool and knit back again "into something more beautiful."[11]

So many posts and so many stories told to me in person return to the body in an emergency, craving things, withstanding remarkable pressures, resisting nudges and disciplines, getting a subject thoroughly caught up in the acts that ought to be so predictable as to be unnoticed. In a particularly humorous, long post, one author tells of being infected with Enterocolitis, from drinking water from forest springs after the city water source was poisoned by the occupying Četnik forces. The worst thing about it, he writes, is that you must stay close to a toilet, since you do not trust your own bottom; you live in fear that you will have soiled your pants before you know it, that the toilet will be occupied just when you need it. The humorous, lengthy recollection of all kinds of small mishaps related to the illness ends with a rehearsal of the lesson learned: "and here a human realizes how the little things in life matter hugely."[12]

Emergency, however, also provided ample opportunities to make money or to obtain valuable items at windfall prices. Trader Sanela, whom I mentioned earlier, collected startup capital piecemeal, smuggling cigarettes across the Croat–Bosnian border by taping boxes to her ties, well-disguised by the many folds of traditional, bulbous pants (*dimije*). Another trader at Arizona remembers well the day when she procured a beautiful red carpet for a bucket of milk. A man came from the city with the carpet roll, slung over his shoulder, looking to swap it for peasant produce. City folk, especially in the first years of the war, took their prized personal and household items to the market—carpets, Levis, jewelry—that were suddenly devalued in the economy where belly carried the loudest vote and sought to swap them for villagers' dairy and agricultural produce.

CRACKING

Peacetime has ushered in different kinds of emergencies while encouraging many to pursue the good life with the doggedness of someone making a reasonable claim, though the circumstances may not favor the endeavor. Or might undermine it, thoroughly.

One such investment stands out in my field notes. It is related to an apartment on the seventeenth floor in a building just across the street from where this chapter began. In the fall of 2006, herbalist Šaha borrowed 4,000 KM (around 2,700 USD), a substantial amount of money in local terms, to renovate her apartment. She had vague plans about selling it later and moving to the countryside. Since the war's end in 1995, Šaha has worked at a daily open-air market in Tuzla. She had begun practicing herbal medicine commercially, however, in the late 1980s, after having left her job with a public company, taking severance pay and an early retirement package, which were offered en masse at the time of intense economic restructuring in the name of efficiency. She supports herself and her disabled son with sales of medicine and with her late husband's pension and thinks that the Bosnian economy is, more generally, sustained by parental indulgence: "Parents would go to the end of the earth for the sake of their children; they give them everything even if they have to pinch money from something else. And most parents don't want their children alone to be poorly dressed in school, so they say, 'fine, we'll spend a bit less on this or that.' I see them shopping here, [making purchases], and . . . whatever the children want they get it for them . . . I am as much to blame as anyone."

Šaha dresses her adult disabled son well: from boutiques rather than the open-air market, although she can barely make ends meet. She finds fault with the logic that values brands and overextends household budgets to meet children's desires, but she understands only too well how compelling is this imprudent spending: "Children learned to ask [also "grew accustomed"; *naučila dijeca tražit*] and we, the parents, to give."

Shortly after her renovations were finished, she invited me over one evening to see the difference her hard-earned and borrowed cash made to bathroom pipes, tiles, and the bathtub. To save money on labor, she and her son had spent the previous week knocking out the old tiles. "Every bit of my body is aching," Šaha tells me, preparing coffee. "What did I need this for? You tell me. Am I ill? Am I mad? Who am I doing this work for? How long will I live to enjoy it?" She answers her own self-doubts in a short while: "It's just that a human [*insan*] has learned to live in a beautiful [*lijepom*], neat [*urednom*] space." Surviving in style makes no sense if it were not for the fact, as Šaha here reminds herself, that it is the only way one knows how to live. When demands for a good life exceed her budget, like so many others, Šaha, goes into debt, grows alarmed, doubtful, remorseful, and self-critical. She also excuses her own and the collective endeavor of attending to beautiful, neat, enjoyable appearances as a learned and historical habit, a proper way to be human.

Within months, Šaha saw the value of her top-floor apartment plummet when the seventeen-story skyscraper cracked just above her window, and a two-ton cement block tumbled to the ground. It crushed a woman passing by and flattened Šaha's faint hopes that the costly renovation was, after all, financially prudent—a long-term investment. Šaha's building is in the neighborhood at the edge of Tuzla, recently nicknamed Sadaka City (sadaka translates as alms—see chapters 2 and 5), alluding at once to the poverty of its residents, the supposedly socialist unskilled labor force of peasants and provincials, and since the 1990s, rural refugees. Like other places in Bosnia, Sadaka City is in fact far more mixed, housing all sorts of people from the once classy, classless society whose world is coming apart, sometimes in small, quiet tears—like a family argument over whose fault it is that the money has run out—other times cracking evidently and irreparably, shattering the very infrastructure of contemporary lives.

The cracking above her window made Šaha miserable. She wondered seriously about her unlucky fate, while it mobilized residents and the urban-planning department around the threat of further deconstruction of all ten buildings on the block that, everyone knew, were built sloppily during the late socialist era when public resources and enterprises were misappropriated, informally sold, or miscalculated for personal gain. Sadaka City was not the only neighborhood in Tuzla where rooftops were unstable or tumbling and which pedestrians avoided in large circles, cautioned either by the official signs of danger or the rumored past incidents.

THE MOST MODERN SEASON

As the concrete resisted gravity, danger signals faded, and pedestrian attention gravitated toward more grounded fields of contingency. Daily traffic pressed on in pursuit of events and markets—outward to provinces and inward to the town centers. Several blocks from Sadaka City, the walkway morphs into a busy route to the public health center, to several technical high schools, universities, and to a small curbside market composed of four picnic tables. Goods displayed here issued colorful invitations to pedestrians with time to linger or in the habit of finding cosmetics, lingerie, or accessories on the go. Alma's table always featured things "most-modern," small accessories, and makeup that captured the fickle attention of hundreds of high-school and university students, many of them daily commuters from nearby villages and small towns. Alma runs her hand casually over stacked heaps of commodities (nail polish, lip gloss, earrings, and rings), recomposing the exposition of hues, shapes, and sparkles, burying some, upturning others, and promising plenty to gaze upon. Even in the grayest winter, fogged with coal-burning stoves and smog, here I find another season: fresh, "most modern," out of tune with the rest of this curbside world, by the smelly trickle of the industrial Jala River. One day, after the afternoon traffic waned, Alma's weary prodding set off a squeaking frenzy of fuzzy, stuffed-animal pendants meant for key chains, bags, and cellphone tags, as she thought aloud: "So many are well-dressed but if you look into their houses, you'll find nothing to eat, not even bread." Next to the students, Alma's clients are women formally employed in the public health center, department stores, banks, and businesses. A refugee from eastern Bosnia and a single parent of a twelve-year-old boy, who spent his toddler years by his mother's side, with a large cardboard box for a playground, she is often critical of people complaining about money and running up debts. Nevertheless, she indulges other people's cravings for accessories, and offers goods on credit, free of interest, when the "date is high" and budgets are low.

THE OPEN ITEM ACCOUNTS

Green gloves—Gloves were purchased and then, sadly, lost. Not so the shared memory of their perfect hue or softness, or of a discreet label inside, claiming Italy as their origin.

Restaurant, "Expres"—The city's iconic restaurant that *Front Slobode* enthusiastically announced opening in the1960s has been running a public kitchen since the mid-1990s. The socialist menus, however, still whet some Tuzla folks' appetites and summon memories of daily specials and some particular cooks' skills.

Alma's stand—In the summer of 2014, shrunk to an open suitcase set on the smallest stool and tucked further away from the main road, on a dirt path between kiosks. She was caught by the market inspectors too many times and spent nights in prison. . . . Besides, she needed only half the income now that her son, all grown up, a teenager, joined his father, Alma's ex-husband, in Germany where he was waiting for "papers" or for undocumented work. But Alma was happy: in love, "like crazy," she said.

Infrastructure, still cracking—In 2013, the outer wall of the building where this chapter starts cracked and shed some of its gray, concrete block surface. No one was hurt. Yellow tape skirted a bottom of the building, directing pedestrian traffic to a supposedly safe distance away from the potential wreckage, until it was, eventually, removed. Not so the possibility of the structure's further crumbling, though there may be only a few of us who are still warily approaching the building.

NOTES

1. Following a protracted arbitration process over the contested town of Brčko, the High Representative (HR) for Bosnia and Herzegovina established it as a district, an internationally supervised experiment in multiethnic city administration.

2. By 1971, however, Horvat was vocally disgruntled with the growing class differences in the midst of national financial crises and noted, wryly, that Yugoslav elites at the Belgrade international auto show would find no luxury car too expensive.

3. The privatization of socialist companies after the war proceeded with massive early and forced retirement plans. Given the fact that most companies, privatized or not, profitable or not, distribute meager and regularly deferred salaries, earning the pension (at either age sixty-five or after thirty-five years of work) is the major incentive for keeping the posts, which often cost employees more money in commutes than they earn in salaries.

4. In his late 1960s ethnography of markets in western Bosnia, Lockwood (1975) describes *šverceri* as a "derogatory epithet to denote all those who sell products not of their own production." Hence the category includes not only illegal but legal forms of reselling. *Šverc*, i.e., smuggled commodities for informal resale at home, grew in popularity outside the market proper as the number of Yugoslav guest workers in Germany rose from the 1960s onward. In the late 1980s, the mass of šverc commodities expanded at the market and many discovered that the market was profitable and joined it. Hana, a trader at Arizona, tells me that her town of Brčko knew her as Hana Švercer. She started her market career with farm produce and moved onto imported commodities. The regional market legend, Hame, is a Tuzla Roma who made a fortune at the marketplaces in the 1980s and whose family carried on the tradition to this day. An entire marketplace, including a very popular flea market, on the eastern outskirts of Tuzla, is owned by Hame's family.

5. A product of Takovo socialist food conglomerate, Eurokrem was advertised with a nurturing line: "Growing up together."

6. Post by Cholina_Lokica, January 15, 2009.

7. Post by "Zeleno volim te," January, 15, 2009.

8. Post by "B.boja," September 21, 2008.

9. Post by "Zeleno volim te," October 23, 2009.

10. Recipes copied in the post by "Zeleno volim te," January 15, 2009.

11. Post by cHupjahalic, September 19, 2008.

12. Post by Giga, September 19, 2008.

TWO

Insanely Generous

Making Wealth in an Economy of Debt

🌿 In Kreka, a regional mental hospital plastered in pastel shades that changed regularly from pink, to blue, to green, courtesy of international aid agencies' money, an outpatient was diagnosed with a peculiar manic disorder: a "giving mania" (*manija davanja*). Repainting a façade was a quick fix, a humanitarian shorthand for aid until around the turn of the millennium, when the budgets for post-conflict psycho-social care dwindled and the façade sunk into a dull olive green. The hospital, located on the outskirts of the northeastern Bosnian town of Tuzla, still figured vividly in the popular imagination of excess, exception, as well as norm. When in the 1990s the hospital swelled with inpatient refugees from the conflict zones, it opened its doors to include in its backyard the neighborhood and main road that runs through it. Patients' daily marches on the streets in search of cigarettes, money, events, or attention became a sign of the more general disorder of the 1990s war. What locals usually refer to as *čaršija*, literally "downtown" or the town center, comprising a cluster of promenades, cafes, bars, and restaurants whose occupants carefully mind everyone's business, recounted particular patients' habits that displayed, in an exaggerated form, more general states of fear and restlessness, impoverishment, and displacement. Since the turn of the century, the popular imagination of the hospital shifted to index post-socialist as much as existential and psychological disorders. Traders and shoppers at the regional marketplace Arizona, some 60 kilometers north of Tuzla, at the crossroads between two entities of the Bosnian state and close to the borders with neighboring Croatia and Serbia, former Yugoslav republics, invoked it frequently. Arizona was massively popular from 1995 through

2000 but shrinking in visits and volume of profits by 2006, to the great consternation of the masses of vendors, many of whom had joined the business of trade after having lost their jobs and savings to the war and the disintegration of the socialist Yugoslav economy (see chapter 3). One winter day in 2006, after Arizona's traders had been weathering weeks of slow sales, accounting in the meantime appreciating debts, one woman among them shook her head at her fellows' long faces and said, laughingly: "All of us here, we are fit for the Blue Hospital." The hospital's name remained color-coded—blue, green, pink—irrespective of the color of the latest façade of the sad-looking building on the edge of Tuzla.

Since the hospital also houses the regional psychiatric practices, and so offers consultations for more general psychological complaints, including everyday anxiety and its associated vernacular complaints of *sikiranje* ("worrying yourself sick"), it spatially bunches together but diagnostically keeps apart quotidian and pathological maladies. This is how the outpatient in question earned his diagnosis, while breezing through the psychiatric ward on the occasion of one of his springtime psychotic episodes. Not a category of mental illness in the *Diagnostic and Statistical Manual of Mental Disorders* (DSM), the American but globalizing psychiatric reference, "gifting mania" is a local doctor's diagnosis of a particular disorder: a compulsion to give carelessly, beyond the sound calculus of one's means, in the generally impoverished economy. The generous man tends to laugh at the time when doctors declare generosity insane. He utters *Bismillah*, "in the name of Allah," giving away with ease whatever he has—the income of his pensioner mother (though she cleverly hides it), with whom and off of whom he lives. He gets presents in return and passes these on, too. He also dispenses pencils, essential oils, his poems, and pastiche books, the production of which consumes him for weeks with the tasks of finding, cutting, gluing, writing, meditating, and praying for inspiration: he sends these into circulation, obsessively, as gifted commodities and "economic monstrosities," as Bronislav Malinowski termed the products of excessive labor of love or love of labor, "too good, too big, too frail," or too ornamented to serve any purpose ([1922] 1984:173). Useless. He quickly redistributes the small pension he gets from the state on behalf of his disability, in front of a mosque, to those gathered, waiting for *sadaka* (Turkism, from Arabic *sadaqa*), which translates as alms, mercy, and merit. In return, some in the gathering sometimes laugh at his turned back, thinking him silly, if not insane. When he has spent all—pension, his mother's money, and gifts given to him—and has, for the time being, contracted all possible debts from friends, family, neighbors, and traders (who give, reluctantly, though they say they know better), he offers a nice word as one should, he says, if one has nothing else left to give.

He takes as well, but selectively, and decisively not the prescribed antipsychotics or tranquilizers. He makes impossible requests for other people's belongings or money. He purchases extravagantly, relatively speaking: choice cookies, ice cream, or foods when the household has run out of money, by the middle of the month, and buys commodities on an open tab at the local shopkeeper's. He invests in things of delicate beauty that he enjoys, shares, or gives onward, saying that one should give what is dearest and what one would rather keep.

MARGINALLY MANIC

This chapter departs from the charged margin of a town and the down-town's common sense, which is a local mental clinic, with an unusual psychiatric diagnosis in hand in order to investigate not the clinical di-agnostic predicaments and limitations but the ways in which marginally manic gifting practices speak of general dispositions toward generosity. One man's extravagance, I suggest, is kindred to the local habit of giving beyond one's means while all along knowing and rehearsing a sense of good measure, and policing and protesting against the excessive gifting urges and expectations. Most concerned observers—relatives, acquain-tances, the neighborhood, and the downtown, čaršija—would agree that the diagnosed man gives too much, not only because he gives all that he has but also because he has so little to begin with, and because he makes no money, holds no job. He gives, in other words, what he himself had received rather than earned. He lives off gifts that, considering his circumstances, could be easily confused with alms, and what he redis-tributes is in an equally ambiguous category. This gesture too, however, of passing gifts onward, of regifting what has been received or gifting on the condition of having been prior gifted with means, is more general and economically significant under the present historical circumstances where a formal accounting of incomes, expenditures, and debts would seem to recommend a tighter hand.

While gifting has a rich ritual history in Bosnia, tied to major life-cycle and social events, from birth to weddings, while charity and openhandedness have been valorized by all three dominant religions (Islam, Eastern Orthodoxy, and Catholicism), quotidian gifting has been practiced with particular abandon since the 1990s' war and peace. When, during the war, shops emptied out, when military, humanitarian, and black market logistics trickled in scarce goods at exorbitant prices, and produce was grown by those who could access land in the cities and neighboring villages, people shared whatever resources they could obtain. Although everyone's need for goods was rather obvious, sharing the surplus of scarce supplies, however obtained, called for tactful offering and persuading of the other into taking. Since the end of the war, when everyday life feels like "surviving," limited budgets are regularly extended with the aid of other people's generosity as well as by overextensions in giving. The project of this chapter is to show the extent to which everyday economics are entangled in gift giving and taking, inside and outside the market.

The market sphere exploded in venues, from open-air markets and supermarkets to neighborhood shops and pharmacies, from itinerant to installment-credit and catalogue sales, all of which have been the busiest sites of income making and spending since the 1990s (see chapter 1). Selling and buying, however, has been greatly facilitated by informal loans of money and commodities that are extended free of interest and with negotiable return timelines. Since personal forms of lending and borrowing presume and enact generosity, intimacy, and tactfulness among the exchanging parties, debt is no simple market instrument in Bosnia. Under the circumstances, though perhaps surprisingly, circulation and accumulation of debts generates a sort of wealth. One trader's puzzling words prefigure this chapter's argument: "I don't have any debts. Never had any. But that's why I don't have anything. I don't owe anything to anyone." I take up this vendor's insight to ask what kind of wealth is comprised of debts. And how do we perceive of "owing" if it participates in the accounting of wealth?

LIVING BY DEBT

The trader who claims to have no debts, Zlata, is a single mother of a teenage daughter. Once an accountant in a socialist enterprise that closed, she has worked as a salesperson in a boutique at the Arizona regional market since the 1990s. On the same occasion, she also said:

> I did the math and realized that I can't afford a loan [*kredit*]. I don't have money to return the interest. If I earn 400 K M and the two of us live off of that, how can I have 100, 150 [K M] to give [in installment] every month? There are people who constantly investigate credit options. They raise several credits [*kredite*, plural]. I don't understand where they find any interest in that. A math professor, a friend of mine, did a calculation to prove that they do have an interest. But I don't see it. I know that I can't afford a credit. But even at the market there is so much of that: this one lent to this one and that one borrowed from the other. Constantly they borrow from one another. And in Srebrenik [a nearby municipal town] even the big ones are failing under [the burden of] credits. There was a wealthy man who made a fortune before the war but raised credits that he couldn't pay back. . . . People live on debt [*ljudi žive od duga*].

Zlata observes a shared existential condition at the new market and narrates herself out of it. Her prudent domestic accounting of incomes and expenditures can make no financial sense of the popular borrowing passions. While the woman's calculus counts with a stash of money that evidently grows with incomes and slims with the expenses, the math professor's formula—if at all related to skillful, real-life lenders and borrowers—must have incorporated the shuffling acts that multiple returning timeliness and interest rates entail as well as the value made in the extensions and deferrals of money in motion that is never properly owned as much as hosted while in transit, promised and owed to someone, and expendable until the due date. In Zlata's common sense, we can read a habitus that trusts hard numbers and prudent economics, and that cannot be simply traced to the socialist habits of either rationing or enjoying the relative plenty. Socialist Yugoslav history is itself marked by sharp turns in national fortunes that variously informed personal spending and splurging (see chapter 1), although the general confidence in the solvency of the Yugoslav economy and the aspirations toward the good and better life on the national horizon wove an optimistic underlining into the late socialist consumers' tactics, from issuing checks without collateral, to skimping on food to save for vacation or clothes, to building food stocks for the crises to come. Zlata's economic prudence seems misplaced in the new economy that appreciates negative numbers, elastic totals, extended timelines, and uncertain incomes.

Moreover, Zlata's telling shifts back and forth between formal and informal lending. She starts with kredit, an institutional form of loan, lent at interest by banks or microcredit organizations (MCOs), which she says she cannot afford. Moreover, the trader says that much the same business of lending and borrowing takes place at the market, though she is describing personal loans that are arranged free of interest and with less rigid repayment timelines. She takes no part in personal lending either and tells a cautionary tale of overextending in loans and bankruptcy that can happen even to the rich and market savvy.

Conflation of institutional and informal loans under the single category of debt, *dug,* is common in Bosnia and speaks to their practical and experiential entanglement. People borrow from multiple sources to run a business, supplement subsistence, and not least to pay installments or settle outstanding informal debts. In 2006–2007, when I spent the longest time in the field observing the markets, bank loans were available only to the few who had a regular source of income and could meet the stringent borrowing requirements. More accessible and, becoming increasingly more popular, were microloans. This sector of grassroots banking grew out of humanitarian responses to the war and postconflict needs, when relief agencies began experimenting with small banking projects initiated with the World Bank's twenty-two million dollars in 1995 for the population with limited access to formal loans. The MCO's stated objectives—to encourage entrepreneurship and postconflict recovery, to improve standards of life, to empower peasants, women, or the young, "to realize a dream"[1]—sound compelling but their image among the population at large was rather otherwise. Since the microloans are often piloted by humanitarian nongovernmental organizations (NGOs), are run by the former NGO staff, and flaunt the language of assistance and service, the high interest rates that they charge (18–30 percent) are read as evidence against their professed humanitarian claims. In the provincial market one day, a trader and part-time beekeeper told me that he borrowed 5,000 K M from an M C O to invest in a honey business and returned 6,500 K M, with a grudge: "They grab you by the neck and use you up. Our human being is constantly indebted." His wife and trading partner adds: "These microcredits, they just flay you. They aren't exactly helping." At the same market on another day I found two employees of an M C O distributing leaflets to a largely unsympathetic audience. A small vendor of gold jewelry, which she brings from Turkey, shouted after them that she was "not insane" (*nisam luda*) to take up a credit that would "break her back," and other traders joined in her voicing of displeasure with the terms of repayment.

The outrage shows that people are taking M C O promises of assistance and dream fulfillment literally and holding them to the standard of the informal, personal loans that are interest free. The insanity amounts to paying back the exorbitant interest rates. And yet people in need of capital to finance a business or in want of money to live decently lean on M C O s and repay loan installments by borrowing informally, including borrowing from loan sharks, when in dire need or at the height of the trading season.[2] In short, trading businesses throughout the region tend to operate with loans of money, institutional and personal, and advances of stocks from wholesalers. In turn, they regularly extend their stocks for promises of later, frequently deferred, payment to clients who, likewise, tend to shop with money borrowed from M C O s, banks, family, neighbors, and friends.

Traders then are habitually indebted, stretched between simultaneously owing and lending to one another: whatever money they have can be claimed in turn by those on whom they themselves count for emergency cash. A trader at her corner of the weekly market of a southern town of northeastern Bosnia, a refugee and a single mother of two adult sons who had once been an accountant in a socialist company, describes the spirit of mutual aid: "When one of us is in a squeeze for a [micro]credit installment, then all of us here help out, with 50 or 100 KM. Especially when the winter comes [and] you can't pay the monthly installment. Here, we help each other more than does the family. When you need some [money] temporarily, here, no problem, I give to you, you give to me." Personal lending between traders often presumes familiar, close relations that are reworked densely as people busily knit together multiple loans, arrange repayment timelines, and traffic all kinds of little gifts and kindnesses in the flexibly extended temporality of the meanwhile.

It was the intimate quality of personal relations between shopkeepers and their clients that kept many a neighborhood store in business even if the corner stores were overabundant, and the supermarkets were usually cheaper and seen as more attractive shopping venues. In the words of a shopkeeper in a provincial capital, Srebrenik: "These shops couldn't work without debt [*bez veresije*]. Everything [here] is 'on debt' [*na dug*]. Working on debt has always existed, but now, that is the only choice. There are some customers who pile up debts and then avoid my street." Each shop keeps a more or less steady clientele of indebted customers who, ideally, settle their past monthly bill, in part or in full, at the beginning of a month when pensions and salaries are due, and start new cycles of shopping in advance of payment. As the shopkeeper makes obvious, however, their customers' deferrals can extend indefinitely, tensing and suspending their relations until the debt is settled or the expectations of its settlement expire.

Pharmacies, which mushroomed following the full marketization of the Yugoslav economy in 1989, and especially since the peace, also took part in the economy of promises until around the turn of the millennium when the pharmaceutical market consolidated into fewer hands, competition intensified, and debt books turned further unprofitable after over-the-counter sales of prescription medicine became more regulated and taxable.[3] Nevertheless, the head of a formerly public and currently city-owned pharmacy in a provincial capital that still used debt books in 2006 was surprised that pharmacies could escape debt: "How can they not have the indebted regulars? This pharmacy at all times has some 3,000 KM in debts: people took medicine but haven't paid yet." Hers was both a moral judgment of pharmacies' general shift to the logic of the new market that treats patients as customers and denies them drugs if they lack the purchasing means,[4] as well as reflecting the genuine question, how does one go about saying no? Genuine, that is, if one keeps in mind the fact that provincial pharmacists often know their clients and patients tend to tell their stories of suffering in minute detail, compelling care. Pharmacists remind the patients to settle their debts in time for the pharmacy's annual financial audit and then let them reopen debt accounts with each new year.[5]

Traveling vendors and peddlers of catalogue-order cosmetics and accessories are likewise counting on their clients' promises of money. A remarkably successful trader, Dragana, complained to me that trading was "a hard work because all you have is in debt [*sve je u dugu*]" (see chapter 1). Shortly after our conversation, Dragana shifted to a safer niche in the debt economy. On behalf of a local clothing brand and for a commission, she toured regional companies to show seasonal fashions to employees and offer items on three-month installment credits. Installments were directly deducted and redirected from the staffs' paychecks. Dragana's new clients reportedly resented and resisted their employers' attempts to set prudent limits to the share of salary that could be extended in advance. A purchase of a 300 KM coat, for instance, amounted to one-quarter monthly deduction from an average 400 KM salary. Some received as little as 20 KM a month in cash after all the various credit payments were met.[6]

Street vendors were entangled precisely in the messy deferrals and negotiations that Dragana had exited. These informal workers, whose market displays hurriedly folded at the sight of market inspectors or police, were not only borrowing or lending from one another and advancing goods to their clients, but often were lending money free of interest to their regular customers who appealed to them for help to finance anything from vacation plans to infant formula to a fancy cellphone. Traders tend to be judgmental about their clients' spending habits but, nonetheless, can be indulgent. Take a very popular street-stand owner, Alma, who tells me about one of her clients: "She carried away 30 KM from me this morning. She already owes me 96 KM and this morning she took another 30 [KM]. She took it to have a good time, to spend it on a [Women's Day] holiday trip. Imagine! What bank?! I'm more of a bank than a bank. . . . But she is honest, she gives back."[7] By extending a loan to a woman with holiday plans, Alma effectively has the pleasure of giving pleasure, which, as I will show later, is the very mark of gifting, and not only in Bosnia. Also, Alma points to an important verbal cue that accompanies talk of informal debts: the debtor does not simply "repay" (*otplati*) but returns or gives back (*vrati*).

Working side by side with Alma is trader Bahrija, with a sidewalk stand dressed for the season—bathing suits in the summer, hats and scarves in the winter, and underwear throughout the year. Bahrija issues commodities in advance of payment and frequently lends money to her customers, fellow traders, and neighbors, overextending her capital with promises that eventually materialize. Her customers, she says, "pay back from paycheck to paycheck. And people live like that. By the time they receive their salary they've already committed it; they are already indebted. But you have to keep your customers, so you have to give on debt." She replenishes her small stocks piecemeal and runs several open tabs with wholesale traders at the Arizona market. Bahrija and Alma complained one day about how difficult it had become to sustain sales on debt:

> Bahrija: "I can't even borrow [*da uzajmim*] any longer."
> Alma: "No one can!"
> Bahrija: "Because tomorrow it needs to be returned [*vratit'*]."
> Alma: "You can borrow, I can too, people will lend up to 5,000 K M, but
>   if one day you lose this [tapping her cheek], when you once lose your
>   trustworthiness [*poštenje*] and then the [creditors] ask 'Where is that
>   woman, where does she work?' and they find you, you may tell them,
>   'Kill me but I don't have [the money],' they'd say 'Why are you cheating
>   me, why did you ask for money [if you can't repay it], live [by your own
>   means] whichever way you can.' No one is insane [*nije niko lud*]."

Insanity in this case consists of lending money if it will not be repaid. The advice is exchanged between two traders working side-by-side and therefore at the closest distance to one other in case one has a cash emergency. The complaint thus also rehearses the expectations that loans will be taken gratefully and as graciously as they had been given, in good faith, without witnesses, without collateral, without paper trails—except some lenders' furtive note-taking after the fact and out of sight so as not to insult the borrower with a sign of mistrust.

GIVING PLEASURE

Debt underwrites and undermines livelihoods, orchestrating lived rhythms and embodied moods calendrically and spatially to the tune of borrowing and lending. Shopping habits plot onto one's debt relations that will lead to or away from a given shop, pharmacy, or trader and will shift with monthly flows and clogs of incomes and fortunes: before the fifteenth of the month shopping for cash may be more itinerant and indulgent. Appetites are not entirely curbed when cash runs out, but indulgencies can easily be traced to someone's generosity, just like one family's monthly budget enumerates ingredients for a cake—butter, chocolate, hazelnuts—to sum up the recipe into an amount loaned by the budget keeper's pensioner mother, herself regularly indebted for groceries to the neighborhood shop. Open tabs in stores and at street stands sustain unlikely debtors: well-dressed, salaried professionals with expensive tastes, who owe for groceries or make-up and buy coffee or mascara for cash only when they have completely run out of the item. Elegance and cultivated tastes are sustained by debt.

Indebtedness, not surprisingly, is worrisome and discomfiting not only to Bosnians. Popular radio and T V shows in North America give air to people's grievances about debt and offer expert (but not necessarily useful) advice on how to deal with the onset of bills due to childbirth, job cuts, and deaths in the family.[8] Ethnographies converge in depictions of bodily experience within the global trend of rising consumer credit and personal loans. Brett Williams (2004) studied North American credit-card "revolvers" (those who pay the minimum due on their credit card statements and are entrapped in high interest rates), students pursued by loan-collection agencies, and the poor who rely on fringe credit instruments and reported a range of complaints that associate debt with everything from physical aches and sleep loss to disability and lost dreams of better life. From a different context of low-income neighborhood in Chile, Clara Han (2011) shows how everyday life entangles money and family misfortunes into a host of affective and bodily issues that "eat one's nerves" and become the object of familial and neighborhood care tactics.

The language we heard at the provincial Bosnian market in reference to microloans ("flaying," "back breaking") does not only metaphorically articulate a critique of usurious terms of lending but also expresses an embodied sense that skin and bones participate in the toil of collecting funds and generating surplus value to pay back the interest. And while for all practical purposes personal debts are easier to handle, they are also especially oppressive since in practice they are surrounded by sensibilities that accompany gifting. What makes debts so distressing is precisely what makes them most gift-like: their noneconomic surpluses. They weigh on the receiver like an unreciprocated gift, inspiring restless desires to oblige and delight in turn, while the receiver dreams of escaping the guilt and embarrassment caused by other people's kindness. To understand the affinities between personal debts and gifts, and the implications of their confusion for everyday life, I suggest that we turn attention to the habitual, most casual and natural but compulsive giving that suffuses social interactions in Bosnia, and not least the encounters at the market.

In Bosnia, people give for pleasure as often as for duty as well as take pleasure in fulfilling an obligation, which requires us to reimagine acts of "duty" not only as ordeal but also as enjoyment of one's compliance with the roles and norms of goodness and decency in a given order (see Farquhar 2005). Marcel Mauss ([1954] 1990) always spoke in the same breath of the pleasure and duty that motivate giving: "Therefore let us adopt as the principle of our life what has always been a principle of action and will always be so: to emerge from self, to give, freely and obligatorily" (ibid., 71). Formal gifts, however, inspire most ambivalence or downright anxiety in the giver. These gifts must be given to kin and friends on important occasions such as birth, marriage, graduation, and religious holidays, and are given within a certain timeline and in an appropriate monetary value, which is regularly above one's means. Ritual gifts can be oppressive for all the parties involved, insofar as they are expensive to the ritual host and may send all the givers and takers into the market, shopping on debt with a particular stand or a shop owner, or borrowing money from kin, friends, colleagues, or neighbors. Nevertheless, the compulsion is often not simply to give, but to give beautifully, to give beyond measure, to give for keeping. This was well articulated to me by two pharmacy accountants, who complained one rainy afternoon in the wake of the Ramadan Eid holidays, just how much time and money giving takes. But then one of them concluded: "This is a very nice custom, isn't it? To me it's very nice, isn't it nice to make someone happy, to surprise and delight [*obradovat*] someone? And I love to buy beautiful gifts [*poklone*]." The other accountant knew what she meant: "Something beautiful and not something just like that. What do I have from giving something that you will throw away?" A gift—*poklon, dar, hedija,* or *milost* in the local idioms—that is less than beautiful fails to give pleasure, to either the giver or the taker, and thus fails. If the beautiful is the aspired norm, the gifting gesture that gropes for it is best depicted by the common act of prudent gift recycling: among the elderly or in case of formal gifts to the extended kin of the wedding parties, never-opened items of clothing—usually shirts or towels—or boxes of elaborate confectionary, become form of currency. They are given on the condition of prior gifting-receiving and they participate in the understanding that to receive is to give back in. The point here is obviously not to give what is beautiful nor what gives pleasure—although in order for the shirts, towels, and chocolates to become a currency they must appear of just the right quality and price—but more importantly, they deliver and redistribute the emphasis on giving rather than keeping.[9]

Quotidian little gifts, however, tend to be specifically useful or random and charming. Although these gifts presume relatively small expenditures, they are passed in the context in which each counts and so border on extravagant and occasion compulsive giving, beautifully and thoughtfully, even on the occasion of a casual visit. Everyday gifts play important, if subsidiary roles, in historical and cultural contexts much different than in Bosnia.[10] Bourdieu locates the "canonical" value of gift exchanges precisely in spontaneous, everyday gifts among the Kabyle, and their comparability to gifts that, he says, the French would recognize as "trifles" that "cement friendship" ("it's nothing," we would say). These small gifts, so easy to give and match without requiring special occasion or etiquette, are exemplary for Bourdieu of improvisations and uncertainties that inhere in the practical logic of gift exchanges. But while Bourdieu describes ordinary gifts as prompted by life-cycle "pretexts," such as harvest or a child's first tooth (Bourdieu 1997:191), in Bosnia the pretexts for giving are less marked, more mundane and incessant. With the massive impoverishment of a population that not too long ago lived fairly well, gifting makes someone's life somewhat easier, more delicious, or more bearable. The choice of items follows considerations of the recipient's circumstances, often quite literally assessing the stock of their fridge, pantry, wallet, drawer with utility bills, or medicine cabinet. The practical confusion of gifts, as giving pleasure and meeting a need, is a further reason why there is no obvious reason that anyone would take what is offered. Giving, then, is a privilege won after persuading someone, who was otherwise reluctant, to take, discounting the value of the offering ("it's just a little something") and explaining yourself ("I know you have, but . . .").

This can turn gifting attempts into a brawl of sorts. At the urban market one day, Daca, an owner of a well frequented boutique stocked with clothing and cosmetics, forced a bag of oranges onto her aunt who had stopped by: "Here, take these!" The aunt looked shocked, almost offended, pushing the gift away, but the trader was faster: "Take it!" she said, shoving the oranges back into her aunt's arms. The aunt protested again, returning the fruits, but the trader impatiently tucked the bag into her aunt's lap and stepped away. Before leaving, the aunt, whose single minimal pension supports three adults, once more gave into taking a gift, this time of makeup for her unemployed adult daughter.

Presents are rushed into the hands of the other: one is gently shoving, annoyingly pressing, while the other is resisting, denying the need of the act or any desire for the article, admonishing the unnecessary fuss and expense, each party moved by and regretting, lovingly, the attention of the other, who has gone out of the way, spent money they did not have or could have used otherwise, in order to give items one could really use or would rather not. Resistance is spirited, even if a learned bodily gesture, which is why giving up and taking the gift obliges the giver. In the provincial pharmacy that runs sales on debt, the manager once complained: "When some grandpa brings me bananas, I get so angry, I wish I can tell him 'take those bananas; why are you spending your money, I don't want to snub your bananas but I know that your pension is small, that you are deprived of bananas; keep them, keep your money, why would you buy them for me?'" The uselessness of some beautiful gifts or plainuse value of others, like bananas, are part of the gift traffic that is moved by desires to give, by other people's needs and your limited means, by the suspicions and rejection of the other's pity, and anticipation of their pleasure and displeasure. Your giving obliges the taker but the taker's taking is a gift to you. She is indebted for your gift but she has graciously treated you by taking: indebtedness is reciprocal.

Mehmed, an herbalist with a pharmacy and a street stand, habitually gifts parts of medicines to his patients or adds medicinal teas and oils as a gift. When it is obvious that a patient cannot afford a recommended treatment, Mehmed gives it away, saying *halal bilo*, meaning let it be forgiven, or else saying, "Oh, you'll bring [money] sometime," but not bothering to take note of patients' names or coordinates. Daca, the earlier giver of oranges, buys gifts for her extended kin whenever an irresistible commodity shows up that someone might like to have; she also treats her regular customers generously with food, beverages, and gifts of cosmetics. For Christmas, Easter, and in the late fall when households are stocking pantries for the winter with pickled vegetables, fruit preserves, sausages, and smoked meats, she is overwhelmed with gifts of homemade delicacies. A great experimenter with dietary supplements and herbal medicine that happen to be in vogue, she passes these onto her customers in response to complaints or at a hint of a disorder in their appearance (say, someone's looking pale, fatigued, worried-sick, disheveled, cold, or flustered). She gives opinions and advice on people's clothing, styles, and hairdos liberally and quite bluntly. Gifting care tends to hurt a little.

INDEBTING GENEROUSLY

Derrida's famous deconstruction of Mauss's ([1954] 1990) classic essay argues that a gift is impossible, because no sooner is it conceived, intended, given, received, recognized, or given back, it becomes its opposite: an item caught in the economic circulation. As such, gifts, like market objects, call forth repayments, returns, calculation, and commensuration, and in the meantime imply debts, domination, self-congratulation, subordination, guilt, or shame. Derrida's objections presume a universal subjectivity, one constructed through rational calculus of ends and means, one whose good intentions toward another stumble upon the self-love that consumes or subsumes the other, hungrily, as if all human appetites were schooled through the cutthroat lessons of competitive commodity exchange. Mauss, as I already mentioned, was far more comfortable with the ambivalence of gifting experience as at once pleasurable and threatening, generous and self-interested. Bourdieu (1990) developed the ambivalence into the theory of gifting practice, shifting attention away from intentionality to embodied dispositions of a subject who responds to a present in the heat of the practice. Generous disposition, according to Bourdieu, is a trait of a shared habitus, the living, historical mode of perception and action, cultivated in an environment that rewards generosity and makes withholding unthinkable, scandalous, revolting, or downright hostile.

Nevertheless, Bourdieu insisted that anthropologists recognize that gifting societies also count on interest and gain. This is why gift inspires ambivalence, which natives recognize very well ("Gift is a poison," Bourdieu quotes Kabyle), as present appears at once disinterested and demanding repayment.[11] The time that lapses between the gift and countergift, Bourdieu suggests, allow the socially real illusion that gift is an event in itself, unrequited, generous, delightful, rather than a snapshot of an exchange that will unfold full circle with future return. This meantime is productive, "inscribed in the body itself in the form of passion, love, submission, respect for an unrepayable," as Bourdieu puts it, growing the affective weight of the act (1997:237). While Bourdieu's analysis posits a rather untenable distinction between two antithetical dispositions, the generous and the calculating, appropriate to two distinct economies, of gift and of equal exchange, gifting inclinations in Bosnia are variously tangled up in the market proper.

The broader economic implications of this entanglement ought to have become obvious by now. Since generosity is presumed and expected in the informal market, loans are difficult to deny. Requests implicate the creditor with considerations of the stated or unsaid but known or guessed existential circumstances of the borrower. Debts are therefore often extended against common sense. Consider this story. A young man, who had made a fortune at the height of unregulated trade at the Arizona market and invested it into an auto parts store and a small ceramics factory, had all his capital tied in investments and advances but was hard pressed for 2,000 KM in cash. In the winter of 2009, he recruited his father's help. The father qualified for a bank loan on the account of his pension from a state coalmine, but they needed a co-signee and so approached an urban couple with a summer cottage next to their estate. At the time, this couple of pensioners from Tuzla had just weathered a crisis related to another loan they co-signed for the love of their friend who then lost a fortune, defaulted on repayment, and disappeared, leaving them to negotiate with the bank. This near escape from financial ruin notwithstanding, they co-signed a bank loan, once again. To my puzzled look, the wife responded by telling me how grateful the father and son were, how the future of the family's children hung by the thread of the stranded business, and how no one else in the village could have helped them.

Such recklessness is not exceptional. A street-trader, Kova, who sells shirts and embroidery at the makeshift market that unfolds over sheets around the corner from the health center in Tuzla, tells me of the very many ways she extends her pension and her truly meager market earnings in lending to others. A friend of a friend in need of money took more than a year to return, begrudgingly, a 100 KM debt, and yet Kova says, "I can't live without [giving] debts." One could hook Derridian attention at the self-indulgence that accompanied Kova's or the above couple's giving, but the price they pay or the stakes they raise cannot be exaggerated when one considers that they have no income to spare and that openhandedness is not a bourgeois gesture of passing small change.

Similarly, debt settlement is not easily requested except as a last resort or at the point where deferral has exhausted all patience and sympathy, exceeded all expectations, and where the creditor feels that the relationship may as well end. To step into a neighborhood store for a moment: a shopkeeper is collecting funds for her monthly microcredit repayment. She owes money to her produce supplier, to the electrician for some recent repairs, and has borrowed an amount from her brother, a municipal employee with a regular and, relatively speaking, high income. Meanwhile, her clients are running expenses on an open tab and some are dragging out the repayments. One woman steps in to get some cold cuts, sweet cream, eggs, and cookies. In turn, she gives neither money nor a spoken promise and before she walks out the shopkeeper says quietly: "Dear lady, did you forget?" reminding her of the unsettled past month's bill, stating apologetically that "our microcredit is due and we just fixed the store refrigerator." The woman shakes her head; her monthly pension is late. When she leaves, the shopkeeper pulls up a debt ledger from below the counter to add an entry: a book disheveled by the handling and shoving in and out of sight, where it stays so as not to embarrass clients with secrets of their open accounts. The debt ledgers, however, do not keep the stock of all secrets that pass between the partners in exchange. The shopkeeper's knowledge of their customers' lives extends to the smallest details—dietary preferences, hygiene habits, spurts of family's fortune, causes for celebration, everyday disasters and disappointments, as well as how people prefer to nurse them: with tightlipped late-night purchases of sweets, snacks, nicotine, or alcohol, or with a circuitous sweep of an open complaint.

Those suspended in the shared temporariness of an open debt incessantly and insistently transact little presents: of their stocks, of homemade food and produce, of sweets and medicine. These gifts are massaging the sinews of intimate ties that traffic debts in the market. Once I found the manager of a provincial pharmacy—the one who complained about a grandpa's gift of bananas—wrapping up a set of glasses, "crystal, very nice," which the staff bought for an elderly woman, "grandma" (nena), who pops in on the pharmacists' lunch breaks with gifts of elaborate homemade dishes or baklava. The grandma has a history of taking medicine in advance of payment or doctor's prescriptions, but she surprises the pharmacists with delicacies whether or not she is currently indebted.

Making ends meet would be barely possibly and life would certainly be a far more painful ordeal without informal loans. Nonetheless, advances of commodities keep traders in business in a cash-based economy, perpetually stranded for cash. Consumers' loyal shopping preferences oblige traders. Informal debts, much like gifts, are reciprocally intimate indebting. No one calls it "generosity," no one but the anthropologist confuses market debts with gifts but the expectations that lending-borrowing and all the acts in the meantime stir are affectively, undeniably related to the forms and values of gifting away from the market.

WEALTH

An analogous and particularly insightful event of reciprocal indebting is the ritual giving of money, *vitre,* during Ramadan, to a fasting, observing Muslim who is obviously in need. It is usually the task of the women in the family to find just the right recipient, collect the money, and give it on behalf of the rest of the members, sometimes even in the name of extended kin, whether or not they know it, who themselves lack the means or even the desire to give it. Vitre (a vernacular transliteration of the Arabic *sadaqat-ul-Fitr*) is sometimes conflated with *fid-ja*, the money that a Muslim unable to fast the month of Ramadan pays for each missed day of fasting. He is said to be feeding someone else's fast. The gifts are calculated at the going market rate of one kilogram of wheat flour times the number of missed fasting days, or in the case of vitre, for up to five days per donor. One evening in 2006 Šuhra receives our vitre and gives us a wish on parting: "Let God give you health and *nafaka*, first of all, health and nafaka [income, wealth, or fortune]." Šuhra herself lives off of nafaka, as I learn from my mother while we feel our way in the dark, down so many flights of crumbling stairs from Šuhra's apartment to ours. This is a clue about Šuhra's beautiful, elaborate clothes; many generous hands have stocked her wardrobe. Her life circumstances, which I pieced together from the neighborhood rumors about poor health and a bad husband, a violent drunk, whose death she still mourns as a great loss (the neighbors think otherwise) and whose idea of marital life beat Šuhra's small frame into a bundle of aches and occasional nervous breakdowns, compel giving to Šuhra and recommend it as sadaka and *sevap* (good deed). Her late husband's minimal pension of 170 KM is simply not enough for one person to survive for a month, but her nafaka provides plenty for the other household members: her unemployed daughter, son-in-law, and a grandchild.

Sadaka is given to those whose need is compelling, patent, and basic; it has been explained to me, by a clever child, as "when you give bread or money." It registers the giver's generosity and merit, although from the standpoint of the receiver, it communicates pity and alms in the least acceptable form—named, that is—unless the recipient is resigned to his position: alms seekers at the markets, for instance, ask for sadaka. Sevap, on the other hand, refers to the merit that any good or kind act generates, whether in response to a patent need or to someone's desire. Unlike sadaka, sevap takes place between equals. Vitre is at once a gift and an alms, a duty and a pleasure to give. I give to Šuhra, who lives off gifts, but she is obliging me for taking the gift of money, wishing me, generously, health and wealth, and, the expectation is, saying a prayer, *dova,* on my behalf (more on dova in chapters 5 and 6). Although these gifts are specific to Bosnian Muslim traditions, and calculus of how much and when to give is prescribed by the formal religious establishment (the Islamic Community of Bosnia and Herzegovina), the sense of the merit generated through both giving and taking is more broadly relevant.

Beggars on the street also promise good health and long life in exchange for your money: "Give, may you be healthy and alive." These invitations to give and these offerings of good wishes are also challenges that are charged, hard to resist,[12] and sometimes sound ambivalent or express open protest. Once on a market day in a provincial town, I overheard a grandma responding, indignantly, to a Roma, holding out his single hand, asking people to give for the sake of their health: "And I used to give [*i davala sam*]." Her response indicated that she was cross at being reminded that it was good to give, or fed up with promises of plenty without getting a break from requests to give. Or another time, a beggar shouted after a woman who passed him by without giving: "May God always give you this much [*dabogda uvijek ovako imala*]." Her wealth in this case is indexed by her openhandedness, and the link between giving and fortune now sounds unsettling: if she thinks that she does not have enough to give, he is then wishing her an eternity of presumed money lack, and if she has but is not showing it, and seems too poor to give, then he is wishing her forever the same appearances. Because it is by giving that one may seek to alter the flagging circumstances of health and wealth, of nafaka, these are not idle warnings falling on Bosnian ears.

A similar assumption plays out in cases of personal debt. Discussing her habit of giving on debt, of granting commodities in advance of payment but also loans of cash, trader Alma whom I mentioned earlier says: "It's not that I'm showing off, but how many people did I help in these years! So many people I helped. But that's why Allah gave me health; I feel that Allah gave me so that I'm well [*da mi je dobro*, meaning that I'm well or well off], that Allah has made things easier for me." Another time she says, "It's been a good Friday. Since this morning, whoever stops, buys something. I've been thanking Allah for it. Thank you, dear Allah, one thousand times thank you for this nafaka. And then a woman returned a 35 KM debt! It's good that she did. When people are overdue, when they are late one or two months, I'm losing. I have to turn over with that [*da obrćem*]. If it's held for that long, I have nothing from that. The money is melting, it's losing value. And I owe all this money as well."

Alma is quite aware that money requires movement and fast turnover in order to act as capital. Furthermore, working on debt makes good business sense—it is the most effective way to draw and keep customers who are stranded for money as well as to obtain commodities when one's own money is tied up in indefinite deferrals and promises. Repayments, as much as they are anticipated, are also uncertain and surprising, as are incomes: it is an everyday miracle when money materializes, against odds. Nafaka accounts for the miraculous, unexpected, and unlikely that always figure alongside the more predictable math of pending loans, incomes, profits, and expenditures. Nafaka is one's singular and inalienable, potential and actual, monetary and material, immediate and future wealth. Its temporality is both immediate, as it has to do with daily provisions, with the number of visiting or paying customers, as well as with contingencies that lose you a wallet or otherwise compromise your monetary and bodily circumstances. Nafaka is the accounting at the most basic level: it registers the number of breaths you have left to draw on this earth. It is said that "no one can take away your nafaka" and that life ends when one's nafaka expires. Nafaka, however, is not a fixed fate; it is not entirely immutable but subject to interventions and alterations. Generosity, good deeds, and supplications (dove) can turn it around, in particular. Trader Alma's sister, a refugee from Zvornik and a single mother employed in a supermarket, tells me:

> I believe in Allah and Allah gives me everything. Whatever I ask for I get.
> I don't know from where it comes; it's nafaka, but he gives it to me again.
> And the more I'm saying it, the more I get. The little that I offer, if I did
> something for someone, the more I get. For instance now, I saw that man, an
> elderly [person], perhaps he's hungry. Well, I can walk home [i.e., give him
> the money she allotted for a taxi ride], I'm young, I can do it, but he? Look
> around [for those in need]! Allah will delight you.

The idea that giving is good and generative of fortune is widespread even if not every account of nafaka counts on God. Giving is promoted and generosity tends to recruit recipients beyond the circle of one's intimates on whose repayment one can (somewhat) count on. Gifting disposition encourages risk-taking—I've witnessed numerous extensions of commodity credit to first-time customers, without credentials and without recommendations[13]—and so extends the reach of the informal market that hinges on reciprocal indebtedness. The giving goodness is not limited to humans, either. A grandma I met at the market was lugging a bag of cat food she bought at the pharmacy; she told me that she feeds cats that come by her house: "I feed birds too, regularly. They aren't mine, they only come by. I feed them because it is sevap. And you should see: nafaka rains on me. I couldn't possibly have more."

This principle of nafaka is taught early and rehearsed throughout one's lifetime, especially at key events of human existence: birth and death. A gift of money customarily given to a newborn "on the forehead" [*na čelo*], kick-starts a child's nafaka. The money used to be touched to the newborn's head, until the bills got a dirty reputation, not least as hosts to germs. Givers these days simply tuck them beneath the baby's pillow, after circling the money around the child's head, wishing it aloud nafaka, or simply luck (*sreću*), and good health.[14] This is a crucial gift that welcomes a child into the social universe and ushers the life-long process of giving–taking, with the gift of money that is unrequited and hence its first debt, and that like all the following debts, including the last debt accrued to the living for funeral expenses after death can never be, is not meant to be closed. From the start, nafaka is a gift of debt (see Jašarević 2012b).

EXCESS

While Bosnians often complained that they lacked money, they just as frequently expressed wonderment that there was money at all in circulation, considering irregular and inadequate incomes, a shrunken labor market, and the seemingly dwindling remittances from the Bosnian diaspora. Remember the aunt who was battled into taking oranges? On one of her visits to the market I wondered aloud how she could possibly stretch a single minimal pension, her late husband's, onto a household composed of three: herself and her unemployed adult son and daughter. "There is some nafaka," she responded, very pleased, "it's luck [sreća]," and went on to explain that whenever she wants or needs something, it just so happens that money comes somehow, from somewhere. It is also worth mentioning that aunt Mirna, who is an observant Bosnian Catholic, speaks of nafaka, as do many others regardless of their ethno-national or religious backgrounds. While nafaka, a Turkism from Arabic *nafaqa*, may seem proper to Bosnian Muslims, it is one of several concepts in the vernacular of northeastern Bosnia that disregard the formal language politics that police the use of ethnically other words.

Nafaka is a theory of wealth that emphasizes the singularity of each person in the business of surviving, living well, or raking in profits, even if each element is part of the larger and palpable market forces largely beyond one's control. Nafaka picks up everything about one's economic fortunes that is left unexplained after the computing of the usual variables: the class position in the given economic field, within the broader historical trends. In other words, nafaka is about the impossible questions—why this particular person, under these conditions, despite the odds, fared this way and not any other. Nafaka shows the extent to which economy is inseparable from ritual and quotidian domains of practice— an old lesson of economic anthropology—as well as the ways in which the improperly economic but shared sensibilities and inclinations vigorously inform the popular economy.

But how do we make sense of something that precisely resists sensible attempts at fixing and rationalizing and that introduces incomputable variables into prudent budgeting tactics? Or is this—incomputable, other than sensible—always already the territory of the gift? According to Derrida, a gift would take place in departures from the economic intent of producing value or accumulating wealth. Gift would not amass but dissipate, not invest but waste. Gift's nature, Derrida writes, is *"excessive in advance,* a priori *exaggerated.* A donating experience that would not be delivered over, a priori, to some immoderation, in other words, moderate, measured gift would not be a gift. To give and thus do something other than calculate its return in exchange, the most modest gift must pass beyond measure" (1992:38). Derrida here takes issue with the economy of "good measure" that ends Mauss's essay, where Mauss recruits the lessons of gift exchanges for mid-1920s France to recommend a happy medium between generosity and self-reliance, and more specifically, between Bolshevik nationalization and liberal capitalism that were the competing economic visions of the day. But Derrida discounts other moments in *The Gift* when Mauss says that gifting is precisely about surplus and recklessness, rather than restraint: you give back to your enemies as much as they had given you, but you always give more to friends. Potlatch for Mauss is only the most extreme example of the tendency of the gift to overwhelm the other, although it is true that Mauss just as often backtracks at the sight of excess ([1945] 1990:69).

The most quintessential irrationality, the most uneconomic surplus with which Mauss endows each gift, however, is the "self" or "time" that the giver must or desires to give to the other. Derrida objects that neither being nor time can be had or given, thus positing rather contractarian expectations on the use and disposal of these two metaphysical concepts. In the vernacular practice, however, people casually or begrudgingly give their biographical and biological temporality all the time and overextend themselves in affects and effects. Insistent givers smother their recipients with given time and attention that precipitate their financial ruin or emotional bankruptcy. The gifting mania in particular meets Derrida's expectations of generosity as an act on the other side of reason and outside the dialectic that affirms the donor subject in mastery over self and others, thus self-composed rather than manic. A manically generous man might attempt to manipulate and violate others with his openhandedness, but his exercise of power is easily distracted by the irresistibility and often ruinous consequences of the giving project.

A medical diagnosis is also a medical pronouncement on the more generally eager or compulsive gift-giving in Bosnia. Significantly, the diagnosing clinician himself is not steeped in the economizing tactics that restrict gifting exuberance to ritual occasions: a committed Muslim, flirting with Sufi mysticism and the politics of the Islamic Community, he practices charity as a form of spending "dear to Allah," a statement one hears often and that is often followed by a clarification: God loves moderation. Amid the practical impossibility of overstretched budgetary limits, everyday giving–taking works against clinical and pious odds: habitual and impulsive, compulsive and insisted upon, violent and calculated (how much can one afford to withhold), the popular practice errs toward excess (see Taussig 1995:392).

Furthermore, the excessiveness of a gift, according to Derrida, would counter productive work; it would be a product of nonwork. He finds such an example of nonproduct in begging, which "produces nothing, no wealth, no surplus-value" (1992:134) and in the figure of the beggar, whose patent needs demand, implore, and condemn French bourgeois society. Beggar, and the nonindustrious poor, Derrida suggests, occupy the space of an exception in capitalist history (see also an interesting parallel in Graeber 2011:389). It is not clear to me, however, what it is that Derrida argues beggars give, other than an instance of an exit from production and accumulation, while exemplifying the squandered potential of labor time. However, in Bosnia, the nonproductive premise of the gift is fulfilled by virtue of historical disasters and convergences: war with the attendant destruction of infrastructure and population displacement, disintegration of the wider federal network of the Yugoslav economy, and the transformation of the global capital and world order that unhooked the region from the world markets and from foreign capital loans under favorable terms (Lampe, Prickett, and Adamović 1990; Plestina 1992; Woodward 1995).

The man diagnosed as manically generous does not work. He produces nothing but "economic monstrosities," which invert the dynamic of commodity form. Instead of socially necessary labor time, his gifts embody squandered time; in place of abstract labor value that generates surplus under the conditions of industrial production, he delivers increments of superfluous particular work. Except for the money, itself given to him by either the state or benevolent donors, which he redistributes, his gifts have little use value. He is neither formally nor productively employed, and has never been. A gifted artist, he has forsaken his art practice and has refused to give lessons in exchange for good money.

But most people in contemporary Bosnia are not formally, productively employed wage workers. They live the predicament of a post-industrial society where those displaced from factories joined the significant surplus labor force, inherited from socialism (Woodward 1996), and the rural population fleeing unprofitable agricultural work. And while alms seekers are more active and visible in the streets and open markets, the majority of people get by through exercising giving and taking. While most Bosnians are working in the service and consumption industries, making ends meet or gaining profits in the sphere of the market, they remember the lessons of the socialist political economy that valorizes production as the only viable source of national wealth. A different kind of wealth, however, is constantly being made and recycled.

NO GIFT ISLAND BUT A GIFT TERRAIN

At the tail end of this chapter, I worry that it may be read as terribly naïve: painting Bosnia as a gift island. I may very well be naïve, but the people I worked with, those who mastered or weathered or survived in the market on the account of the economy of debt, cannot exaggerate nor misconstrue—at least not for long—the conditions that have kept them afloat. Listen to this exchange between two Arizona traders: Mirna: "All we have is in debts." Djemila: "I have no debts, but that's why I don't have anything. If I had debts, I'd have something to wait for." The two women speak from experience, with the authority of those who skillfully navigate the new market—their families' existence depends on it—and speak to the historically new economic practice in Bosnia that generates wealth through social obligations and deferrals.

I investigated the kind of debt that was being generated and contract-ed inside and outside Bosnian markets, but there were so many other ways to present a snapshot of Bosnia's post-socialist economic present, not least by attending to the features of "primitive accumulations"—particularly the alegal or downright criminal processes of privatization, which are opportunistic rather than "generous" and are rarely local but, rather, involve investors and speculators from across the entities and states of the former Yugoslavia and wider Europe. Reindustrialization of old factories and technologies—for steel, coke, or leather in particu-lar—under the new conditions for flexible capital accumulation, with lax labor laws and mere lip service to environmental protection, also gives a much different portrait of Bosnia's new economy. Privatization, foreign investments, and international interventions have very much shaped the Bosnian economy since the 1995 peace, through the mixed tactics of post-conflict state-building and post-socialist market transition, con-spicuously planned by the IMF, World Bank, EU, and USAID (US Agency for International Development) (see Zupčević and Čaušević 2009). Also, a fuller account of Bosnia's socialist history of industrialization, heavily reliant on Western capital in grants and loans, and on the markets in the

East, West, and global South (Woodward 1995, 1996; Lampe, Prickett, and Adamović 1990), would have tied Bosnia, via Yugoslavia, more obviously to the same laws of global capital accumulation while showing how local contests over economic policy (see Horvat 1970) undermined Yugoslav socialist self-management and rendered it utterly vulnerable to the global crisis of the 1970s.

The expansion of trading venues in Bosnia's informal markets and the shrinking volume of trade that was so palpable in 2007, can be likewise compared to the proliferation of trade in other post-socialist contexts (Burowoy and Verdery 1999). The downward trend can be explained by contradictions of a consumption-based economy reliant on a few, external sources of money and capital, from remittances, to the civil service sector, to international aid. Bosnia shares many predicaments of post-socialist European economies, with some significant differences: the credit card industry and formal bank loans are still far less prevalent, although they were on the rise in 2014.

Finally, neither Bosnia nor post-socialist states are alone awash in debt. Rising indebtedness is a global trend that has attracted the analytical and historical attention of many scholars, among whom David Harvey's stands out as most prolific and thorough critical theoretical engagement with the conditions of the global present (1989, 1991, 2003, 2010). Harvey predicates the global rise of debt on the financialization of the crisis tendencies in capitalism, especially since the 1970s.[15] Put simply, he expands on Marx's theory of money and speculative capital to explain a host of tendencies that led to the 2008 "subprime mortgage crisis," including the widening gap between value, generated in production, and money and credit forms, created in the sphere of circulation and speculation. The gap is ultimately corrected by defaults, bubble bursts, bankruptcies, and the return to a more sound monetary basis. Harvey rereads the third volume of *The Capital,* where Marx describes societal forms of insanity whereby accumulation of debts—bonds, interests, and profits—appear as the accumulation of wealth ([1982] 2006:269). Marx's point is that it takes a mass delusion of sorts to mistake monetary or promissory forms of appearance and future claims for the expression of real value, in necessary labor hours. Harvey takes this point to its logical conclusion to propose that "fictitious capital" refers not simply to speculative endeavors but appears more generally, "whenever credit is extended in advance, in anticipation of future labor as a counter-value" (1991:266). Any investment that counts on future surplus value is fictitious; fiction is enabled by the money form that readily carries imaginary surplus above and beyond labor value. The rising consumer debt extends the circulation of fictitious capital across social classes and so broadens the popular participation in the "collective insanity" that constitutes wealth out of debts.

My survey of the paths not taken or taken for granted by this chapter is only partly a nervous, last-minute show of basic familiarity with more critical and comparative terms of thinking through the economies of debt. Nor am I only building up momentum to chime in the typical ethnographic note—which rings true—on yet another example of local particularities that do not get to be properly anticipated let alone explained by the more systemic and, I think, politically most progressive accounts of world-historical contradictions of value in capitalism. Rather, my rushed references that make Bosnia inseparable from other contexts of global capital are mostly keen to establish that I am telling one among many possible stories of the Bosnian economy, a story that doesn't strive to be historically or economically comprehensive so much as angled toward the sites of peculiar wealth production, through debts. Whereas this chapter gave the most obviously market-based account of informal lending and borrowing, the rest of the book returns to the problem of intimate debt as it figures in various guises across a range of quotidian sites and practices.

NOTES

1. In 2007, an advertisement of one influential Bosnian MCO read: "You have a dream? You want to start your own business and need the start-up means? Mi-Bospo has a solution. Absolutely everything for young women entrepreneurs."

2. And then there are unlikely loan sharks as well. One, for instance, is a single mother who borrows from microcredit organizations and then lends the funds at a very high interest rate. Her clients emphasized the fact that giving business to her, interest rates notwithstanding, was an act of merit making (*sevap*).

3. In 2001, tighter legal regulation and more-regularly enforced market inspection limited the unregulated sales of pharmaceuticals and curbed profit opportunities. Moreover, the pharmaceutical market has become far too tight for the expanded number

of wholesale suppliers, and with the more-regulated import procedures, their needs for liquidity dictated faster cash turnover. Similarly, town pharmacies had to maintain a certain turnover minimum in order to prove their viability to the management of the municipal board. However, debt practices continued in pharmacies until at least 2003 and it was not rare that pharmacies, like groceries, closed down, with unsettled clients' debts.

4. Patients also contract debts in prescriptions for subsidized medicine. Each canton in the Federation of Bosnia-Herzegovina decides on a list of "essential medicines" that are subsidized according to a ranked plan and issued on color-coded prescriptions. Monthly supplies of subsidized medicine are usually lower than the demand and patients try to procure them while the supply lasts, promising to bring prescriptions to their pharmacists at a later date.

5. This particular pharmacy is the prime example of the intimacy of informal debt exchanges that I am describing in this book. Debt accounts are maintained alongside with concerned exchanges of health advice, complaints, and often inquiries about family and life in general. Traffic in small gifts is ongoing, but hugely contested on behalf of pharmacists. A grandmother, once a debt customer, regularly bakes baklava and other sweets and brings them over to pharmacists just in time for their lunch or coffee break. The pharmacists give medicines "on debt" to their regular customers, people they know don't have money at the moment but have sources of reliable income (mostly pensions) or seasonal gains (help from the outside, from children, during the holidays). The pharmacy also sells drugs piecemeal—a number of pills to tide a patient over for just a few days. It still happens, however, that a debtor does not pay the debt and disappears altogether. The staff has held meetings on the issue of debts many times and have agreed to keep debt accounts running, but now instead of pulling up everyone's resources to pay the defaulted debts they initial debt entries in the book so that each pharmacist is responsible for settling particular advances they extended. A pharmacist told me: "You give on debt, running a risk. But something always saves you."

6. Draga's career is closely tied to the war economy. She started traveling to Turkey in 1994, the second year of the war, to procure cosmetics, clothing, wigs, lingerie, stockings, and accessories, for employed women in need and in possession of disposable money during and after the war. Her clients also included sex workers who serviced the UN and then NATO peacekeeping troops.

7. This is a tale of a more complicated and very telling encounter. The client, Džana, in her early fifties, was lingering at Alma's stand for a while. Alma was telling us about a mutual acquaintance who took 23 KM worth of makeup on credit earlier that morning: "Just for the holiday, just to have a good time. Imagine! I wouldn't take so much makeup just for one holiday, ever." Džana: "And just yesterday she returned the debt and today she took away on debt again." Alma, laughing, said: "It's true, so true. But I don't give to everyone. I've learned over the years [to give] only to those I trust." Džana: "Right, you know whom you can give." Alma: "After all these years, they can't just cheat me like that." Some girls approach the stand to look at the display. Alma: "And to me, it's the worst. Kill me, just don't ask me for money. Ask for anything, everything, here, have my soul if you need it, but don't [ask for] money. Because I earn it with such hardship, to give it to someone just to spend it to have a good time, I can't." Džana: "Don't ever

give to people like that. Just to have the good time. You have nothing, no weekends, no holiday, no break." Alma: "That's right." In a while, Alma says: "So, you are going for the celebration of the 8th of March?" Džana nods. Alma: "When? Tomorrow morning? And how long are you staying?" Džana: "Two days." Alma: "So nice, two days, you'll have a good time. And where was it that you are going, I forgot." Alma is saying all of this in a casual, amicable tone, dividing her attention between Džana and the girls who are checking out the lip shimmers on display. "Very nice. God willing you'll have a good time. And who organized that, the company? And how much did it all cost you?" Džana: "Ninety [KM], with everything included." Alma: "And did you have to pay all at once or in installments?" Džana explains that they gave a deposit and the rest will be settled in installments." Alma: "Do have a good time, God willing you'll have fun." When the women part, Alma tells me that Džana borrowed money from her for the holiday trip that morning.

8. Matt Sapaula, the host of a Chicago-based radio show and the "money smart guy" is a shining example. This ex-marine is sympathetic to your troubles but confident that you can do better, no matter how bad the economy, if you color-mark your expenses, budget prudently, and give up the five-dollar morning latte, for example. His radio show is aptly named, "Living the American Dream," and Sapaula offers financial couching from within the dream world, certified by a university degree in financial planning.

9. In 1960s Bosnia, William Lockwood (1975) noticed such recycled gifts of confectionary. In 2000, a trader at the market told me of the care she takes to mark the provenance of gifts received for wedding and childbirth, which she intends to recycle. Once she received a gift of a shirt she herself had previously gifted due to the negligence of the recipient to keep track of what comes from which giving hands.

10. Levi-Strauss similarly describes the spontaneous gifting of wine that takes place between strangers sharing a table in restaurants in southern France (1969:60). Nancy Munn (1986) also points to the importance of ordinary, nonritual gifts, *skwayobwa*, that sustain Kula, the highest domain of value generation and transaction. Malinowski ([1922] 1984) describes similar exchanges, such as *gimwali* and *urigubu*.

11. Gift economies, according to Bourdieu, rest on the irreducibility of the double truth of a gift, the experiential truth that it is a generous gesture and the objective truth of its strategic, interested character, which is maintained by a collective "misrecognition" of this contradiction, which everyone knows and does not want to know. This denial of the economic, Bourdieu suggests, became dispensable and indeed too costly in time and labor to maintain and was consequently abandoned in the societies with "undisguised" economic self-interest (1990:198).

12. To inspire and frustrate desires is generally considered unkind, unfair, or unhealthy. Desires and wishes, in other words, have their potencies. A shopkeeper, Zlata, stuffed my groceries in an opaque bag so that no one could see them—or else "someone would sigh after them" (*uzdahnuće neko*).

13. A great trader at Arizona, Beguna, who estimated the value of her debtors' defaulted debt (*propalo duga*) at 8,000 KM, tells me she swore more than once never again to give on credit (*na veresiju*) "because this is not flour, not bread" and describes shortly after how earlier in the morning she gave goods on credit to a woman from the Serb Republic whom she saw for the first time: "This morning a woman came; her name

[nickname] is Lepa [Pretty], and she wanted two "series" [a full range of sizes of an item]. She said 'I have [money] for one and for the other one I don't have.' So I gave it to her. 'You'll bring it.' I know her name is Lepa and that's that. She'll bring it." When I ask how Beguna can know that, she replies: "It is felt on the human level [*osjeti se na insanu*]. Sometimes you feel some kind of a fear, then you don't give [on credit]."

14. Birth is also an occasion for extended gift-giving (*babine*) to new parents and between in-laws. Customs vary from one region of Bosnia to another, with *na čelo* and babine being either separate events or folded together. For the first forty days the mother, the child, and the paternal family in the case of extended households receive visits and gifts, after which time the baby is taken for the first time to the mother's natal kin and her husband's family accompanies them on the visit, loaded with gifts. The three major ethnic–religious traditions in Bosnia hold the term, babine, in common for very similar gifting occasions (see Filipović 1982). Also, Vlahović (1972) describes similar gift-giving rituals organized on the third day after a child's birth, when the child's fate is expected to be settled. Guests are treated to a feast, they gift the child with clothing or money, and engage in several rituals that aim to improve the child's fortune.

15. With the critical categories of value and money in mind, he attends to some unfinished parts of Marx's theory of speculative capital to suggest that "credit-fueled capital accumulation is a condition of capitalism's survival" (Harvey [2010], 112). Credit solves the problem of effective demand and of capitalist reinvestment. Under the conditions of depressed wages since 1980s, consumer credit kept the American economy afloat, 70 percent of which is rooted in consumerism, itself sustained at the larger scale by the US borrowing, at the rate of some $2 billion a day (12–13; 16–17; 29–30; 34). Given the growing industrial competition that lowered prices since the 1990s, surplus capital has been most profitably invested in speculation that was absorbing the surplus liquidity. Banks' internal trading and increased leveraging went out of control, until a few scandals spurred de-leveraging and bailouts. In case of production, credit reduces the turnover time and facilitates circulation of fixed capital (1991:263–265).

THREE

On the Edge

Worries in Common and Circumstantial Communities

↙ From the backseat of an informal taxi I listen to a woman complaining to the driver about the past week's poor sales. We are on a two-lane regional highway, traveling from Arizona, once the reputedly largest open-air market in southeast Europe, now curtailed and almost a shopping center. I have finished a day of fieldwork at the market stands, and the passenger, as it becomes clear, has taken off from work early, in frustration. I join their conversation. The elegant woman was once a technician in a socialist leather factory in eastern Bosnia, which she fled during the 1990s war. A refugee in the region's capital, Tuzla, she found employment at Arizona in the middle of that decade when the market was the site of a thriving "black" economy, trafficking all sorts of goods, from unregistered, bootleg, or outright criminal to plain but eagerly coveted after years of war privation, across the porous borders of the Bosnian state newly established by the 1995 peace agreement. By fall 2007, where this story begins, a series of interventions had mostly cleaned up the criminal stocks at Arizona and transformed the anarchic open-air exchanges into an ambitious shopping mall project, courtesy of anonymous foreign investors and the Brčko district administrators, who keenly managed the image of this independent administrative unit within the two-entity state (see Jašarević 2005). As elsewhere in Bosnia, however, much of the trade was still variously informal: service workers were undocumented, goods and profits unregistered or underreported, loans and investments personally negotiated, rarely with a paper trace. Evasive business tactics were common and commonly excused as the only way for the small entrepreneurs to make ends meet or make a profit in an unfavorable economic climate, where taxation added to an extortionist percentage of the incomes. Nonetheless, compared to the postwar years of exuberant commodity traffic, trade was generally slumping in the markets across Bosnia and the informal debt economy that sustained it weathered steadier deferrals and slower turnover capital.

The trader in the cab was personally fed up with work that "boiled down to sorting through the stocks of made-in-China underwear," hoping they would sell. When I asked what work was like at the market, she answered by opening her purse: "Look! I'm full of medicine!" she said and rummaged through the insides to identify various bottles and boxes of pills: "for calming down" (*za smirenje*), for cholesterol, for sleeping, and I lost count of what else. This was not an unusual response to a question that I was in the habit of posing during my fieldwork. Another trader at a market further south, who sold shoes and accessories while fondly remembering her career as a business accountant with the Yugoslav industrial giant Energoinvest, also gutted her handbag to answer with a fistful of medicine: "Here, here is how it is, write it as you will, but this is how we manage. Working here burdens you physically and psychologically [*psihičko i fizičko opterećenje*]." She reported suffering from kidney stones, high blood pressure, and recovery from a recent minor stroke. A single mother of two, she said she could not support the lifestyles of her teenage sons: whatever money she gave them was too much for her and too little for them.

This chapter picks up the challenge that the two women shoved into my ethnographic face: "Here is how it is, write as you will." How is one to write this answer up anthropologically if a fistful of drugs for all sorts of medical disorders is a response to the seemingly unrelated question— "How's the work going?" To begin with, the women's answer perhaps seems a typical description of the more general bodily experience of precarity in late capitalism. Ethnographic descriptions abound (Williams 2004; Han 2012; Stewart 2001). Together, these works undo the fast and clear distinctions between bodies and economics, between collective affects and class circumstances, while threading together intimate tactics of caring, borrowing, splurging, dreaming of fortunes, and suffering disappointments and injuries to a tangle that cannot be expertly handled by either political economy or biomedical science.[1] The following pages carry on with the task of descriptively undoing such categorical distinctions while suggesting that market is a thoroughly bodily affair, in contemporary Bosnia as well as elsewhere. If the market is an object of health experience, however, the chapter further asks, how might we conceptualize processes, grounds, sites, objects, and consequences of experience? How is experience had and narrated, and by what kinds of subjects? How is it shared? And how do histories, politics, or biographical idiosyncrasies figure in the event of undergoing an experience? In the pages that follow, I explore these questions that have always been at the heart of the problem that experience posed to inquiry. I do so by revisiting briefly a few returns to experience in anthropology, as well as by reading through Martin Jay's (2005) reappraisal of experience in Euro-American philosophy and social thought.

Popular complaints about struggle in the market and poor health were still more complex as they tended toward worries about death: one's own, one's intimates, and of relative strangers. Consider the following field fragment:

In spring 2007, I was spending time at the "new Arizona," a marketplace that had opened up on municipal grounds adjacent to the original site. My hosts were clothing vendors in one cluster of small wooden stands, each of which spreads out with goods onto open doors, showing mannequins, mobile shelves, cloth hangers, and scaffolding that props fashion displays. At the end of the working day, a stand folds back into a single storage room. The people at this corner of the market were at the time preoccupied with the deteriorating health of one trader's hospitalized husband. The neighbors would join forces in comforting the wife on her daily visits to the market stand, run by a hired saleswoman, asking for detailed updates on the sick man's condition: his diet, skin color, bowel movements, and the doctor's latest diagnosis. Long after the woman left, the traders would recount the signs of ravaging illness that she described, as well as anxiously add up the reported costs (such as 50 euros for a daily dose of medicine, literally a fortune in a place where an average salary was no more than 170 euros), and the hidden ones that, everyone suspected, involved securing the favors of the public hospital staff. Djulzida, a kind woman with a sound reputation for common sense about business and life in general, bears her arms to show us goosebumps, exclaiming: "How the worries of others affect me! I have had enough of funerals and misfortunes. The organism must have collected too much of such stuff." She and her husband lost most of their family in the 1990s war in eastern Bosnia.

Within weeks, the trader's husband passed away. Neighbors were not so much mourning his death as repeatedly and collectively imagining his wife's and his family's pain, the troubles that await them, the costs accrued by the illness and the funeral. A week after his death, we are sitting in front of Djulzida's stand, gathered around for afternoon coffee, when she reports feeling a heaviness whenever she walks into the mourning wife's stand. "It affects me so much; it's not good for me; I know it isn't but I can't help it," she says, admitting that "I asked them to take the obituary notice off the door. I just couldn't bear to see it any longer."

Djulzida's feelings about another's death and another people's mourning are too intense to bear. This kind of empathy is more than she can withstand. It is unwise to have, but she cannot help it: "it affects me." Perhaps, she speculates, her own "organism," the organic frame for all the interrelated vital, anatomical, affective, biographical being that is Djulzida, has good, historical reasons for resonating so readily, so unwisely, and so irresistibly with "the worries of others." No body proper would be compromised by feeling so much of the affairs of another; the individual body anticipated by the allopathic medicine or modeled by the economics would have a more prudent calculus underlying its affective economy. Nor is the organism as spelled out by the lexicon of modern medicine quite the fitting model for this empathetic engagement insofar as it delineates a contiguous living system of any sort, but the contiguity begins and ends with the single life form. Instead, Djulzida's and many stories that follow paint an extended contiguity of a living human that thoroughly involves the self with the other, when it comes to concerns over health and death. What I describe is neither porosity—a bodily materiality that seeps into the environment—nor a blurring, where the boundaries between one and other are indistinguishable, dissolving. Rather, it is a contiguity of living bodies that are always already extended and further extendible with and among the others, but the lines and points of contact of each singular being cannot be blurred or subsumed. In the intensity of feeling for another, people imagine how it must feel;

they feel relief that the misfortune did not affect themselves nor someone closer and dearer still. This is a disposition learned at the level of thoroughly historical bodies, which constitutes, disturbs, and transforms subjects as well as composes intense but fleeting assemblies that I will explore, with Jean-Luc Nancy, for their political potential.

FONDLING THE LIMITS

Ethnographic materials collected here speak of a widely shared sense that lives are lived on the edge: compromised, every day, by market trends, general indebtedness, and ample evidence that people are falling ill and dying unnatural deaths. Crises that people report are recurring according to a monthly schedule of incomes received, expenditures made, bills paid, nonnegotiable due dates for installment credits, and the looser micro-rhythms that contract, extend, and defer informal debts. Accidents, of course, happen and their poor timing charges them with existential angst, whether it is a matter of a store refrigerator breaking when there is no money to fix it or replace it or a health disaster that portends uncertain and costly medical interventions. For the most part, however, the kinds of crises that I attend to here are at the scale of the ordinary, especially compared to recent historical events that have made this region among the prime spots to research the extraordinary experiences of war violence and its medicalized traces, from trauma to PTSD. The crises described in this chapter are also ongoing, day to day, partly anticipated and variously managed—not least with medicines—but never quite habituated.

Conceptually, this is already a problem. Social thinkers have tended to make a distinction between an ordinary experience, had by the common lot, and usually suspected as creating habits and regular forgetfulness, not least of the experiencing body or the political-economic conditions of the experience, breeding boredom or complacency, nurturing tastes that are rarely critical or self-reflective and more often obliviating, anaesthetizing (see Highmore 2001 on the problem of everyday experience). A different matter altogether are the expert sorts of experiences, which require a cultivation of senses and disciplining or compromising of the body, a finer mind or an adventurous spirit that deliberately probes the limit to what can be experienced and withstood. This kind of extraordinary experience—mystical, transgressional, or sublime—that scrambles bodily integrity, that intensifies senses and the textures of the real, that feels the limit of life and death, is transformative of the experiencing subject and is potentially more: disruptive of the wider contexts that favor experiential moderation and prescribe norms for healthy, decent, sane, or salutary beings. Not surprisingly, neither the uncritical commonness nor elitist virtuosity entailed in this antithetical model of what experiences are possible recommended the term to scholars of the social who were interested in more generous descriptions of quotidian lives and popular imaginations.

Martin Jay (1995, 2005), for instance, worries about the theoretical split between the common and the "limit experience," but he nevertheless articulates a defense of the concept of "experience" against the general post-structuralist mistrust of the term (especially Joan Scott's 1991 objections). Put simply, Jay is keen on keeping, rather than resolving, the tension between the experiential encounter (what is withstood before or besides being verbal and known) and subsequent reflection and narration of an experiential event. He revisits the writings of Georges Bataille and Michel Foucault, two thinkers who fantasized about transgressions and pursued life experiments that underwrote their texts. Experience for Foucault is something that happens to change the subject radically and is recounted after the fact; in that sense, he considers all of his books as experience-books (Foucault 1994:241–246; Jay 2005). Bataille gives an incoherent, ambivalently mystical account of "inner experience" as a dangerous pursuit that disrupts constitution of a self-knowing, coherent subject in a negative dialectic that at once denies interiority and exteriority (Bataille [1954] 1988; Jay 2005). From Bataille onward, limit experience is defined as a dangerous pursuit, a refusal of reconciliation and relation, with either self or others. Its very premise, however, holds a contradiction, as Derrida (1967) points out, since the modes of experiencing the limit—vulnerability, laceration, torture, and pain—render the subject utterly exposed to the outside and others: "superficial" (Jay 1995).

The superficiality of the subject and exteriority of experience are at the heart of Jean-Luc Nancy's rereading of Bataille. It is Nancy's phenomenology that this chapter reads and pairs with ethnographic instances and vernacular imaginations of surfaces and limits as sites of experience for singular beings and sites that bring beings together, around an experience in common. Nancy extends the bodily being onto the outside, unfolding layer by layer what is usually conceived as "interior" and incorporeal: thinking, reading, sensing, wishing, and feeling faculties. It is because my body is an outside even to myself—I can only ever touch myself along the skin—that the experience of self is by default the experience of a being among, with, and for others (Nancy 2008a:128–129). Self is regularly displaced to one's self, lost: not exactly here, where I am pinching, nor in the expiring utterance of an "I," nor fully in the remainder, guttural or mental, that said it. To exist, according to Nancy, is to experience this kind of an "exile." Since exile and exposition define a being, the plains on which we exist among, with, and for others are touchable up to a point, which limits the proper grasp and a full appropriation. Here is a different articulation of a limit that makes it integral to any experiential encounter: limit is the point of meeting and separation, a site without depth that puts in contact, but keeps apart, the senses of the body touching and the body touched, of the being sensed and the being groped for. Derrida, a close reader of Nancy, elaborates on the elusive, persistent quality of surface: "Even if one touches an inside . . . of anything whatsoever, one does it following the point, the line or surface, the borderline of a spatiality exposed to the outside, offered—precisely—on its running border, offered to contact" (2005:103).

The extensity in Nancy's thought goes beyond the skin-to-skin contact as he thinks extension of singular bodily being through reading, listening, and witnessing. "Bodies don't take place in discourse or in matter," he writes; "They don't inhabit 'mind' or 'body.' They take place at the limit, *qua limit*: limit—external border, the fracture and intersection of anything foreign in a continuum of sense, . . . of matter" (2008a:17). The experience of existence, one's own or another's, takes place on the surface and along its disruptions, some more alarming than others, all formative of what we are and how it feels.

Anthropologists may be skeptical of philosophical tendencies, poststructuralist or phenomenological, to abstract "the experience" from local historical and carnal materialities, from political and cultural proj-

ects that produce subjects and collectives. Nonetheless, anthropological returns to experience have always been variously flirting with philosophy while at the same time negotiating the discipline's own fashions
of thought. An edited volume by Turner and Bruner, *Anthropology of
Experience* (1986), was an early attempt to bring together anthropology
and phenomenology, and specifically Wilhelm Dilthey's phenomenological hermeneutics and William James's radical empiricism. The volume introduced collective interest in "experience, pragmatics, practice,
and performance" (Turner and Bruner 1986:4). Together, the authors
asserted the primacy of experience, defined as an encounter between
individual consciousness and phenomenal reality. Starting with an individual experience as an interior mind-bound event, these authors raised
a recurrent phenomenological problem: how can scholarship transcend
discrete experience to grasp it as an object of study and an object of
shared knowledge? Their answer pointed to aesthetic expression of collective meaning in ritual or theater.

A decade later a volume edited by Csordas, entitled *Embodiment and
Experience* (1994) reacted against the emphasis on representation that
reduced the body under the anthropological gaze to a biologically universal and symbolically expressive vehicle of cultural meaning. Situating
the analytical centrality of the body in "late" consumer capitalism, this
collection revisited the problem of experience in the light of techniques
and technologies that reconfigured the ideas of physical, emotional, and
collective existence. Central to the volume is Thomas Csordas's proposal of "embodiment" as a field of investigation complementary to the
"textuality" but different inasmuch as it starts from phenomenological
"being-in-the-world": a subject's present and sensory engagement with
material reality. A focus on embodiment starts with the pre-objective
sensory encounter, before the subject of consciousness and the object
have been formed and distinguished, and emphasizes that the locus for
understanding a culture is here in the intimacy of one's self, intuited
rather than known through the objectifying distinctions to everything
else. Being-in-the-world, nevertheless, the volume argues, is thoroughly
cultural and historical, contingent on global trends and local forms of
knowledge. The emphasis is on the body as an agent and a part of the
general flux of epistemes, commodities, and relations. While the volume

aspires to leave behind the conventional distinctions between nature–body–object versus culture–mind–subject, by siting both nature and culture in the existential immediacy, the contributors are still somewhat preoccupied with lives of the mind, mental states, and emotional pain, with meaning making, psychological disorders, and traumas. It is partly the "fault" of phenomenology that it encourages a certain forgetting of the body's bodiliness, since one's body is the starting point by default (Merleau-Ponty [1945] 1958), and rare is a phenomenologist who has patience for the carnal life.

A more recent volume, edited by Margaret Lock and Judith Farquhar (2007), emphasizes the materiality of social life and embodied subjects. The editors take it for granted that the textual, epistemological, and political are hard to separate from the flesh of the living subjects. Lock and Farquhar trouble the idea of the body proper, presumed by the many standardizing global regimes, from the pharmaceutical to the legal, while inviting a rereading of classic and contemporary texts. The obviousness of the biological body used to make mundane or technical questions, such as those referring to gut cultures and digestion habits, unlikely and uninteresting. The editors, instead, paint the world of a multitude of local bodies whose insistent physicality cannot be shoved under a symbolic blanket. The authors are not proposing a unified theory of experience but point to the relevance and efficacy of experience in constituting bodies as well as local forms of knowledge that people live by.[2]

My work, too, is stimulated primarily by the suggestive quality of the ethnographic materials, including the various theories, anatomies, and practices of my interlocutors: therapists, traders, taxi drivers, patients, pharmacists, shoppers, and other people I encountered. From this local archive I play up the resonance between vernacular and philosophical imagination. The everyday circumstances prompt people to experience other people's misfortunes and I am most interested in thinking how experience is so readily shared or, perhaps, plural and shared to begin with. Nancy's thought has dwelled on the existential events that at once expose ontological plurality of each singular being. Moreover, there is a striking affinity between collective readings of obituaries in public—I will describe them closely—that take place across Bosnian urban spaces, and Nancy's proposition that events of death, which for him take place in the existential register of finitude we have in common, signaling neither the community of mourning nor the question of possible transcendence, draw together intermittent communities that are "political" in the most inoperable—and precisely on account of it—most hopeful sense.

HEALTH SCARES

In a tight little neighborhood of market stands at Arizona, some traders and I are sitting around at an early afternoon coffee break, usually an event everyone looks forward to and to which they eagerly contribute desserts, crowding the picnic table with offerings. Coffee is thick, served in small round cups, meant to be sipped leisurely. It is a break from work or from nonwork that more and more takes place between the usual peaks in shopping schedules and seasons. The staple of today's conversation is unpleasant, but the collective mood, nonetheless, skirts close to providing simple pleasures—warmth of the cups, wakefulness of coffee, sweetness of sugar, the glow of a daily ritual. They are discussing the long trend of slumping sales, which, one trader declares, qualifies 70 percent of market vendors for admission to Kreka, the infamous regional mental health clinic. Rahima, a relatively successful trader in the group, goes on to explain how trade leads to mental disorders: "You go to the market [the wholesale Chinese market in Budapest] and spend 3,000 euros on fashions which then turn out to be old-fashioned or unpopular. Then you watch them collect dust. The bills, meanwhile, keep piling up. You can't return the commodities, nor can you pay rent with them. I get a headache, but I can't take a pair of pants to a pharmacy to buy a Kafetin [the most popular brand of headache medicine]. So then you start selling below the purchasing price, just to pull some money out of the whole misfortune."[3]

Since the 1990s, the market in Bosnia has been commonly perceived as a vital site of opportunities, to make money or to obtain goods, whether or not the money is in hand, and a serious threat to health. Living on scarce money and overextended incomes is a source of constant strife, shortages, unexpected circumstances, chances missed or met just barely. Wherever commodities are trafficked, from pharmacies to tombstone shops, from neighborhood stores to produce markets, from open-air to flea markets, people share alarming evidence that everyone's health suffers the market "nowadays." Moreover, there is a popular consensus that health is assaulted by corrupt or careless medical professionals in both public and private medical institutions (see chapter 4). People's stories constantly intertwine the subjects of the disordering market and unreliable medical care, fanning general anxiety about health.[4] The fact that post-socialism made pharmaceuticals into market commodities that are often prohibitively expensive, while they used to be prescribed free of charge, is only adding to the sense that medical worries are historically justified, "in these times" (*na ovom vremenu*).[5] In a pharmacy where I was stationed on Tuesdays, the municipal market days, a man waiting in line said to no one in particular: "I think that pharmacies now profit the most [*najviše zaradjuju*]." Another man rejoined: "No wonder, when everyone now uses medicine, there is not one person nowadays who doesn't use medicine." The first man: "They [pharmacies] even run out!" The second man: "Pills, syrups, teas . . . such are times [*takvo vrijeme*]." Thoughts on "nowadays" and "these times" can be rehearsed for the sake of anyone, especially if the people gathered are strangers under uncomfortable circumstances. Such thoughts are timely especially because those gathered presume to know what it is like to be waiting for pharmacists to fill prescriptions, hoping that the subsidized medicines will be on stock, wondering how much the drugs will cost, whether they will bring relief, whether they are right for the condition, and whether the pharmacist—who exercises far more counseling competence in Bosnia than, say, in the United States—will be able to evaluate it or complement it with herbal remedies. Additionally, given the fact that municipal market days are significant events, most people in the pharmacy have either arrived from the marketplace or are heading to it afterwards (see chapter 1). Shared therefore is also the trajectory that regularly takes people from the sites of market to the sites of medicine, while connecting both with the practical issues of not having enough money and worrying about health.

As I show throughout this text, people insistently link the new market and visceral affairs. Points of body and psyche, of nerves and blood pressure are variously presumed to be contiguous with budgeting or missing business deals, with borrowing and lending, promising, deferring and expecting, overextending and miscalculating. Signs of disorder are legible in, what seemed to me, some surprising signs. Traders, for instance, scrutinize each other's appearances for proof of disorder; finding or suspecting them, they ask each other, obliquely, whether they are hot, cold, hungry, underdressed, or tired. At the end of one coffee session at Arizona, one trader gently asks another whether she is cold. She is not, she responds, but the other trader insists that she seems to be cold. The woman wonders why she appears this way, unless, she proposes, it is due to the messy state of her hair, which she did not style that morning. Perhaps, the trader responds, but you still look as if you are cold. After a pause, the woman admits: "Actually, I am nervous [*nervozna*]. There is no work," and the other trader accepts this as a straightforward answer to his question.

The traders read into disheveled appearances and the slightest signs of unease. Given the shared predicaments of working at the market they suspect troubles. Queries about health are insistent and invasive. They initiate and lubricate an intimate traffic of health advice and remedies, and hands-on, immediate, or practical meddling, from touching-feeling the head or the back of another, to offering a drink, a seat, a massage, or a word of advice: to take a break, to calm down, to eat better (and quite specifically, to eat this or that), to dress warmly, to style the hair, to touch up one's makeup, to try a remedy, a recipe, a therapist, in short to take better care of oneself or to get oneself in order (*čuvaj se, sredi se*). Open concerns about the health of others regularly make personal and familial circumstances everyone's business, leading easily to shifts into an exchange of business recommendations, informal loans of money, or advance of commodities.

That same afternoon at Arizona, shortly after the above exchange, another trader joins our group, who are still lingering over empty coffee cups. People exchange kisses, handshakes, and lavish compliments on the woman's style (she clasps a huge, gold-colored handbag; gold is in vogue this season) and her weight loss. They have not seen her in a while as she works as an elementary school teacher in a southern municipality and has hired a salesperson to cover for her during the school year. The teacher, it turns out, has come to Arizona on an important business mission: to negotiate the sale of one of the boutiques she otherwise rents.

The deal, however, fell through. She blows off steam. Silence settles in briefly, before one trader asks the teacher whether she is feeling cold. No, just nervous, the teacher replies promptly; she then proceeds to talk not about her disappointed financial expectations but about her husband's recent medical issues. In the course of what was supposed to be a routine medical examination, which was required by his prospective employer, a coal mine in the south, he was found to have elevated liver enzymes. The traders promptly speak up, asking her to calm down (*smiri se*), to not worry herself sick (*nesikiraj se*) and they listen, approvingly, while she rehearses plans for scaling down the business and getting herself and her husband in "order."

Taking the cue from her interlocutor's question about her immediate discomfort, the teacher paints one emergency after another that have shaken her up: a failed sale, overextended business and personal resources, her husband's new medical condition and, possibly, due to it, a lost employment opportunity. Here medical alarms trail foreclosed economic opportunities, leading the conversation to the general consensus that the teacher's weight loss makes obvious her overall "ruin" (*propala si*).

In all of the above encounters, the terms of health experience are of common sense to everyone. This intelligibility is presumed by the man who complains to his fellows waiting in the pharmacy, by the trader who evaluates the general mental health at the market, by the listeners who expected their inquiries to solicit a story about the troubles of health and wealth more broadly. The intensity of sharing, however, can grow further still through acts of close, carnal listening, reading, and imagining.

WORRYING—SICKNESS

At the end of a provincial market day, an unlicensed taxi I flagged is full of visitors returning home to the neighboring suburbs and villages. The woman sitting up front is the driver's acquaintance. He inquires about her health, and she sighs deeply in reply and then complains of a headache. Her shopping bag sits between me and two other passengers in the back, stuffed with medical purchases, a faucet, and a wall mirror that she worries might break and often turns to check. When she repeats how poorly she is doing, the man next to me, sitting with a sack of flour on his lap, suggests: "Well, all that has to do with the fact that people are psychologically burdened [*opterećeni psihički*]. Nowadays, even the young are dying." The driver nods in agreement, and the man continues his point: "I don't want to worry myself sick [*neću da se sikiram*], but who can live without worrying these days? One has to be insane not to be worried sick [*nasikiran*]."

I want to rephrase slightly what seems to be obvious to my fellow travelers: existential worry is the norm in today's Bosnia. The vernacular term *sikirancija*, literally "worrying-sickness," is a category of health disorder widely recognized by traditional, conventional, and alternative medicine and is associated with a whole range of symptoms, from irritability to indigestion to insomnia to visceral malfunction, as well as to a host of signs legible in medical technology. Among the most common shorthands for sikirancija are laboratory test results for cholesterol, diabetes, and blood pressure, whose metrics are tokens commonly given and taken in the course of a verbal exchange with the expectation that anyone listening will easily plot the cited pressure bars, sugar levels, and cholesterol percentages onto the scale of what is normal and what is out of control.

"We can't take care of our health; we must live," a shopkeeper in Tuzla says, telling me in fact that living is unhealthy. For the shopkeeper's family and her customers, subsistence entails negotiating multiple deferrals, including informal debt deferrals, and collecting funds, by whatever means, to repay bank and microcredit installments on time, as well as to settle debts with wholesale venues in order to keep deliveries coming. Then there is the lending to and from friends and family and advancing goods to clients, while subtly reminding them of their dues. "So how can you not worry?" she asks rhetorically, "How can you not worry yourself sick?"

Work and health are regularly interwoven, as when I ask a taxi driver about his health and he answers by telling me how poorly the work is going. Earlier in the year he had a stroke, he says, and "all of a sudden everything gave up: my blood pressure jumped up, blood sugar, cholesterol . . . But all of this," he adds, "is from worrying myself sick [sikirancija], stress. With this work and everything else. No wonder." Shortly after, he hints at what "everything else" entails: utilities and central heating in the winter alone cost some 260 KM, he complains, and his pension is no more than 408 KM.

US—SHARING

A very popular stand in the old town marketplace of Tuzla is shaken by an accident one day. Run by Daca and her employee, Fikra, the stand extends over foldable desk surfaces loaded with hair accessories and makeup. Against a display of tall fragile screens of quivering earrings, a gendered population of legless, headless, sometimes breast-full mannequins feature the latest fashions. This is a vibrant spot in the market that attracts a steady flow of visitors and shoppers, with blasting music, cordially hosted coffee and sweets, and delicious pieces of news and gossip. A visit by a young woman and her parents creates a stir, drawing traders and shoppers from surrounding stands, who shower her with kisses, hugs, and questions. Daca turns to me, excited, to explain: this is a sister of a girl who had *that* motorcycle accident a few weeks ago—haven't I heard about it? As I have not, the traders take turns to describe the collision of a young couple on a motorcycle, and the trailer truck whose driver was either fatigued or drunk—it was undecided. The biker lost a leg and his girlfriend was still in the intensive care unit in the regional hospital, which was perched atop one of the hills surrounding the city. Daca concludes the tale by saying: "When I heard about it, I cried for two days. Did I get worried sick! I couldn't come to my senses. I know her, I know both sisters, since they were children in the neighborhood." When the family leaves for the next stand, the crowd still lingers, discussing and disbelieving the accident, while Daca stutters from one person to another, repeating: "When I first heard of the accident, I almost expired [*kad nisam crkla*]." I watch Kaća, the owner of the stand now hosting the family, as she listens intently to their tale. She presents a figure of care: clasping hands on her chest, then throwing arms in the air, and touching the daughter and the mother gently and often.

With the family gone, Kaća comes by Daca's stand and reports that she was getting goosebumps (*ja sam se ježila*) while listening to the girl's father. "What a catastrophe they weathered! Look, I've got goosebumps again." Stroking, absentmindedly, the massive belt buckles on display, she says:

> A human cannot imagine how a life can turn around in a second, in one second. How did she change their lives! I got worried sick again. That's how I feel with the people. Because I know how this family lives. How their life was stirred! A human only puts herself in their position. My son too has been through a car accident. He was unscathed but I worried that he got so worried sick, because what you experience is stress [*doživiš stres*]. And you can just imagine how it is for his parents [of the young man who lost a leg in the motorcycle accident]. That's how a human dies too: there's a stroke or an accident, and [life] is cut off as if by an ax, finished. But no one thinks about that, no one. And you are writing all of this? It seems that you too were shaken.

Daca and Kaća were the neighbors of the visiting family and so were, understandably, familiar with the accident and more personally involved. But judging by the excited gathering that the family's visit drew, the news about the accident had traveled far and involved many more people, from superficial acquaintances to perfect strangers. The accident provoked intense visceral responses that, at first, I found surprising. To Kaća this is only natural; after all, she assumes that in listening and taking notes about death the ethnographer could not be otherwise but moved, "shaken," and also stressed out. She considers other peoples' misfortunes closely until her thought unhinges from the particulars to extend to the general fact of physical frailty and finitude. "How must it feel for them?" Kaća wonders about the parents of the young couple involved in the accident, stretching her imagination to probe the sense of other people's death and misfortune. This sort of question turns other people's problems into issues that concern "us," that perform a common ground for thinking the commonalities of being—worried, ill, mourning a loss. In the course of the fieldwork, I learned that events of misfortune recurrently staged collective participation. Death was the limit to which this empathic imagination tends.

WE—LISTENING, READING

At a used books stand one morning, I am listening to a talk about a young man's death. The bookseller is a retired teacher and refugee, "once the most elegant lady of Srebrenica [eastern Bosnia]," she said, "always the first one to street-walk the latest vogue," but now, she shrugs, sighs, and illustrates: an old friend walked straight past her the other day, failing to recognize her. She sells books every day in front of her building, handling them with more or less reverence—a 1960 copy of the Koran, for instance, is brought out only for the sake of the most promising customers, and then wrapped up like a baby on a cold day, whereas a collection of worn-out porn magazines is stacked messily in the corner of the stand. Her interlocutor is a regular visitor, also a pensioner, who fondles the books on display this morning, as ever (he never buys any). The two are discussing a young man's suicide in details that were not given in the obituaries that were posted on the walls, trees, light posts, and announcement boards throughout the city. Obituaries in Bosnia are placed in public spaces following a death to announce the mourning and upcoming funeral to all those in the city who might have known the deceased but are not immediately related. Newspaper obituaries are published only later, commemorating anniversaries of death (see also Rihtman-Auguštin 1988). The bookseller is sad, "worried sick," and sorry for the young man's parents. She clasps her face tightly between the palms of her hands while retelling the young man's story. Her friend, too, is upset, angry even. He says: "There's no longer any order in dying! If there were a [petition] to reinstate the order I'd be the first one to sign it." It is not so much suicide as a premature death that they find unnatural and make indicative of the more general disorder.

At another street market, Selma's, a regular customer is looking through the latest items on display, while she explains to the trader how her entire office took time off from work to attend their colleague's funeral. Selma wonders whether the deceased was one of her clients; learning that she died at the age of forty-eight, she shakes her head disapprovingly: "Young, so young . . . Was she sick?" The woman responds: "No, it happened all of a sudden. Stomach." Selma keeps shaking her head, worried: "Nts, nts, nts." The woman gives more detail: "This is a sister-in-law of a man whose wife hung herself last year." Selma, appalled, adds quickly: "gluho bilo" (literally, let it not be heard). "Look how cute these are!" says the woman diverting their attention with a finger pointing at brittle bead earrings. Selma is unclipping the pair to better show them.

A young woman, pushing a baby stroller, who was silently listening to the conversation while browsing through the accessories on display, concludes aloud: "I too will have to start drinking Lexaurin [a popular brand of tranquilizers] when I get this worried sick. I don't take anything now, but a human must, must!" Selma remembers another misfortune of the day (worthy of a tranquilizer): "And the market inspector wrote us a fine again this morning."

What is remarkable about the deaths featured in these marketplace stories is that they are rather ordinary. They are neither the gory deaths that are the stock of sensational journalism nor the overly politicized deaths of the war martyrs or genocide victims mired in the tragic stories of mass killings, exhumations, and reburials: rather, it is the premature deaths and suicides of ordinary people that preoccupy the impassioned listeners. My hairstylist, one day, for instance. She consumes a tranquilizer before attending to my hair and explains herself: she learned earlier in the day that a younger son of her colleague was found dead in a bathtub. "A nice, quiet woman," the hairstylist says and proceeds to tell me that she cried her eyes out and could not go on with the day until she bought a box of Lexaurin. "My age," she chants, "my age, and her children are the age of my children. I can only imagine how it is for her, for the mother to bear. I immediately think of my children, God forbid something like that. How is that mother going to survive? She's better off dead." After the haircut, my sister and I take leave, asking her "not to burden herself" (ne opterećujte se), but she replies that it cannot be helped "when you hear such things" and earnestly urges us, as if we are in imminent danger, to take good care of ourselves. We part with mutual concerns for each other's life and well-being, exchanging excessive fears. One could get into the habit, I realize, of dreading a misfortune, imagining an accident, making every random death a glimpse of how it might feel to bear a death.

OURS—ADVERTISING DEATH

I noticed people's attention to obituaries (posmrtnice) in the early days of my "return" to Bosnia as a researcher, while I was still feeling awkwardly foreign in the familiar place I left in 1997 to pursue education, and was learning how to make it into my "ethnographic field." I observed the understated omnipresence of obituaries in the urban landscape and joined the readers that their publishing would draw around a notice board, a tree, a building entrance, a corner wall, or a utility pole. Readers would pause before a small image adjoined to a large bold print of a name, father's name, and surname of a deceased followed by a small-font list of relations in mourning, and would regularly comment on the deceased's age ("so young! my age!" or "the generation of my so and so"), the causes of death ("so sudden"), and the information about where the funeral would take place.

The obituary gatherings are recurrent, tight, and small (the largest I counted was of eight people, around the death of a child), often silent but for sounds of disbelieving ("nts-nts-nts") the fact of death all should know but tend to forget. The text of the obituary is short but people pause longer than it takes to read the legible before they disperse and others take their place. Those at the fringe who are unable to see over the posting hands or reading heads, ask impatiently for a preview, as one man, for instance, panicked: "What is it? Who? Is it a child?" The lively readership gets "worried sick" over the death of people who are rarely absolute strangers and more often than not traced (so incredibly often in this city of an estimated 180,000 people) to intimate relations of friendship, kinship, (ex-) work collective, and neighborhood, or else are kindred by coincidences that make no one a random human, but born in the same year, suffering the same illness, buried at the same site as someone of one's own. Throughout the town, and further across the region in cabs, in shops, at the market or street stands, people retell stories about posted deaths and about their bodily experiences of reading or listening. Reading and retelling reportedly raises people's blood pressure, disturbs blood sugar, upsets stomachs, gives goosebumps, disrupts the ability to carry on with one's day, and stimulates the use and sharing of medicinal teas and remedies or anxiolytics.

My "field" was home, more so than any other place I ever lived, and my ethnographic luck would rarely have me forget this fact. Too often, I got to exercise our trade of "participant-observation" beyond what was comfortably researchable. I have no taste for autoethnography and would like to remain tangential to this book's project, yet the inquiry could not turn away what I was presented with, by the virtue of being at home in the field. One day, I got to announce a death that was "ours," my family's, and to invite others to mourning. I stumbled onto the streets of Tuzla early one morning in June to help my mother's brother's son (*rodjak*) tell the city that my mother's brother (*dajdža*) and his father's brother (*amidža*), had passed away. We walked the city from inside out, from the center to the southern and then the northern end, choosing the best places to post the obituaries. The bulletin board in the town's center was smooth with loan advertisements and vacation deals—people in Bosnia regularly take loans to afford a vacation—whose summer mood we easily spoiled with a few pieces of tape fastened at the corners of the obituary, smack in the middle of the glossy surface of the featured Adriatic Sea. The boards that followed were far more gritty. With globs of glue, shreds of paper, and films of urban dust, the surfaces resisted the tape, pushpins, and our eager thumbs. With a sense of relief we found expired notices of other deaths and funerals; they proved to be most easy to replace, corner for corner, with our death. We learned that empty bulletin boards were always blank for a good reason; they were unreceptive to tape or pin, pressure or adhesive. It was easier to post over past announcements about death or notices and advertisements about the good life that multiple busy hands had posted and stripped, dressing the board with a thick skin.

We pinned an obituary to a great tree at the crossroads that leads to the central open-air market, but we found nowhere in the marketplace to announce our death in writing. News of death travels to the market by word of mouth. As elsewhere, a readership followed the course of our work, reading across our shoulders over and around our hands holding, fondling, slapping, sticking the body of the text. Behind our backs, two women and a man were reading and despairing, over the death in general and a premature death in particular. One said: "La ilahe illallah![6] What is this? These days, the young are dying and we, the old, remain."

In the neighborhood of Slatina, we found the best wall spot on the corner, where we could capture the busy health-related traffic. Positioned across from the public health center, adjacent to an informal street market, and surrounded by no less than seven pharmacies and a popular herbalist's stand, the site guaranteed readers. As we tended to our task,

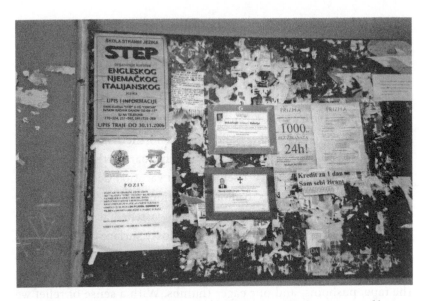

Figure 3.1. A bulletin board along a well-traveled street of Tuzla. Announced here are foreign language classes; an invitation to a commemorative meeting of the People's Liberation Struggle of the Second World War (topped by the image of former Marshal Tito); a handwritten herbal remedy advertisement (an inexpensive fix for warts); 24-hour hassle-free loans; and obituaries. *Photograph by the author*

people already were gathering at our backs, raising voices: "Who died?" "Oh God, oh God," "My generation, my generation."

We stepped back to make room for others to get a closer look as well as to see how it all looked from afar: the story of our death, the reading public, the moment after the work is done. Sadness welled up. I picked up a scent of dill, always a bit unnerving to my senses but stranger still right then, drawing my attention to bouquets of feathery leaves that a grandma was selling nearby, at a fringe of the street market, two for one KM.

OBITUARY—GATHERING

Publishing obituaries initiates a sharing within a network of people somehow related as well as with a broader community, yet-to-be formed around the announcement but already addressed and invited to take part in the collective thinking and feeling of death. Obituaries incite communication on the occasion of a particular loss and tragedy and then expand beyond by word of mouth and by the power of imagination trained to take each death personally. This communication and this community spatialize across multiple surfaces, bodily and thingly. Take our death. The text of the obituaries came printed on a paper body that had to be negotiated onto the textured corpus of the most visible planes of the city. Our hands and fingers attached obituaries: skin was the limit at which we pressed and pounded the paper to adhere to our mission, and the limit to which we could sense the power that the familiar photo in the corner of the text exercised on us, palpable but not to our employed hands. With obituaries we sought to reach and touch the readers, and beyond them, their listeners.

News of death travels from one surface to the next, with reported effects: raised blood pressure or sugar levels, increased heart rates, depressed breathing, erected papillae and hairs, welled-up tears, and heightened worries or fears. This efficacious assembly of surfaces calls to mind Nancy's exposed being inclined toward others, disposed toward gathering into a fleeting, experiential community. Nancy imagines a community that has no essence (human, class, national, or ethnic), no transcendence (spirit, body, cohesive identity, institution), and no project (such as mobilizing action or producing value). Such community has nothing corporate or bonding, has no fixed markers in place or time. Instead, it springs up spontaneously around shared events and disbands just as quickly, without a trace (1991:30). It is composed of "singularities," which are neither subjects constituted in a dialectical move of consciousness through an outside object, nor individuals, each an atom, a world onto its own. Singularity is composed in the spontaneous inclination of one being toward the other. This is the plural, social core of each being. In order for there to be an experience—in order for us to perceive and feel anything or anyone, including any sense of the self—there must be a community. Our senses, our selves exist only by virtue of the fact that we are "being-with" others, for others, in exposition to the others, likewise exposed to us. Such togetherness is an experience not that we have but that makes us be and can be evaluated only from within the experience of the community of singular plural beings (Nancy 1991:27, 2000:98–99).

This community is "perhaps inaccessible," as Nancy tentatively admits, and it infinitely frustrates some anthropologically minded questions, such as where and when is this community, and why think an impossible community in the face of so many really consequential and perplexing political realities, not least in the complicated postwar Bosnia. But to disregard a certain convergence between the ethnographic and philo-sophical would be a wrongheaded kind of political realism that would decide ahead of time what kinds of concerns and mobilizations matter and, most of all, what constitutes an effective mobilization or action. What takes place at various meeting points, in pharmacies, at market stands, or around bulletin boards is a gathering at once arranged by his-torical, economic, and social circumstances but also decidedly spontane-ous and recurrently empathetic, caring, and sharing, effectively making a difference in how it feels to live on the edge, every day. In intimate gatherings over poor health, accidents, and deaths of others we can find what Nancy calls "the politics of the political if the political can be taken as the *moment*, the *point*, or the *event* of being-in-common" (1991:xl). Political here is defined by a shared disposition that brings community into play, a community of disposition that takes place within formally constituted politics (of nation, class, ethnicity, etc.) as momentary, spon-taneous, and recurrent potential, potent for as long as it escapes any formal recruitment.

THE POLITICAL—SURFACING

But still, why should we look for such sights and ideas of the inoperatively "political"? Why should we search for the possibility of a community in the seemingly anecdotal, in the ethnographic, or social, and why would we ever do so in Bosnia? The simple answer is that invocation of the oth-erwise "political" would earn more serious attention to the material of everyday life that eludes and exceeds the formally political grasp of state and nonstate institutions. Post-foundational politics would offer at least a modest conceptual counterweight to the otherwise overwhelming sway that formal ethno-nationally-marked politics wield in the region.

Another reason for seeking the "political" in the unlikely places of quotidian, existential emergencies would be to appreciate experiences that exceed the formal or formally imaginable conditions of possibility. In Bosnia, people say they are just surviving and that they strive to live relatively well, both on the account of informal and intimate economies that circulate capital as well as from access to and advice on medicine and health care. The informal practical orientations and spontaneous, collective inclinations are closely related and grounded in the concerns for good life, health, and wealth.

The most compelling reason to me, however, does not invest so much in the "political" as in the idea of an effective community that it exposes. Nancy's political thinking is inspired by a wish to recover the idea of "community" from disenchantments with communism and from the exclusionary politics of the Right (1991:9). The elusive, inoperative, impossible community that he invents is resistant to thought as much as to organized action. The gathering-dispersing of strangers around "surviving," not least the death of another, is intimate, recurrent, and intermittent, taking place alongside many other forms of relations and political alliances. The obituaries on display also regularly reference these other orders of value. They come in significant colors and bear one of the available marks: Orthodox or Catholic crosses, a secular garland, a partisan star, or Islamic crescent moon and star. The list of proper names of people in mourning speaks, even if ambiguously, of ethno-national belonging, and in case of the obituaries in Tuzla, of the ethnic plurality of urban relations of kinship and friendship. The chosen burial grounds index preferences, not always nationalist (see Jašarević 2012b). However, no one political platform can claim or recruit the obituary (or health) gatherings for its cause, would think of drawing these anarchic passions into a party fold, would know where to begin mobilizing the unruly, unstable body to dress their sentiments, buy their votes, or even to sort through their mixed composition.

In Bosnia, where peace has been predicated on the constitution that safeguards ethno-national communities and where postwar politics are founded on policing the difference and separating territorial entities, public institutions, ethnic histories, and national interest, I kept bumping into places and events that made the dominant politics beside the point. Following Nancy as much as taking a cue from these popular gatherings, it seems that death and health anxiety make obvious the limits of identity politics that presume a fixed, transcendent essence that serves as the radical marker of alterity and affiliation. Nancy's writing on the "inoperative community" is marked by an exigency, Bosnia's as much as global, which he underscores by providing the context of one of his texts: the summer of 1995, a list of conflicts over identities around the globe, and the besieged Sarajevo, Bosnia's capital, as the iconic point of reference for nationalist politics.

Reduced to pure identity so that it could become a clear military target, the otherwise "political," Nancy suggests, must be considered precisely because it seems possible to identify "some substance or presence by this name, a presence measured by the yardstick of the 'national' or the 'state,' [a proper name, location] a body-symbol set up precisely in order to create body and symbol where there had only been a place and passage" (2000:146). The next chapter, following in the footsteps of people searching for genuine healers and real cures, takes us even further into the domain of common experience and pressing strangeness of lived bodies and further away from the bodies of essence presumed, counted on by identity politics.

NOTES

1. This is not to say that biomedicine and political economy do not bring bodily or psychological health and economic wealth together, but they do so on terms that keep the categories apart. "Health and wealth" thus is a frequent subject of economic discussions that correlate life standards, poverty, quality of health care, and public health policy with the individual or national states of health (see Lindh de Montoya and McNeil 2003). Similarly, biomedicine recognizes "stress" as a bodily and psychological reaction to threats, not least to one's economic security, under the rubric of "psychosomatic" illnesses that tend to posit a clear division of labor between mind and body: mind fools the body into feeling this or that. Patients with such complaints are, accordingly, often dismissed or treated pharmaceutically for imagining things (for a critique of psychosomatic "corrective" in the biomedicine, see Lock and Gordon 1988 and Lock 1993).

2. Lock draws on her previous studies of clinical categories and bodily states—from menopause to death to Alzheimer's—that have been transformed historically across a range of practices, from clinical medicine to pharmaceutical industry, from medical ethics to pop culture and transnational legal regimes (1993, 2001, 2008). She suggests no simple social construction of reality but an ongoing production of difference in medical objects and biological and biographical lives. Farquhar brings a related interest in bodily life and life-nurturing principles as they play a part in the gathering of civic, urban communities and relate subjects, through a myriad of everyday practices and appetites, to the history of "the people" in China. Forms of medical knowledge and daily exercise routines, ways of inhabiting a street or one's kitchen, are all mundane habits that link

up social beings with the public space and the various attempts at its ordering—deliberate, effective, popular, coming in and out of vogue: advertisement campaigns, cinema worlds, popular metaphysics, and ten thousand other things (see Farquhar 1996, 2002, 2005, and Farquhar and Zhang 2012).

3. Rahima's complaints show that the market is not troubling only small or informal businesses and their struggling customers but is affecting people more generally, including many professionals, state and private business employees, and successful entrepreneurs. Rahima works with average turnover capital of 20,000 KM, a considerable amount in contemporary Bosnia, and collects rent from a number of market boutiques and stands. Yet she describes the work at the market as surviving, a "nervousness" and a "worrying-sickness" that has earned her stomach ulcers. When the work is slow, she says, her stomach contracts, "a sickness in my stomach grabs me: a nervousness [*nervoza*]. It wasn't always like this, but since I started working at the market. Nerves is the number one illness in trade."

4. Public health coverage is contingent on registration of employment or unemployment with the employment bureau. Employers, however, in an effort to evade contributions due to the Public Health Insurance and Retirement Fund, rarely register their employees. Given that the contributions amount to 40 percent of employees' salaries, another strategy to minimize operational costs is to register staff with the legally minimal salary and informally negotiate higher remuneration.

5. Not all life-saving drugs are marked as "essential" and thus subsidized, nor are subsidized medicines available in sufficient quantities each month.

6. This is a local transliteration of the Arabic for "There is no god but God," the principle statement of Islamic faith. In the vernacular, the expression also highlights one's astonishment, dismay, or otherwise strong feelings.

FOUR

Medical Detours

Materiality and Magicality of Quotidian Cures

🌿 Who knows how the jar got there, but for as long as I can remember visiting one darling *nena*'s (grandmother's) home, it sat at the far corner of the kitchen table, out of the way, veiled and unveiled by the curtain dancing to the summer wind's tunes, in the canopy of a true indoor garden, by the side of a salt and pepper shaker, as inconspicuous as the shadows on the wall. Look at the photo: it is a quiet moment in the life of a curative mushroom, stuffed tightly in a recycled jar, partly submerged in sweetened water. Nena thought its name was *Japanese mushroom* and she had heard it was good for lowering cholesterol, regulating blood sugar, and more generally, "good for everything" (*dobra za sve*). A quiet moment and a manifold mystery is withdrawn within the transparent glass: What was it called, properly; what was it, properly speaking; did it really work and, if so how; and how did one ever know that it did? By what circuitous routes, by means of what intimate exchanges and conversion rates did it get to nena's kitchen and her dietary regimes? What did it do to her bodily being? She had received it, with recommendations, from a neighbor who in turn somehow had gotten it as a gift, she does not know from whom or where. The mushroom was one of many remedies on trial in Nena's kitchen and in her diet, paired with daily pharmaceutical staples (diuretics, blood pressure pills, and blood sugar medicine) for no particular condition other than the infirmities of old age and an ongoing complaint about stomach pains that clinical and lab examinations could not definitively decipher. The mushroom was also on stock with many other comestible and herbal remedies that this kitchen and a pantry, like so many across Bosnia, hold for daily treatments or just in case they were needed.

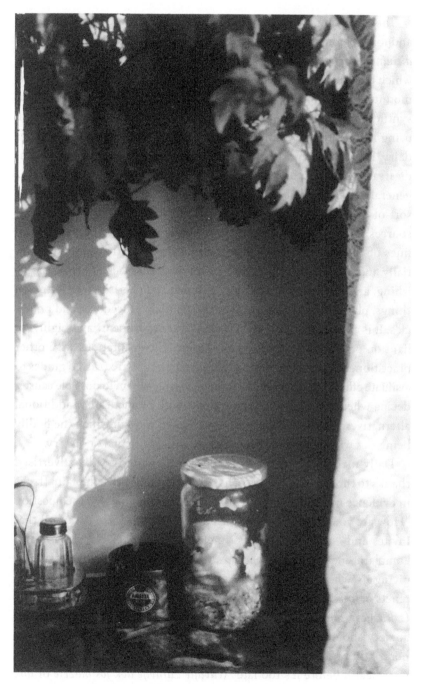

Figure 4.1. A fungal corner of a grandma's kitchen. *Photograph by the author*

There is a long, rich, and practiced tradition of using medicinal herbs and folk or home medicines (*ljekovite trave, ljekovito bilje, narodna medicina, kućna medicina*) across Bosnia and the wider ex-Yugoslav region, which include "wild" vegetal items (*divlje*) collected from the meadows, mountains, and forest, as well as *domaće* produce cultivated without synthetic fertilizers and pesticides and prepared at home or in the yard, using labor-intensive, time-consuming techniques. Domaće includes dairy, fermented vegetables, vinegars, fruit preserves, juices and brandies, sauces and tinctures, all of which are meant to be delicious as well as generally healthful (*zdravo*) "good for you." This is a diffused, vernacular sort of tradition that references a handful of legendary, encyclopedic sources, that consults trained experts—well-established herbalists with lines of commercial products in pharmacies—but that most substantially and matter-of-factly informs everyday practices of eating, nourishing, and nurturing health. It is a domain of cherished, well-known things, plants, flavors and ingredients, familiar procedures and potencies. It is a domain widely open to practical experiments and highly reliant on personal observations and informal consultations with other practitioners. Subjective and collective experience are trusted guides to evaluate efficacies, sort through influences, trace them to possible causes, decide when to complement treatments with biomedical or additional alternatives, and to monitor the complicated ways in which the bodily being as a whole responds to treatment, be it medicinal or dietary.

Daily medicinal experiments tend to be more broadly advertised thanks to the popular culture of health care and health complaint that is in evidence in many ways, not least in the commonness of the question "How are you?" or "How's your health?" (*Kako si? Kako zdravlje?*) that invites and—whether one has time to spare or not—solicits a health complaint more detailed, perhaps, than one is comfortable hearing or giving elsewhere, and in North America especially. Moreover, one of the tenets of folk and home medicine is that "health is the greatest wealth" (*zdravlje je najveće bogatstvo*). Tirelessly repeated, the maxim rings with anxiety about poor health and health threats, particularly in contemporary times, as well as goads the one listening or reading to "preserve your health before it's too late" (*čuvajte zdravlje dok još možete* or *dok ga imate*). Preserving health has much to do with eating well. Another staple saying drills this message—"health comes through the mouth" (*zdravlje na usta ulazi*)—especially for the sake of those who seem to be forgetting the point. When it comes to health, those who practice or subscribe to folk and home medicine in Bosnia are unabashedly intervening, advising, recommending, diagnosing, and readily evaluating each other's medical and pharmaceutical regiments: health and illness are not private affairs. The experimental and experiential character of folk medicine and healthy diets opens it up to ever new trends, renewed optimism about the old, tried items, embracing, inflating, and either routinizing or forgetting new fads. While I observed, particularly from 2006 to 2007, there came and went the following items: Hawaiian Noni juice, silver water, cranberry everything, Aloe juice, Royal Jelly pills, Japanese quail eggs, black cumin oil (*ćurukot ulje*), and many other exotic remedies or regular ones in commercial guises, promising enhanced benefits. Some items entered more permanent positions on well-stocked home pharmacy shelves, renewed each season with fresh herb bundles, bottles of syrups and juice, more *zambak* and *čuvarkuća* oil tinctures (the last two for burns or scars and earaches, respectively). A small number of medicinal mushrooms had been flowing through Bosnian households since 2006: notably tea-based and dairy-based fermenting agents, which people commonly called *gljiva* or *gljivice* (mushroom, singular and plural) and sometimes more precisely kombucha, Tibetan mushroom, mushroom from the Caucasus, and kefir mushroom. Unlike these items that quite engaged the popular imagination (see Jašarević 2015), the mushroom in nena's kitchen was more obscure, showing up just here and there in conversations, and its local curative career was short-lived. That the grandma would take it in and drink it diligently, for a while, is remarkable, given the mushroom's limited fame and odd looks—unlike kombucha, this fungal form looked like it could be growing by the side of the road and seemed misplaced in a jar. But nena's confident trial of the obscure mushroom is also telling about curative promises and medical expectations beyond her kitchen: informal and vigorous health concerns opened up routes to propositions that were less than obvious, pointing to therapeutic practices and introducing remedies and routines whose influences were indiscernible until one embarked on tasting, testing, listening, and taking note.

MATERIALITY, MAGICALITY, MEDICINE

This chapter takes off from the corner of a grandma's kitchen table to pick up questions that issue so readily from the jar if one attends closely, with voracious curiosity, to some seemingly simple matters or simply amusing domestic and dietary habits. Such attention prods questions concerning the materiality of medicinal objects, from remedies to technologies to the bodies, whether or not human, intervening or intervened upon. What interests me are various things that enter and exit popular health-care practices as well as the circumstances that promote their therapeutic relevance, that discern potencies, that make remedies available—promising, potent or mute—and that shape treatment regimes while nurturing, relating, and recomposing bodies. The objects are many and of all kinds, a therapeutic clutter, perhaps more diverse than ever, although medicine in the region was plural at least since the arrival of allopathic technologies in the nineteenth century. On stock in the medical cabinet are some quite ordinary items—such as not more than three leaves of fresh *kadulja* or *žalfija* (sage) that many of my interlocutors were in the habit of chewing, or earnestly recommended doing so, first thing in the morning, on an empty stomach. (It fortifies the organism, cleanses blood, and is good for the stomach.) Included also are items backed by formal clinical evidence and secured through the trial of navigating the public health system or visiting more accessible but more expensive and sometimes doubtful private clinics: obtaining referral forms (*uputnica*), prescriptions, and pharmaceuticals. These sorts of items may seem obvious and plain, compared to some edgier devices in circulation, such as the so-called "bio-pyramid," a handheld form that promises good vibrations for the needs of every person, business, or a home—but ethnographic as well as vernacular scrutiny render them just as intriguing. Pharmaceuticals can at once be persuasive, make a difference in an instant but also create long-lasting, sticky attachments, and leave consequences that are legible between the lines of the descriptions of side effects that make many drug users wary (Healy 2002; Hacking 1995; Whyte, Van der Gist, and Hardon 2000). The bio-pyramid, on the other hand, resides in what may seem as the medical fringe, available at the fancy premises of a clinical center for alternative medicine in Gračanica, northeast Bosnia, and by mail order, if you follow instructions advertised in *Aura*, "A magazine for healthier life. Culture of Living. Alternative Medicine. Personal Fates." Fringe medicine skirts no strict center entrenched by authority, commonsense, safe assumptions, and reasonable doubt, but runs like an ornamental trim across the whole, wider terrain of treatment possibilities. People in Bosnia themselves are symmetrically inclined and an anthropologist only needs to follow their cue in order to practice what Bruno Latour recommends as an analytic strategy (1993, 2005): to bring comparative descriptions without privileging obvious, official epistemologies. *Aura* regularly advertises biomedical clinics, more conventional herbal medicine, and healthful diets, side-by-side with CDs and DVDs of Koranic suras recited for protection against *sihir* or *nagaz* (see below in the "Listing" section of this chapter). On *Aura*'s pages Islamic medicine practitioners rub elbows with bio-energy experts, seers, and talented healers of old, new, and reinvigorated afflictions: arthritis, high blood pressure, cancers, heartbreaks and jealousy, spells and black magic.

But if the symmetrical attention hailed by Latour and like-minded scholars of science, technology, and of knowledge practices more generally is meant to correct the outdated anthropological mode of highlighting some native, non-Western, nonmodern alterities, the symmetry that I am interested in here plays up rather than tones down the oddity, making us wonder again about the materiality across the board. A wondrous materiality, even, when we consider that on stock are medical things cherished because their provenance puts them outside human control—wild crab apples tiny and sour, hard to find in the forests—while long labor and old technologies (*torkulja*, a massive wooden fruit press; a cauldron over open fire) process them into rare substances. Or humble, steeped, submerged matters of plant and bacterial-yeast collectives, at work fermenting and transubstantiating microbial, vegetal, human forms. Or when mobile phone technologies—SMS—effectively act as vital extensions of the therapists' and the patients' bodily being, intersecting them in consequential sympathies that enjoy the more global name of "bio-energy." Fermenting and texting are nimble, banal activities that work everywhere on tacit assumptions about the matters at hand, but when they are deployed for medical treatments they urge a second look, a speculative inclination, and a dose of literally minded inquiry to fully appreciate their implications for the phenomenal and ontological fabric of the real and for forces and efficacies that make a real difference.

Medical advice and complaints trafficked from within and between kitchens and across the broader textually and commercially mediated terrains that *Aura* issues traverse, I suggest, register substantial bodily and thingly indeterminacy—still unknown but incrementally knowable, unpredictable but speculated. Radical responsiveness and vulnerability to influences that need not be understood to be felt, need not be visible in order to be credible, need not be credible to be evident. Therapeutic as well as pathological action were authoritatively and more narrowly defined by socialist modern medicine, which never eroded the value of folk and home medicine nor alternative, traditional, or Islamic medicine, but successfully married progressive modernity with scientific rationality of clinical medicine and socialist humanism with historical (secular) materialism. Because socialist allopathic medicine stood so clearly for all things promoted as sane, proven, certified, and developed, as well as for the common good, practiced for the sake of a human while bettering the life of a socialist nation as a whole, many traditional and alternative treatments, let alone explicitly religious or magical practices, may be denounced as backward, peasant, irrational and may embarrass all those associated with it, pathetic patients and cunning charlatans alike. Nonetheless, since the 1990s war and peace, the field of plausible efficacy is more widely open to exploration and speculation, the field that, I suggest, is intricately related to home medical trials and lessons learned from personal bodily experience. Put simply, what I noted while following health concerns of people across northeastern Bosnia, is, on the one hand, a certain expectation, even comfort, with a fuzzier play of conditions, causes, and effects, and on the other, a habit to speculate on what caused a health condition, how cures and how bodies work. Potencies thus might be highly promising but indiscernible; potentially pluripotent but unknown as of yet; perhaps effective, but who could tell in the tangle of treatment threads, obscure and simmering in a potential. Performance of pharmaceuticals and clinical technologies is only somewhat more predictable but not reliable—I have not encountered anyone who leans entirely on formal interventions, particularly not to treat a composite complaint. Finally, patient bodies themselves are highly un-predictable, notoriously particular in the ways they register interven-tions, take time to respond to treatments, interact with drugs or make drugs interact with one another, manifest signs with liberal improvisa-tions on standard bio-medical diagnostic categories and experience. Let alone when a shared cultural sense about what makes a body does not evacuate biographical detail nor soul from physicality and when multiple practices act on plural etiological hunches, while converging on some privileged anatomical points (such as the stomach) or a life-historical and nutritional sense of vitality.

MEDICAL DETOURS

Contemporary health matters in Bosnia may be plural or etiologically and epistemologically muddled to the extreme, but my point is that they also speak more generally of the extent to which biomedicine, anywhere, is the domain of supreme uncertainty. Its definitive authority is con-tinuously unsettled in patients' experience and subject to coincidental and circumstantial details of each particular case that may be bracketed only to a point. Procedures gone wrong, inconclusive diagnoses, recov-eries progressing remarkably well or unfolding a jittery course, signs of ameliorative difference made by remedies snubbed or discredited by the medical profession, unwelcome drug interactions or a snowballing spell of medicalization that targets symptoms as much as drug side effects—these are among the prime events where the contingent and unknown trumps predictive confidence. Because the object of health care is not a universal body proper (see Lock and Farquhar 2007) but contingent bodily lives, and because efficacy of drugs and technologies is unresolved rather than precise materiality, that which figures in medicine is never far removed from certain magical qualities. If, that is, "magical" can be repurposed to grasp a broader and looser sense of quality of what is un-known, what evades secure grasp but leaves plenty of traces and clues to follow, of what is intensely attractive to pursue or explore, irresistible even, and what makes us wonder, as well as doubt. In one powerful essay, Isabelle Stengers (2003) argues that among modern sciences, medicine is particularly anxious about its scientific standing and enjoys a precarious claim on rationality precisely because it has had to distinguish itself from many competing curative traditions while decisively denouncing compelling powers of all sorts of practitioners—charlatans—whose captive subjects are strangely responsive. The clinical trial becomes the trusted technology for asserting the rationality of medical procedure where subjects and objects not only enter some replicable conditions of controlled influences but are themselves first of all reductively defined, stripped down to relevant faculties and qualities. The clinical trial becomes the central stage to distinguish fact from artifact, and a rational procedure from irrational influences, that work only due to excitable human imagination. "Imagination" here is the power of interference, a disruptive, unreliable power, essentially tied to the fantastic charm of the charlatan, which is controlled for with the placebo. What distinguishes modern medicine from the charlatan, in Stengers's story, is the shift in attention from curing, which may be affected for a wrong reason (as with Mesmer's famous tub fluids), to the evidence-based treatment that emphasizes the rational, fully explicable, predictable treatment procedure. The figure of the charlatan thus stalks medicine, according to Stengers, who suggests a "radical disjunction" between sites where the hunt for the charlatan persists and those sites where it is a matter of curing, not clinically proving (29). The proof that sustains curative arts does not conform to the experimental protocol but uses "theoretico-experimental practices" to glean insights from real life and from the medical object, which is the suffering body (28–29).

Stengers is a philosopher of science and her investigation of modern medicine is part of a broader, critical but "diplomatic" (2000: 14–15) inquiry into the conditions of scientific knowledge production as well as into the sciences' ambitions to finally articulate truth claims and relevant questions. Stengers is an unusual philosopher insofar as she remains a committed "daughter to a practice responsible for many divisions," including between knowledge and belief, materialism and animism (2012:1–2), and yet she often turns to sources that may be considered on the fringe or dismissed as enchanted—from Virgin Mary pilgrims (2010), to neopagan Wicca, to Vandana Shiva's impassioned activism on behalf of local knowledges—precisely to trouble scientific confidence about "knowing better" (2012). She is in the habit of posing annoying

questions, such as "What is matter?" The answer is to be found in no
particular science but rather in an "interpretive adventure" that "must be
defended against the authority of whoever claims to stop it in the name
of reason" (2011:372). Stengers puts forth some key items on the agenda
of a new materialist inquiry: divergent and plural practices; adventure
and wonder as means of being surprised and asking questions; and the
ongoing struggle over the meaning and relevance of knowledge.

I want to pair these keywords with cues from popular practices that
I am familiar with. Unlike a philosopher, an ethnographer is perhaps always already granted a license not only to tread but also to take seriously
into account epistemologies from the street, from the marketplace, from
the curbsides of formal speech. Present-day Bosnia reverses Stengers's
problem of modern medical competence insofar as public spaces are not,
or no longer are, stalked by science nearly as insistently as they used to
be at the height of Yugoslav scientific socialism. On the contrary, official
medicine has never been less obvious, challenged by elusive disorders,
and compromised by the difficulty of access to public health facilities
as well as by entrepreneurial interests of medical professionals (see the
introduction to this book). Whereas the search for a cure, whether or not
scientifically valid or rationally explicable, has long been a reasonable
thing to do (see below), and the quest nowadays is wider—practitioners,
practices, claims, and disorders have proliferated—and more complicated and more unsettling. Searching for a cure entails following recommendations, traveling, trying, hoping, consulting, despairing, trusting
someone's advice or regimen and growing disappointed, mistrusting but
going along anyhow, arriving by chance, pondering coincidences, getting
cheated, accruing debts, exchanging gifts, and juggling many propositions, hints, hunches, fragmentary theories, explanations about what is
the matter, what matters, how things work. It entails an "interpretive adventure," indeed, and long detouring to arrive at an effective treatment,
to find relief, to make sense of an ailment, to discover genuine healers or
real doctors. Moreover, the search for a cure demands criteria according
to which all kinds of medical practices are evaluated, including those
practiced at pharmaceutical and clinical establishments.

The best way to tour the new medical field in Bosnia analytically, I
propose, is also to detour, following people's own meandering routes,

projections and disappointed arrivals, multiple trials, bold experiments and desperate ones as well. The rest of this chapter therefore is detouring as it tries to, on the one hand, mimic the gestures I observed. I will thus tell stories collected on the go, while traveling by train, eavesdropping on a bus, shopping at the market, visiting a few home practices, and waiting in the pharmacy, or hanging by an herbalist's stand. On the other hand, in order to take stock of the therapeutic clutter and to wonder about the materiality of medical things, I will perform several close readings of sources available in and guiding the health journeys. Finally, because the field of health care is at once mundane or domestic, wide-open in treatment possibilities, and curatively promising, and potentially a slippery scree, overwhelming and outrunning one's ability to figure out what is the matter and what exactly to do, I will compile a mixed listing of afflictions and of items for remedies. The stories in the "Open Accounts" at the tail end of the chapter pick up a few items from the selected readings and listings as they figure in specific therapeutic encounters and theories.

AT HOME, IN A GARDEN, IN THE VILLAGE

I found Franka following an advertisement she placed in the cantonal classifieds in the *Mali Oglasnik* (Herald) offering gifts of kombucha and kefir grains. A retired cook from a local university dining facility, Franka spends most of her time in the country, where her small house is surrounded by a garden overflowing with fruit trees, plants, and herbs, just south of Tuzla city. Bound by no work schedule and wishing to stay close to her daughter, a physical therapist at the regional clinic, and to help raise her granddaughter, Franka prefers the village over life "on asphalt" these days. Here, she produces her domaće foods and remedies; her daughter consumes them gratefully but is too busy to make any herself. Franka's love affair with herbal medicine —for one must love herbs, she tells me—began early. As a child, she says, she would fall asleep curled up with medical reference books and herbalists' manuals that her father bought "on credit." She got serious about it, however, when, as a young woman, she became anemic. Preparing half a liter of freshly juiced beets a day—the taste was not exactly pleasant, she adds, but it improved her blood in one summer—led her onward to prepare tonics, ferment vegetables, and concoct wild fruit syrups. Since then, her days start with the first among the herbs, which is žalfija or kadulja, exactly three leaves that she collects on her morning stroll and chews on an empty stomach. It's also good to peel a leaf of downy, plump čuvarkuća. I heard this advice often and followed it sometimes. It is good for everything; it cleanses the liver and restores the organism. Franka's herbal knowledge was composed over the years, sometimes through feverish trials, as when she managed the stress that her daughter's suicide attempt caused her and while nursing or nourishing others, her ailing mother for a while and her daughter's family now. Other times, she learns more leisurely, listening and exchanging tips and recipes with other home medics and cooks. Like so many households, Franka's holds books on herbal medicine by three venerable herbalists in the region: Sadik Sadiković, Vaso Pelagić, and Jova Mijatović.

READING: A REFERENCE GUIDE TO HERBAL MEDICINE

"I am not a learned man nor am I skilled at writing," Sadik Sadiković humbles himself in the opening lines of his *Folk Health* (*Narodno Zdravlje* or put otherwise, People's Health), alerting his readers to the fact that "although I have searched Arabic and Turkish books for knowledge on curing people since my youth, my entire work is mostly founded on long years of experience and research [*pronalaženju*] of medicinal plants, which are plentiful in our land. I think that I am not mistaken if I say that experience is sometimes better than high science." Published in 1928 and reprinted twelve times in the "Library for Every Home" series, this classic guide to herbal and home medicine and medicinal meals by a legendary herbalist from Herzegovina is still of practical use to experts and dabblers in domestic curative arts.[1] To an anthropologist, it offers precious insight into a number of health-related issues of persisting relevance today, from the imputed merits of experiential knowledge to the commonsense about the composite nature of the human body, to the specifics of efficacies and potencies of foods and herbs.

"Health is the greatest wealth in the world and woe to those who do not know how to care for it," Sadiković spells out on page 1, a saying that is of equal currency in present-day Bosnia. Moreover, illness is a

physical-metaphysical condition as is appropriate to an ontological multiplicity that is a body: "Illness makes a human brooding [literally "dark"
(*mrk*)] and crabby, illness clouds his soul [*dušu*] and sways his thought,
makes him reluctant to work, picky in eating." (1988:9). Illness is so much
more grave if the patient grows scared, hopeless, pessimistic (*malodušan*,
literally, with a loss of spirit/soul) for "a body puts up resistance in vain
if the soul has succumbed to the affliction" (10).

Sadiković recommends that his readers seek medical doctors (*liječ-
nike*) who know a lot and can help, provided that they studied consci-
entiously, and are especially effective in treating illnesses responsive
to modern medicine, such as syphilis and diphtheria. Where doctors
are not to be had, he continues, people have long treated themselves
or sought the advice of experienced folk doctors whose knowledge was
passed from father to son or was learned through long experience and
study. Moreover, Sadiković suggests that "an ill person seeks health, and
it is all the same where he will find it. This is such an obvious truth that
some medical doctors have also come to me for advice. I have strived to
help them and can now boast to have sincere friends among them who
can correctly evaluate my selfless work . . . they are good practitioners,
full of knowledge, and so are aware of the fact that 'only all people can
know everything,' as the saying goes, and so they do not look down upon
my experience" (12). Selfless service is neither an immodest nor a rhe-
torical remark: Sadiković is still remembered as the genuine healer who
practiced in a room above a town café in his native town of Ljubuški,
from morning until late at night, without charging a fee. Hailing from
an affluent landed Muslim family with a long paternal line of curing
gifts, he asked for "nothing" from his patients but added that those who
felt inclined could donate money to charities, whose vouchers he had
on hand. At the peak of his fame, he allegedly attracted upwards of
15,000 consultations a year, a traffic that reportedly caused car accidents and prompted the town officials to improve the roads. Likewise,
he earned infamy and slander among those who disbelieved his "curing
and seeing" arts, accused him of fraud, and scolded the credulous patients who sought him out. In turn, a whole number of "cheats" (*varalica*)
and "charlatans" (*nadriljekari*) were cashing in on the regional currency
of the Sadiković brand and were denounced in the newspapers and im-

prisoned for impersonating the man himself, or claiming to assist him or to have studied with Sadiković, side-by-side "with some Brazilian and Indian folk healers"; apparently, even Sadiković's fame could use propping with the elsewhere exotics.[2] Contemporary medical advertisements in *Aura* cash in on such embellishments, as we will read shortly.

Recursive invocations and denunciations of charlatanism are as amusing as they are overdetermined, given the mass appeal and impressive curative record of a practitioner whose resources are the occult skills of "observation and experience." Sadiković admits this much in the book's introduction: "questions arise on all sides: how do I tell the various illnesses. Most of my patients declared me a seer [*vidovitim*]. It is difficult to respond to these questions . . . it takes knowing not only the external signs of illness but knowing the patient soul and knowing the human from around here" (11). Earlier, he writes that "afflictions related to the soul pains [*duševne boli*] together with physical ones leave obvious traces on one's face, in the eyes, in the muscles and on the whole body," (10) and a very similar sense of bodily legibility of discomfort guides contemporary practice: people scrutinize each other's looks readily and admit, wearily, that try as one might, deep hardships and troubles cannot be masked, but are left hiding in the gaze of open eyes.

Experience is the valued source of knowledge that guides more than just Sadiković's diagnoses. It instructed him in composing recipes for some "excellent medicines," many of his own making and especially designed for a book in wide circulation: the ratios of certain plants, he writes, are conservative so that not one of the recipes listed can hurt; they can only help. Sadiković invites his readers to exercise their own experimental attention: to "test personally the effects of a medicine and then adjust them," whether increasing or reducing their intensity (11). Precise dosage cannot be set for everyone in advance: what will cure one person needs to be "multiplied ten times to affect another." Vital idiosyncrasies need figuring out. Readers should also be able to tell for themselves the difference in medicinal potency between herbs grown in the wild (*divlje rastu*), especially in the dry, rocky mountains (*iz krša*) and the ones cultivated in the northern lands—go ahead, he impels, take a dash of chamomile from such two places, make teas, and you'll smell and taste the difference (10).

Finally, an acclaim for weeds and a plea on their behalf, which ought to be cited at length:

> When on a hunt, sometime, somewhere, you marched through an over-grown field, how angry you must have been picking off the small fruits of *čičak* [Burdock flower], sticking to your pants! Or if someplace, by an old building, a leaf of hidden stinging nettle burnt you, how scornfully you must have scolded the negligent caretaker, cussing him for letting such weeds spread out. And yet, you were wrong to do so. These despised herbs like hundreds of other unseemly ones and wild ones hold a miraculous power to preserve and restore health. Let each one of you protect, nurture, spread, and collect them. Our people of old have cured with them, great heroes tended their wounds with them, their power was sung by the old folk poems where you will hear how mountain fairies applied them to wounded heroes. After all, they are the cheapest remedies and accessible to everyone." (11)

LISTENING, IN THE MARKETPLACE

Under the anemic sunshine of an early spring, trader Zineta tells me about her daily medicinal diet of five raw Japanese quail eggs. They make her thirsty and nauseated, she says, making a face. We are at the weekly flea market in Lukavac, a small town with a major air-pollution problem that has only grown worse since partial privatization handed over the management of its industrial coke and by-product complex to a subsid-iary of the global Ispat Group. Zineta travels with wares to the markets around the region, one town a day, and the ethnographer often lingers at her stand. Since Zineta began consuming the eggs, the lab tests have shown an improved blood count, but also a spike in her cholesterol and blood sugar levels. Her blood pressure too, which used to be low, jumped up. Her doctors "will not admit that the eggs might be causing it. They say this is just from my being worried-sick [*sikirancija*]." She doubts it and so refuses to take medicine prescribed for high blood pressure, cholesterol, and blood sugar. Nor will she run any further tests before she takes a vacation at the seaside. She has been planning this trip with her girlfriends for the longest time and does not want to ruin it with more test results and medical prescriptions: these would only make her worried-sick (*nasikirali bi me*). A customer who has been searching through a pile of clothing on Zineta's stands is curious to know what

Japanese quail eggs are good for, and Zineta replies: "Well . . . for wom-
en's illnesses [*ženske bolesti*]," which is a sometimes vernacular code for
problems with reproductive organs, anything from menstrual cramps
to infertility to bladder infections to uterine and ovarian cancer. Zineta
alludes to the latter conditions when she next says, "I was supposed to
undergo radiation but didn't."

People come and go, tune in and out of her health history. She speaks
of her latest trials in public and private clinics and her failed attempts to
secure funds through the Center for Social Care for two costly cancer
therapies, which she is receiving in private clinics: freezing and radiation.
She finishes on a different note, though: "But what is this; no one's buying today?" "But people have no money. It's the fifteenth of the month," a
granny reminds Zineta of the shared calendric condition of being strung
between the last and the next income infusions (see chapters 1 and 2).
Zineta just underwent cryosurgery, *zamrzavanje*, "freezing," she calls
it, explaining that it exposes tumors to extreme temperatures, "to kill
off their sprouts [*klice*]." The only clinical treatment left to try is radiation, but the doctors are convinced that if freezing failed, "it's 99 percent
certain that radiation will do no good either. So why should I bother?"
The experiment would cost 1,200 KM. "If only," she adds, "we could get
it on installment credit, like we did the seaside vacation. But how are
we to come up with that money at once?" The public hospital staff also
have been telling her lately to try *whatever* comes recommended (*štagod
čuje*), to seek *everywhere* (*traži*); that she has *nothing to lose in trying*. These
are code words that will sound throughout this text on popular health
travels: they signal the critical point where clinical science declares defeat and joins other, nonprofessional voices in licensing a broad quest
for cure. The case is hopeless unless there is a miracle cure. Stories are
told of such finds against the odds and there are plenty of leads to point
someway. Someone suggested that she becomes a vegetarian, someone
else mentioned a medicinal petroleum, which she had to procure from
abroad. At the advice of one medical doctor in a private practice, she goes
to medicinal sulfur spas in Tuzla, twice daily. Zineta changed four or
five doctors in the last months and explains: "I'm trying everything. You
know how it is: when you're drowning you grab for a straw. Each time,
you hope that someone will tell you something different."

Just recently she incorporated an alcohol infusion, recommended to her by an herbalist she encountered in the markets. Since we insist, she dictates the recipe to a few of us who are listening. "You soak forty-two flowers of *neven* [marigold] in a *domaća rakija* plum brandy, for ten days, discard the flowers, add *domaći* honey, and drink a shot, three times a day." The recipe is "precisely for that," the herbalist told Zineta, and what "that" is, is precisely vague in her stories. A woman fingering a collar of a shirt on sale she seems to fancy, asks: "And what is this recipe for?" Zineta replies, as earlier: "For women's illnesses." The remedy lowers her blood pressure, however, putting her quickly to sleep, which is why she only takes it on her way to bed. Zineta talked with a woman whom marigold infusion "greatly helped" and whose number the herbalist passed to her with the recipe. Over the course of the day, Zineta mentions other items in her domestic pharmacy and diet, including some potent api-therapeutics. Her attention darts between the relevant details of her health history and potential sales, speaking of grave matters but also interrupting to point to some good brand names or to say "shirts on the cloth hangers are 3 KM. Or two for 5 KM." She makes no excuses for shifting between precariousness and practicality: banal, basic matters of health and clothes, life and beauty, promise and risk hang tightly together, casually or else purposefully, like the bargain clothing items on the hangers.

In the late 1990s, Zineta, a newcomer to the new market, earned enough to finish her house construction, which had been ongoing since before the war. In 2006, however, her income was not sustaining her, especially given the costs of her medical treatments. The cryotherapy procedure alone cost her 100 KM. Her medicine is not on the cantonal list of essential medicines and must be paid for in full: some items cost her hundreds of KM. Even accessing the subsidized medicines was difficult. She was instructed to take a single costly capsule to "protect the organism," within twenty-four hours of cryotherapy. Although the drug qualified as essential, the private practitioners cannot prescribe it. With a note from her service provider she turned to the health center to ask for a prescription. The doctor there, allegedly, first declared the handwriting on the note illegible and when Zineta returned with a capitalized transcription, courtesy of a nearby pharmacist, the doctor said flatly that she should finish her business where she started it: in the private sector. At that point, Zineta says, "she lost it"—"it doesn't take much these days, anyhow, I'm on the edge, quivering with nervousness"—and told the physician off: "Now, listen! I didn't give away 100 Marks [for the treatment] because the bills bothered me in my pocket. I went to a private doctor because the public system does not have this technology!" She got the prescription and received advice about asking the social care center (*Socijalno*) for assistance with her medical costs. She did. The staff there told her that they fund "just such cases," but have run out of money. A potential customer, picking through the cosmetics on the stand, lifts her head from the nail polish display to intercept: "And when did they ever have money for someone? They only *take* money [in taxes]." Zineta: "So true." The woman: "And good luck trying to remain indebted to them for something [*de ti njima ostani dužan*]." Zineta wonders aloud about how difficult it must be for people without public health insurance; the woman could not agree more: "How? They alone know what it is like. They get ill, suffer, suffer, and die." Zineta shakes her head.

Zineta is "going everywhere," "trying anything," but also, sometimes, second-guessing the advice she receives as well as attending carefully to clues about the success or failure of remedies. With treatment so multiply threaded, involving so many items and potencies mutually interacting and interfering with her body, Zineta is regularly speculating about causes and effects. Speculating, she does not reduce the multitude of efficacies to a single outcome nor does she bundle all symptoms to conveniently discrete labels: sikirancija, on the one side, and cancer on the other. The choices opened further with the doctor's statement: she has nothing to lose. Her life is at stake. Multiple efficacies, however, muddle into signs and traces, with no definitive lines of action or connection: What could have increased her cholesterol levels, for instance? Certainty is still sought and desirable ("it is 99 percent certain . . ."; a phone number leads to a woman who benefited "greatly" from a home remedy for "precisely that"). But uncertainty is also productive and comforting: it keeps open the possibility of things happening and turning around or turning up, unlikely things, things unknown or yet untried. Hers is a keen sense that everything somehow, more or less, matters: the marigold infusion (which puts her to sleep) as well as the individual ingredients used to make it: not any brandy or honey, but domaće. The items arrived at her pharmacy by many routes. Some exotic ones are mass-produced and marketed at local supermarkets (quail eggs), some are brought from abroad through networks and kindness of kin and friends (petroleum), while others are secured through the hard work of collecting referrals and prescriptions. Yet others require careful sourcing from trusted producers of domaće or honest beekeepers.

And money matters run the course of health talk: costly treatments, poor sales, "high dates" (marking mid-month steep rise in borrowing), installment credit and subsidized medicine, payments up front and money missing, bills not chafing in the pocket. Gifts are expected, found and denied: the herbalist issued the marigold recipe, free of charge. Installment credit acts like a gift in this story because it gives time, which is a generous advance if one is long-dreaming of a vacation. The clinic and the social care center, however, are reproached for being on the outside of the gift economy.

WAITING, AROUND THE CORNER FROM
A HEALTH CENTER ON STRIKE

Public health professionals went on strike in 2007 in the Federation part of Bosnia, and over the course of six months gradually withdrew outpatient and, by and by, clinical and emergency care. Eventually, the staff demands for paid overtime and better wages were met, no small feat in a state where strikes are common and commonly ineffective, even if they are dramatic. Media, government, and nongovernmental agencies, as well as the health workers themselves, treated the strike with an air of indifference as the winding game of shifting responsibilities unfolded between different levels of administration: municipal, cantonal, federal, and state. About a month into the protest, the public health staff staged thirty-minute daily walkouts before returning indoors to sit but not work.

Around the corner from the health center in Tuzla, by the side of an herbalist's street stand, I observed the staff gathering to protest, to have a smoke, to chat. The sight was largely lost to the public, as the media had soon lost interest and patients were away (patients were waiting for the strike to end or else were lining up in the hallways, hoping to ambush nurses or doctors on their way back from the walkouts, to ask for exceptions: a drug prescription, a referral, or an exam). Herbalist Mehmed is popular and well-situated at the junction of many health routes, between the health center, emergency room, and a cluster of five major pharmacies. His is also a lone-standing structure in the midst of an ephemeral market that spreads out on sheets over sidewalks, exhibiting small, inexpensive wares (socks, shoes, clothes, and underwear) that can be folded, fast, at a sight of the police or market inspectors. As the strike slowed down the patient traffic, so did the small market wane, causing vendors to explore other outlets. Not so Mehmed: people tend to swing by and linger at his wooden kiosk, to consult him about possible treatments, to share health updates, as well as to complain and gossip about medical doctors and pharmacists, never more vigorously than during the strike. One day I came too late to catch an event that Mehmed's interlocutors were eager to retell: having been denied a medical consultation in the health center, an elderly man waited for the right moment to up-stage the health workers' protest with one of his own. Using the white-coated workers as his audience, he turned around, bent, and dropped his pants—the "full monty." This quintessentially Rabelaisian act took place a few steps from the marketplace and brought the professional claims to the vernacular bottom line, seeking to ridicule, to embarrass, to enrage. In subsequent days, the story's retelling butted in on the official speech of the health workers (that the people are behind them) and on the texts of the strike's posters (that the strike was for the people's sake). People throughout the region complained less bluntly and suffered the consequences: paying for drugs that would have been prescribed, missing regular checkups, seeing private practitioners, and after the strike, waiting through the backlog of appointments to schedule a visit.

On the day of the grandpa's protest (elderly man are commonly addressed as *djed* or *deda*), two men were lingering at the herbal medicine stand before its closing. One inquired about black cumin oil (čurukot ulje), which Mehmed recommends as the "Prophet's medicine" (*Poslanikova medicina*) and combines with herbal teas for a host of disorders. When the man mentions his previous consultations with bio-energy healers, Mehmed laughs dismissively; they are good for nothing. He is equally skeptical of most folk and Koranic healers, whom he suspects to be cheats, although the Koran itself is medicinal and "real imams" can help: he himself had been cured by one from a sihir. Mehmed begins a preparation of each of his herbal remedies with a *Bismillah* (in the Name of God) and imbues these remedies with supplications, dove (*naučim*, see chapter 5). He does so in the manner that is only more earnest but not different in kind than consulting his friends among the medical doctors for clarifications: "You must explain cholesterol to me," he once said to a hurried doctor in passing; "people ask me what it is and I can only cough in response." He believes in the kind of science that reconciles the active mechanisms of his herbal remedies, Koranic suras, and pharmaceuticals. He often makes gifts of his herbs and creams and extends them in advance of payments.

The second man at Mehmed's, it turns out, has also been searching for treatment and trying out different therapists, but has nowhere to go in the health system since doctors turned him down this morning, even though he is recovering from recent heart surgery. Unbuttoning his shirt to show a scar running across his chest, he says: "Imagine! They will not see me. They're on strike! And how can *I* go on strike about my 240 KM pension? Who would listen? They should be ashamed. I would fire them all and move folk medicine into their place [pointing to Mehmed's stand]. I went to the clinic and the doctor told me, 'I would see you but my boss won't let me.' Terzić [a leading cardiovascular surgeon at the regional clinic, who was building a private clinical center in 2007] told me 'come see me privately' but I have no money to pay 85 KM for an exam. I spend 284 KM for medicines alone every month." With his war-disability check amounting to 130 KM and his military pension, his monthly income is only slightly higher than his pharmaceutical bill. The man continues: "And who's asking me how I manage? And you, Terzić, make up your mind; you're either in private practice or in the public system. Make up your mind! He is an expert, I know that, but I have no money to see him. You [Terzić] used society to get free education, to get specializations, and . . . now you say thank you society, so long, off I go to work privately. One nurse gets 700 KM salary!" Before his anger runs out of steam, Mehmed interrupts him calmly: "In their hearts is a money fetish. When they see you, they see a summer vacation, winter holidays;

you are only a means to them, to point you to a pharmacy, to have you buy medicine, and they get money from that."

Stripping off one's pants or unbuttoning a shirt are grievances articulated at the level of a body, dressing down the politics to banal matters—heart and bottom, care and neglect—and dressing up the banal with vital importance. These acts address two kinds of audiences. One is presumed to be sympathetic, to know how it feels to seek care and not find it in public health spaces, which are deemed public in more than one sense: accessible to everyone, and built by a history of collective contributions and deductions. After all, *health center* is an inaccurate translation of what socialist history in Bosnian, Serbian, Croatian (BSC) calls "Home of Health"—Dom Zdravlja, the same concept of a familial, nurturing, people's-own institution that organized other social needs of socialist humans, such as the Home of Culture, the Home of Residential Community, the Pensioners' Home, the Mountaineers' Home, and so on. Public also means bound to selfless service by the gift exchange that underlies the medical practitioners' public university education. The second is expected to care and yet is perceived as negligent and arrogant; far from removing institutional medicine from relevance, professional slight only inflates people's commitment to medical humanism. The Hippocratic Oath is taken at graduations from Bosnia's medical universities, and whatever its status in the value schemes of contemporary schools, the fact of its existence and its precepts are stubbornly invoked on the streets.

People were also frustrated by the tepid official response to the health strike, considering the stakes, but this was one in a series of disappointments with the Bosnian state. It is not that the new state is a lean, neoliberal machine, simply withdrawn from public investments: some 20–30 percent of the central budget is spent on social provisioning. This is a fact that the World Bank, part of the economic task force in charge of Bosnian economic planning, regularly regretted (International Monetary Fund 2004; Pugh 2005) and local voices criticized as a political strategy for ensuring the (ethno-national) voting loyalties of social care beneficiaries (notably war veterans and the families of war victims and martyrs).

It does not help that contemporary Bosnia administratively and legally enfolds constitutional ills to the point where its ongoing state of becoming and undoing inescapably and creatively reproduces and amplifies its original faults (see Hayden 1999; Gilbert 2008; Kurtovic 2012). Formally, it is comprised of two and practically of three entities, each with an ethno-national majority (Bosnian Serbs, Bosnian Croats, and Bosnian Muslims) and pockets of ethno-national intermingling. The lived landscape is frequently messier because cities, in particular, have remained ethnically mixed or regained ethnically plural populations (notably Tuzla, Sarajevo, and the Brčko District) while ethnically cleansed areas are designated for refugee return, which does not always happen according to plan. When it comes to the sites of economic and medical exchange, however, formal politics that are exclusively concerned with ethno-national terms and electoral stakes are mute and rather irrelevant, not least because health and wealth pursuits are largely ethno-nationally irreverent and, if anything, strongly determined by governmental micro-sites: cantons, municipalities, districts, particular offices, particular officials' penchants, and the relative power of networked influence to work around formal entries and exits.

FOLLOWING, ON BOARD A TRAIN

On board an old train, whose door compartments' furnishings are faded except for the glow of metal handles, shining dimly a socialist history of gripping and polishing by the collective hands of the commuter labor force, I meet nena Mevlija. She is headed to a bio-energy healer in Brčko district. The train conductor (who issued local stop tickets at the price of full fare to Brčko, the last stop, and pocketed the difference) lingers to tell us about the recent celebrations of the railway's sixtieth anniversary. People were not the only ones dancing, apparently, as the wall portrait of President Tito went up and down and up and down in the spirited manner of an unresolved argument—and spirits, probably, represented in more than one way, as no party is complete without plum brandy, domaća—over whether socialist Yugoslavia meant the good old times (up with Tito!) or was it just as well that those days have passed (down with Tito!). Mevlija wears a busy headscarf and countless layers to keep warm. She feeds me an apple sliced in her lap with a pocket knife and indulges my curiosity with stories that drift from economizing tactics during the war, when she sold produce at the market, to the various herbal and folk therapies in hers and her family's medical history. Putting the knife into her purse, she pulls out a "good recipe" for lowering cholesterol—would I like to photocopy it?—sent to her by a dear friend, a refugee in Norway since the 1990s. Its title is reassuring, "A Surgery without a Knife: Liver Cleansing Recipe by Dr. Hulgi Clara," and the instructions promise a cleansing without major cost or hassle. Mevlija is eloquent, funny, and in the habit of casually referencing the titles on her reading list, from the Koran to *Communism in Ambush*. The latter she quotes in response to the conductor's story about festive indecisions about Tito's legacy, told not without fondness for the historical figure, stating serious concerns about communism and, especially, about Mao's Zedong's global imperialist designs. When I suggest that Mao has passed away, she doubts it: "The *Šejtan* [devil] can never die."

I accompanied Mevlija to her bio-energy therapy for several days, and over the course of the year we kept converging, by chance, along the regional pathways of market and medicine. I learned about her fixing, finally and on her own, her ill-fitting dentures with a pocket knife, after three different dentists in private practice failed to help but made considerable money trying. She reported on a new back-massage device, "a Russian invention." She admitted losing control over her headaches and frequented several *strava* practitioners.

This is Mevlija's second visit to the bio-energy healer who, she explains, is based in Vienna but operates a visiting practice in Brčko several months a year. She watched him on TV last night igniting a gas stove at a distance with a hand merely suspended above it, but this was no news to her. A year ago she learned firsthand about his touching without touching and, potentially, his stirring without intention: apparently, "you must wear cotton around him or else he might set the clothes on fire." After about ten minutes of the first therapy under his hands, never in contact with her skin, certain points of her body warmed up. When her back snapped loudly, the therapist was pleased by the remedial sign and discharged Mevlija with some cream to apply for twenty-one days to her hips, spine, and shoulders. Mevlija says she knew that the treatment was working because shortly afterwards, she began discharging excessive phlegm. "That's how sick I was!" she says, taking bodily responses that biomedicine would dismiss as "side effects" as proofs of therapeutic efficacy.[3] The therapist further concluded that it was "no wonder" she experienced headaches, since he detected spondylosis and poor circulation, while also diagnosing her with a weak nervous system, rheumatism, and bronchitis.

When I ask what "bio-energy" is, Mevlija readily defines it as "an energy, which has to be spent, so that he who has it treats even free of charge. If someone has no money he'll do it for free." Last year in the therapist's office she met someone who could not pay but was treated nonetheless. Bio-energy was hotly discussed in the marketplace of health. Its credibility was disputed and defended but consistently described in terms of a vital power that everyone has, but that some have in excessive supply, in which case it must be lavishly expanded, lest the bio-energy therapist suffers the surplus of "life." Symptoms include great discomfort and pain, headaches in particular, high bodily temperature, or nervous breakdowns. Such an extreme embodiment of therapeutic power and of an urgency to divest it advertise the popular ideal of medicine as a genuine gift and medical care as a disposition that is not only irrepressible but also pernicious for the therapist to withhold.

On our way back from Mevlija's bio-energy treatment the following day, she briefs our friendly conductor on the progress of her treatment and offers him a leaflet from the therapist's office to copy (and offers her reading glasses too, for the conductor is squinting at the text. "Magical" she laughs, "they suit everyone. From the store." As the glasses fail to improve the legibility of the recipe for the conductor, she diagnosis him with myopia). The conductor would like to visit the bio-energist about some nagging aches of his own but worries about the price. Mevlija reassures him: "Three treatments cost 40 KM. It's less expensive than the thermal baths for which you have to pay 400 KM, and I did it last year, but this has helped me more. Well, the baths helped me too. My bones came about afterwards. Everything has its own efficacy [*sve ima svoje*]. Every ailment has its cures, and these are many."

Detouring uncovers the many sources and forms of local knowledge, from TV advertisements to eclectic reading references, and from revelation to conspiracy, while exposing its limits ("Mao is [not] dead") as well as its generative possibilities. This is a practical kind of knowledge, circulated in recipes and handled confidently, as with the pocket knife, the same one that peels an apple to share with a fellow traveler. It passes with critical judgment and enthusiastic recommendation with eyes on price and curative effects. It is intrusive and imposingly intimate in a way that presumes quite a bit of prior forgiving and forgetting: the conductor pockets small change at the expense of a struggling public railway system, neither hiding from nor winking at us—he presumed us for accomplices, while nena shoves her eyeglasses into his hands and counts on my liver needing this kind of help. Significantly, the vernacular medical knowledge is at once caught up in the local histories and contested memories and open to the worlds beyond, consuming them, incorporating them into people's thinking, tasting, therapeutic diets. The recipe that made it from Norway to Mevlija's purse misspells the name of Hulda Clark, a controversial medical doctor with worldwide fame, and infamy, whose alternative medical inventions, devices, recipes, and texts sell widely—Amazon in the United States carries them. And while denunciations on quackwatch.com and elsewhere pull no punches ("bizarre," "phony"), her book *The Cure for All Cancers*, and her idiom of everyday toxicity loads are familiar to many health-conscious mainstream and underground publics. The conductor may or may not have gone to therapy himself but he most likely passed on the recommendation to other passengers, family, friends, or whomever he might have heard complaining about poor health.

EAVESDROPPING ON A BUS

A woman boards the bus in Sarajevo, the capital, bound northeast, to Tuzla, with a small boy in tow and a kitten in a cardboard box. She seats them together, across from me, the boxed cat on the boy's lap, both very quiet, and strikes a conversation with another woman, which will last the course of the three-hour winding ride. Shortly after the introductions, their talk turns to health, which the ethnographer silently appreciated and took note of.

The woman's interlocutor, it turns out, is a trained pharmacist but is employed as a dental assistant in a private practice in Brčko. It also turns out that she works in the suburban district where the woman, the boy, and, soon, the kitten too, live. The dental assistant talks enthusiastically about a new clinic in Banja Luka, the capital of the Serb Republic, one of the two administrative entities of the Bosnian state. The clinic, according to the woman, features the "most-modern" (*najmoderniju*) equipment and a staff of experts from across the former Yugoslavia, which, combined, produces "an accurate diagnosis, something that you don't find easily these days. A comprehensive exam costs 500 euros." She describes the abdominal scan that she underwent at the price of 100 euros, when the boy's mother interrupts with a complaint: "I recently tried to fill a prescription for my child but in every pharmacy they told me the same: the cream shouldn't be used on a child. But a doctor prescribed it to him, for pain! My son's legs are hurting. He played soccer [on a school team] but we stopped that. . . . He can't sit still. But he doesn't have chronic pain, why did he give him the cream?" The dental assistant suggests: "It costs 35 euros for a child to get x-rays [at the Banja Luka clinic]." The woman, who fiddles with the box to make sure that the kitten has enough air, thinks that money is not an issue: "When it comes to health, one would give the last dinar," the old Yugoslav currency that still is iconic for money in general, especially money not had. Local health talk inevitably rings with the tunes of ultimacies: the last dime, the last chance, the odds between life and death. She is reminded of another story: "You know that man who opened the auto parts shop in the city center, next to the health center? Well, his son got ill. Their only son. He is wasting away. They are taking him everywhere. To think that they just pulled their lives together nicely, and now this. There are some strange illnesses nowadays." She pauses, ponders this common but rarely casual-sounding saying and adds: "Maybe the doctors don't want to say what is the matter with the boy." The dental assistant: "They would say, why wouldn't they, but they don't know it. It's not so easy to come by a real [*pravu*] diagnosis these days." The women next compare the prices and expertise of several pharmacies in her home district and the conversation slows down—the sun has already set and darkness veils us to each other—before it takes another turn.

The passenger traveling with the boy and the cat initiates it: "Do you know about that woman who makes spells [*ona što čara*] in D. [a district

town in northeastern Bosnia]? What do you think? Can she really help?"
Dental assistant: "That one? She sells fog! And makes big money, too. I
called her at home, and she got angry, started shouting at me, as in 'why
was I bothering her?' But her number was advertised! She then told me it
would cost 100 K M just to make an appointment. If she were someone for
real [*pravi neki*] she would just help. But she won't do it without money."
Her interlocutor guesses that "people probably do anything in order to
see her. They borrow money." Dental assistant: "Her advertisement was
constantly running on T V; she's a real Gypsy."

My ride on the bus lasted long enough to catch this moment in the
conversation that narrated a swerving course of medical uncertainty
and the search for cure from the "most-modern" clinical center equipped
with current technologies and staffed with pan-Yugoslav experts to the
widely advertised charms of the rude, "real Gypsy" spell-maker. The two
forms of curative expertise return us to the anxious opposition between
the doctor and the charlatan, showing at the same time how their appeals
are effectively constituted through a jarring juxtaposition of two alter-
authenticities and a pairing of affinities: both technologies are highly
specialized and possibly divining the real diagnosis, which is otherwise
elusive. Regional folklore has long regarded Gypsies as masters of black
magic—marginality tends to earn a reputation for occult potency—
even as Roma fortunetellers and spell-makers have lost the prime place
in the magic market proliferating with all kinds of experts and democra-
tizing in a number of improvised and do-it-yourself techniques. My point
here is not simply to stress yet another case of the familiar, constitutive
interplay of modernity and magic (Meyer and Pels 2003) but, rather, to
point at the long-winding but casual turn of conversation to the subject
of a woman with a high-profile business in sihir. That the dental assistant—who is attracted to the clinic in the Serb Republic because it guar-
antees "accuracy"—not only knows about this *shiribaz* (a dealer in sihir)
but has already inquired about her terms of treatment speaks loudly
about the popular, symmetrical inclinations to compare treatments on
equal terms, expect accuracy, and, in the process, uncover and generate
constant confusion: Can doctors know, will they tell, does this woman
really help, can she help if she makes money, and if she helps, but makes
money, what does that make her?

READING: *AURA*, "MAGAZINE FOR HEALTHIER
LIFE, CULTURE OF LIVING, ALTERNATIVE
MEDICINE, PERSONAL FATES"

I am leafing through the April 2008 issue of *Aura*. The contents do not
nearly capture the abundance of stories, testimonies, issues, questions,
puzzles, advertisements, and practical advice that fit into the eighty-two
pages; my leafing attention will be equally superficial. The issue begins
with several pages of an herbal medicine lexicon, titled "What to Glean
and What to Use for Medicine in the Spring" (5–7), with photographs
of herbs, flowers, blossoming branches, tasseled growths, and arboreal
fruits and descriptions of uses, potencies, and suggested recipes that
vary in breadth from extensive to brief. This reader was surprised to find
out that "Lovely Scented Violet" is used to treat "neurosis, insomnia,
conjunctivitis, bronchitis, asthma, . . ." and that there are instructions on
how to treat each with violet tinctures, oils, or teas, specifying how long
to steep, with what to cure and boil, and how best to consume. Included
are also dandelion, willow, white pine, *podbjel, imela* ("regulates both
kinds of [blood] pressure"), and birch. The next few pages hold brief
life histories, whose trajectories teeter between tragedy and remarkable
achievement: a fourteen-year-old published author who writes, despite
many challenges, mostly realist tragedies, inspired by her surroundings
in an impoverished central Bosnian village, and a seventy-seven-year-old
djed whose three life wishes came true, but two of them not exactly as
he had hoped they would. The article on the next couple of pages investigates "Botox—Dangerous or Miraculous Cure for Wrinkles," starting on a cautionary note, hailing moderation as the wisest approach to
cosmetic treatments and citing an investigation that the US Food and
Drug Administration initiated at the request of Public Citizen, a "repu-
table consumer association." Turning the page, I face a large, colored
advertisement of a western Bosnian herbal pharmacy for an upcoming
product, "The Honey of Life" (*Med Života*): "A natural product made of
honey, herbal extracts, and propolis. Recommended for immunity and
regeneration of the organism." This last claim, just as it sounds, aims
at being comprehensive and so includes treatment of the following:
blood composition, bronchitis, kidney infection, inflammation of the

liver, spleen, and urinary tracts, stomach ulcers, and "ženska oboljenja." Featured below Honey of Life is the cream Psorex, "for skin disorders with a great record of [treatment] success [*velikim procentom uspjeha*]." The herbalist is smiling a beautiful, well-made-up smile and holding an *Aura*-awarded recognition for Phytotheraphy. Skipping a few pages to another article I find the story of one woman's health history around a promotion of another line of honey products, Eko Med, concocted by a Sarajevo-based beekeeper. Beekeepers across Bosnia tend to also be well-versed in medicinal herbs, which they combine with bee products for a variety of therapeutic uses. The featured patient is grateful to both "conventional and alternative medicine" clinicians in Mostar and the beekeepers, whose joint interventions, she says, helped her defeat large intestinal and stomach tumors. She underwent surgeries and six chemotherapies but "managed to keep her hair," and checked the cancerous growth with regular use of Eko Med. This line of "natural medications" is recommended by her stories as much as by small but concise advertisements that run a list of illnesses treated, phone numbers and addresses, and a claim, highlighted in red, "Our proofs are cured patients—ask them about us." Next to the email address and web page is a note to patients planning a visit to the beekeeper-apitherapist: they must bring along their medical records. Honey reappears twice more before this issue of *Aura* ends: in a story about a beekeeper in northeastern Bosnia who worries, on behalf of all the members of his municipal apiculture association, about "counterfeit honey" in the market; and in a sober article that discusses the widespread use of insecticides in beehives that are suspected to have carcinogenic effects. I will skip over the article on the many health benefits and medicinal recipes for čurukot (black cumin oil), never mind a yoghurt diet that gives you a perfect figure in ten days, and will overlook advertisements for a number of handy items, not least for little pillows made of "buckwheat chaff " for "healthy and pleasant sleep," in order to glance quickly at the text on a featured bio-energy healer. It starts promisingly, with: "Those who do not believe in miracles, only have to stop by a Kakanj [central Bosnian town] bio-energy healer … to change their mind after only a few moments in her company." The *Aura* reporter steps into this practice with a former patient who turned to bio-energy when doctors recommended urgent spine surgery; the prose continues enthusiastically: "Čarobne ruke" (magical or wondrous hands), is a subtitle of the section that describe how the bio-energy healer won the affection of the patient by getting up from her breakfast to attend to the woman in pain and, waving hands, made the pain instantly subside. The bio-energy therapist in question is said to cure herniated discs "faster than a dentist pulls out a tooth."

Leafing backward to an irresistible feature, a recurrent one in *Aura*, I linger on the coverage of Ahmed Srabović, looking as sharp as ever in the photographs, including one above his advertised phone numbers and the title "Dr. of energy, natural, and spiritual medicine." *Aura* introduces the figure of Dr. Srabović, familiar to all readers, anew, each time. This time it focuses on one of his inventions—Bio Piramida (see below, in "Listing")—that adheres to a particular theory of secret causes at work behind many common health complaints, from headache to tension to fatigue and insomnia. "Harmful radiations" of various objects and infrastructures—some of them distinctly modern (computers), others ancient and not necessarily man-made (underground water networks)— are all counteracted by the engineering ingenuity of pyramids, which were the source of inspiration for this device (24). Dr. Srabović can be counted on for his interesting theoretical propositions; here he draws attention to the fact that "harmful radiations" are still "taboo topics" in Bosnia, although slowly "we too are catching up with the West," invoking here a different sense of the West, one where the alternative fringe runs right though the center of the iconic trendsetter of its more Eastern and Southerly observers. It is also not surprising that Dr. Srabović highlights an added benefit of the bio pyramid: "it establishes harmony in the soul and body, as well as opens up energy points" (25). A brief paragraph reintroducing this practitioner does not do justice to the portfolio of his practices nor to his habit of operating across therapeutic traditions, easily adopting their cross-translations though fully aware of what they betray. For instance, the paragraph describes him as "a successful practitioner of parapsychology, Reiki, bio-energy, exorcism, telepathy and chromo-therapy." I doubt that Dr. Srabović would object but, given time, he would painstakingly explain each component of his practice, would contextualize his computer-diagnostics technology within broader alternative trends, particularly European ones, and would speak of psyche as inadequately holding the place of other components of human be-ing: soul and spirit. He has spoken and written about the metaphysical aspects of his treatment—I only heard him speak of it. When it comes to treatments for uncomfortable human–nonhuman intersections, he speaks bluntly of reciting relevant passages from the Koran [*učenje ruk'je*; see chapter 6]. This does not preclude him from translating his theories into more global terms, palatable to the alternative medical assemblies he attends across former Yugoslavia and beyond. He is pragmatic about it. For *Aura* he states: "I want to demonstrate by means of a personal example that alternative medicine has to receive its proper place in our country, the place it belongs to in almost all European states" (25).

Aura ends with a familiar genre of illness and curative histories. From one issue to the next, these speak of a still messier, pernicious world, a world of malice and malignant powers, of disastrous encounters with and last-minute rescues from powerful nonhumans—jinn—who some-times act whimsically and other times self-defensively in response to human irritation, or, worse, act at the bidding of another human, who is an expert for contracting the nonhuman services. The experts are said to "make sihir" (*naprave sihir*) onto whomever their clients want healed, harmed, or otherwise charmed and responsive. And the list of clients usually runs contrary to the appearances to compose a close circle of intimate betrayals: old friends, next-door neighbors, former or slighted lovers, business partners, colleagues, in-laws. It is a world that would make one panic. Names, places, and case histories paint a multiethnic, transnational trade in ill will and envy, variously occulted and medi-ated, mostly known as sihir—the word registers both the craft and the artifact for malevolent action at a distance, with a wide range of precise afflictions—as well as a motley field of long-distance healing interven-tions. One woman speaks of suffering for years with a negligent husband ("he said he went to see his dentist, when in fact he was seeing a lover") and an abusive mother-in-law. It was not until her sons were estranged from her that she sought and found treatment from an imam—a well-meaning friend had recommended him. In turn, she now recommends him to readers who can find his photograph, address, and phone num-bers displayed on the page (68–69). A few pages earlier is a story with a few significant differences that speaks volumes to the regional readers: in contrast to the previous sihir patient, a veiled woman, this one features a woman by the name of Maria who had been a kleptomaniac for decades until she was arrested; embarrassed, she sought the help of a young veiled healer, whose numbers are also featured together with a bullet-point summary of specialties: "bio-energy, recitation and healing by Koran, searching and finding sihir by means of prayer beads [*tespih*], removal of all kinds of black magic [sihir] and custom talismans (for home, person, or business)" (65). This genre of health stories and medical advertisements is particularly alarming to read—partly because it suggests the most intrusive and corrosive influences to be had on porous bodies; and partly also because it paints a world in which everyone is possibly to be mistrusted and every slight may be consequential beyond one's wildest imagination.

The last page of *Aura* is typically crammed with two kinds of relief items. One is a handful of advice on how to prepare natural beauty treatments, titled "Avocado for Beauty." The lower half of the page carries the avocado green hue into the background of an advertisement for two-volume do-it-yourself hard-cover guides, promoted as "original, simple and practical," and titled "Protection of People and Homes from Jinn and Šejtan."

Listing: Afflictions

Sikirancija: Most common complaint and disposition, to worry excessively, with thoroughly visceral effects.

Šećer (*visok, nizak, skočio, opo*): Blood sugar, high or plummeted.

Nervoza, nervi: often used interchangeably with sikirancija, nervoza is the state of being jittery and profoundly agitated, nervous. Nervi, nerves, is a shorthand. Sadiković's index distinguishes many kinds of nervousness and afflictions of nerves: nervous dizziness, nervousness, nervous tremors, nerve inflammation with aches, distraught nerves.

Visok, nizak pritisak: high or low blood pressure. People track these with blood-pressure gauges and interpret them readily to each other.

Sihir: Affliction caused by nonhuman agents, working out arrangements made with an expert (who may be healing or harming, but

who can tell) and contracted by someone jealous, slighted, ambitious, or otherwise motivated. The afflictions may manifest as
various aches and failures of the body, as affective and cognitive
disorders, as obsessive and imprudent habits, new and inordinate
desires, or misplaced affections. See chapter 6.

Strava: excessive fears and worries, see chapter 5.

Struna: see the open items, below

Listing: Remedial Things

Kuran Časni: Islamic Medicine or Prophet's *a.s.* (*allejhiselam*), most
explicitly, although other traditional and new forms of healing
variously incorporate Koranic suras in the treatment. They do so
either inconspicuously or flamboyantly.

Domaće foods: fermented cabbage (*kiseli kupus*), apple vinegar
(*sirće*), *pekmez*. Raw milk, unpasteurized cream, whey products.

Caffetin (or *Kafetin*): painkiller brand produced since 1957 by the
Macedonian pharmaceutical powerhouse Alkaloid Skopje,
blanketing the ex-Yugoslav region and beyond. A mixture of
paracetamol, propyphenazone, caffeine, and codeine, it is medicine for headaches.

Mobile phone, particularly SMS: a means for achieving eco-technics,
especially in case of a medical emergency. See the open items account, below.

Lexaurin, Apaurin (anxiolytics, brands of benzodiazepam): It
would seem that the two drugs are indispensable even if I
rarely met anyone not concerned about their side-effects and
habit-forming powers. Many women have an emergency supply
handy, in their purses or at home—and men of the household
depend on them too (see chapter 5). Apaurin sounds a deeper
historicity and wins the confidence of patients who might remember its appearance in the 1980s. Lexaurin is a newer brand
by the Bosnalijek pharmaceutical company and is perhaps more
popular among younger consumers who have coined a cute
nickname for the drug, a diminutive: *Lexić*. Facebook friends
circulated a sweetened image of Lexaurin, spread onto an icing

of a cake. The text on the lower side read: keep out of the reach
of children![4]

Gljiva, gljivice: "little mushrooms." *Aura* featured an article in its
June 2012 issue, meant to inform and clarify "What Actually Is
Kombucha?" (See Jašarević 2015).

Žalfija/Kadulja: many domestic medicine experts recommend this
for cases of inflammation of any kind, as a "natural antibiotic."
Salvia officinalis, sage, earns a beautiful description in Sadiković's
lexicon of herbal medicine (1988:170) and figures as an ingredient
in recipes he provides throughout. Among the uses he mentions
are the following: to keep teeth clean and white, to strengthen
the blood and nerves, to cleanse the liver, to counter nighttime
flashes, to improve digestive juices.

OPEN ITEM ACCOUNTS: STRUNA

One day, a dear woman—I spoke of her in chapter 1—is screaming in
pain; rolled up into a ball, nursing her stomach like a baby. She has not
slept nor eaten for days; painkillers do not help. I want to take her to
the emergency room but she thinks otherwise. It's a *struna*, a stomach
neurosis *(stomačna nervoza)* for which doctors are helpless. They don't
know it. They would keep her in a hospital for days, run tests, charge her
for the bed, and dismiss her with inconclusive diagnoses. It happened
before. So we are driving to her *tetka* (aunt) Hava's for help.

In the car, groaning in pain, the woman is trying to guess what caused
the struna: Carrying an overload (moving heavy things is known to
cause it)? Sadness (memory of heavy soil weighed on her mind since her
brother's burial)? Anger (a disposition hard to disregard, though she
tries)? Or another budgetary crisis, since she ran out of money in the
family purse and "the date is high," midway between the last and the
next income?

"Struna," her tetka diagnoses her a little later, hovered above the woman's body, an imposing figure of care and calm. "You might have carried
something too heavy, you might have caught a little cold (what did you
eat that's cold, an ice cream? That's not for you!), maybe all of last week's
stress and sadness, or maybe it's from nervousness, which you tend to put

in your stomach, though it cannot digest it, the anger." She adds, unable to resist: "You got a stomach like that from your father's family. They all suffer from it," says the aunt who is the woman's father's sister, referring to "the wandering stomach and bad temper."

Tetka Hava lowers her fingers, scrunched up like the legs of a spider, into the woman's bellybutton to listen to the stomach. "Here it is, just very distressed, [*rastrešen*], disseminated [*rasut*], restless [*nemiran*]. It's knocking, like a human being, from below." Aunt Hava recites Koranic suras while massaging the sides of the stomach gently inward toward the center. She prays for it, listening, guiding it softly back to the center where it can calm down and settle. She has me feel it: my fingers press the dimple in the belly, which is like an ear hole to a hand listening for the visceral underworld. The surface collapses to a depth, and the depth is subject to skin-level influences: fingers massaging, suras reciting, the circumstances—be they cold meals or mourning sadness—profoundly upsetting. Next, Tetka Hava places a piece of pressed bread on the bellybutton, sticks a few matches in it, lights them up, and with flames still burning, cups the assemblage with a round coffee cup (*fildžan*) turned upside-down. Instantly, a vacuum extinguishes the small flame while quickening and sucking in the belly folds. She then secures the cup in place with a headscarf and an elastic bandage. Tetka recommends that the woman stays lying down "as calm as a bug," to speak in whisper, to think not, cry not, and to eat something light, just so that the stomach keeps busy with a task. Otherwise, "the stomach is like a little ball; it will again slip and roll off somewhere." The aunt also recommends some medicines, a syrup that she has been drinking for a while to manage her own stomach neurosis—she shows us the bottle in her purse. The woman refuses the medicine but changes her mind the following day when another woman in the family, known for her commonsense, recommends the very same remedy.

PHONING THE CURE

The cell phone, I found, is a significant therapeutic technology. Practitioners use phones, as these communication devices have been intended for business: to receive inquiries, dispatch advice, and make appointments.

Among very popular ones, some strava nene among them, cell phones rang off the hook (see chapter 5). Cell phones, however, have also been put to more immediately therapeutic uses: as devices of invited, intrusive, and intimate intervention. Remembering earlier semantic histories of the word *device*, which my friend Caryn O'Connell, a trusted source on promiscuous English etymologies, told me, brought together desire and invention, cell phones were reinvented among certain medical publics as desire-devices, extending calls for help and sympathetic responses between therapists and patients. Whether in a conversation or, more likely, in SMS messaging (since pretty much everyone was economizing on phone credit), cell phones connected parties consequentially, bringing together complaint and comfort, announcing reported bodily alterations, engendering generosity, generating debts. I bring here side-by-side snapshots of two therapists whose repertoires and dispositions toward medicine could not be more different, to offer a deliberately tenebrist sketch of bodily and telecommunicative extensities. In thinking touching, Jacques Derrida's imagination goes pretty wild and poetic as he describes the plenitude of absence brought up by a phone call, which extends voice across the distance between intimate speakers, "lovers, separated for life. A tragedy" in his brief tale, and in doing so effectively plays up the viscerality of the phoning experience, shared, in the closeness from which, nonetheless, the two are forever weaned. Derrida appropriately calls this visceral-technological embrace "eco-technics," and argues that it is "originary," insofar as all bodies, all of the time, are intersected by some inorganic but intensely sensuous technologies, those that, like language, always come from and reach beyond us. Convincing, perhaps, except that in case of therapeutic uses of mobile phones, the ecotechnics ought also to account for an unlikely play of desire and invention, in such a way that rather than "originary," technologies are especially developed by a kind of expert, and if anything is more generally shared, it is the embodied receptivity to interventions and desire: to heal.

Herbalist Zijo is famous, well-advertised, and expensive. With his base on the outskirts of the central Bosnian town of Zenica, the infamous capital of new industrial air pollution, he tours the region, setting up one-day practices in local conference rooms. Regular and new patients learn of his visits by word of mouth, spread by phone calls and text messages, and gather in numbers to see him. Zijo treats all kinds of ailments, from nervous disorders to imbalances of blood sugar and blood pressure, to skin conditions, to cancer. According to him, good health essentially hinges on the state of the stomach (*želudac*). In this etiology, which is prevalent beyond Zijo's practice, the stomach is the most exposed bodily surface. It literally stomachs the existential and environmental circumstances to the point where it develops lesions, ulcers, excesses, or deficiencies, as well as affects "the nerves" causing restlessness, sleeplessness, nervousness, aggression, or depression. Zijo treats stomach and nerves as one visceral-affective-existential bundle. "Nerves, nerves, nerves!" he says "People come to see me for nervousness, psychosis, nervous breakdown, stress, fears, troubles, when they have nightmares. There are people who come here and cry to me, cry to me!" Zijo, however, has no patience for people's money complaints and he travels with armed bodyguards. Poised against popular expectations that he should practice generosity, he does not project the image of a healer "for real." In his late sixties, he has limped since a traffic accident in the 1980s left him with a broken leg and blood poisoning; that accident, however, inspired his "love" for herbs (*voljet bilje*), which, he claims, saved a leg that doctors wanted to amputate. Our time in his office is constantly interrupted with phone calls that Zijo juggles simultaneously, and with his placing of prescription orders through a hole in a wall behind a shutter, which he slides open to frame, tightly, the ready face of his assistant, a cousin who works in his dispensary. In addition, Zijo's *bratična* (brother's daughter), who processes herbs in a mechanical press that Zijo invented, comes in to consult with him, and Zijo's wife comes once to ask what would he have for lunch, and once more, to ask him to open a can of okra. Zijo's is a family business. Work is interspersed with household routines, and the wealth it produces is invested in his home and children. In his compound Zijo enumerates his prosperity, spreading his arms widely to embrace the yard in our field of vision: "Look at my houses! All from herbs. I schooled my children, bought them apartments in Sarajevo, all from herbs. But one must love, love herbs." Zijo is on the phone. Reviewing a list of orders, he says to a woman on one line: "One tonic for anemia, one mixture for bloody stool, honey for digestion, black cumin oil, and some oil for vaginal application." He pauses to listen. "What?! Well he should listen to you, he should respect you as a woman. Fine, let me speak with him." Zijo repeats the list to the husband—the medicine is for both him and his wife—and gives orders: "You must listen to your wife, do everything she tells you; you must, this is not a joke! And no smoking in the house!" After pausing to listen: "I know that she's weak but these medicines will strengthen her. Does she have heartburn? She does? Then I'll add this tea for her. This all will be 140 [KM], but since you are a regular customer, it's 100 for you. You want another one for anemia? Then 120 everything." At this point, another phone rings and Zijo answers while still holding the first line. After a while, he says to the new caller: "In chemotherapy, are you? Women's illnesses? Send my regards to those doctors of yours! You've neglected your stomach, your nervous system. . . . Your doctors cannot cure you." Now the landline rings and Zijo puts the other two lines on hold to answer: "What? The lungs? Why did they have to operate, take out a lung? They had to? So are you better now that you are in chemotherapy? No! The medicine cannot cure it. Did you lose your hair? Right! I've been banned from TV for saying such things. I said that I cure lung cancer without surgery."

In the quieter setting of a small high-rise flat in Tuzla, you will find Lazar. You will stumble upon him by means that are best left to chance, he says, which inevitably takes you where you need to be, although it helps to make an appointment. Lazar heals with a range of therapies, from spiritual technologies developed by a Belgrade-based, globe-trotting inventor and teacher, Živorad Slavinski, to crystals, herbal medicine, and Reiki, and finally, with devices and recipes developed by Dr. Hulda Clark. Most effective, however, are spiritual energies cultivated through years of meditation, focused and channeled with prayers. A follower of a South Indian holy man, Sai Babba, whose popularity in Bosnia is growing but is limited to urbanites with means to travel to the guru's ashrams, Lazar lives off of alms and a check earned for early retirement from a civil engineering position with a socialist company that privatized and downsized since the war. He professes financial ignorance, has no savings, claims to have no belongings, and he takes the flower I bring to him only as far as the altar in his living room, with Sai Babba's photo, Buddha statuettes, Muslim prayer beads, crosses, and crystals. Lazar

understands the therapeutic mechanism of the healing crystals, of bio-
energy, and of Slavinski's PEAT (Psychic Energy Aura Technology), but
God knows how the prayers work. "When I send a prayer, a person heals,"
Lazar says, and describes a case of a man, recovering from a stroke, whom
he saw earlier in the afternoon of our encounter. Lazar had prayed by
the man's bedside until the patient's attack of dizziness and nausea sub-
sided. The prayer, Lazar explains, has to be genuine, whereas "for many
it's an ordinary ritual, like having coffee. But it needs to be experienced
[*proživit*, literally 'lived through']." Our conversations are occasionally
interrupted by an SOS SMS arriving to Lazar's phone. One, for instance,
sent by a friend and patient, a regional public figure, stated an urgent
complaint of sharp chest pain and a plea for help. Lazar SMSed back: "I'll
try to help. Send ok when better," closed his eyes, and holding the fingers
of his left hand close to the base of his nose, settled into a silent prayer. In
a while he opened his eyes and resumed our conversation. "Everything,"
he says, "is a consciousness and energy combined into varied degrees of
materiality. Everything is energy. With a thought from my heart, I pray.
The thought goes around the Universe. Spiritual power is an awareness
and channeling of that cosmic energy." His cell phone beeped a new
message in his inbox: an "ok."

NOTES

1. A blog entitled "To Good Health via Nutrition," *Ishranom do Zdravlja* (blogger.
ba.com), still lively at the time of writing in 2015, ran a post in December 2009 on Sadik
Sadiković, reproducing the entire introduction to *Folk Medicine*. Upon rereading Sadiković, "whom, I believe, you all know" a blogger named lillium decided to share the
selections, asking his online fellows to ponder the message of this noteworthy man. The
fact that it was written in 1928, lillium says, adds additional charms to the text (http://
djuliman.blogger.ba/arhiva/2009/12/30/2392695). This blog itself offers a good vista on
popular health concerns and repertoires in cyberspace, featuring citations and commentary on Prophet's Medicine, on benefits of fast (and types of fasting), on the miraculous
Amazonian plant *graviola* (soursop), and a long archive of contributions on various food
staples, plants, seeds, treatments, and disorders, from "tennis elbow" (*Lateral epicondili-
tis*) to stress and depression to beauty tips and treatments.

2. A local historian of Ljubuški composed a remarkable biographical sketch of Sadiković, which sings praises to the "king of folk medicine." The official webpage of the
town of Ljubuški featured the story when I last accessed it, in January 2016. See http://
ljubuski.net/1222-sadik-ef-sadikovic-kralj-narodne-medicine.

3. Whereas contemporary global clinical practice considers side effects as "unfortunate extras to the specific effects of a magic bullet" (Healy 2002), in humoral models of disease, treatments mimic the body's own efforts at self-healing and induce diuresis, purging, vomiting, rashes, fevers, or blistering (see also Harrington 1997; 2007 and Kleinman 1980).

4. Thanks to the anthropologist Larisa Kurtovic, who brought this photograph to my attention.

FIVE

Strava

Distant Bodies at Hand

🌿 I admit: I too was caught up in the search for a genuine healer, a healer "for real" (*pravi*). Perhaps I should have known better, given my schooling in academic disenchantment and in an anthropological sensibility that much prefers the grittiness of vaguer statements, imperfect improvisations, and practical inconsistencies to the ideal promises of all things authentically real. Authenticity, like presence, counts on a plenitude of sorts that is immediate and accessible, only given the right grasp, but which in the lived and historical circumstances never fails to disappoint—because the matters are still more plentiful or simply otherwise. In the previous chapters, an anthropologist following popular quests for the real healer across northeastern and central Bosnia was well advised not to expect to arrive, finally, to the place everyone hoped for, but to appreciate, instead, detours and stops that people take along the road to better health, ever arriving at tentative achievements, temporary reliefs, and regular deferrals of effective cures. Moreover, practitioners who are less *real* than expected, which is to say practicing with openly commercial ambitions and efficient but ambiguously curative crafts, can sometimes be just as effective and hugely popular. New medical practices, authentic or not, also tend to be more broadly consequential for how economic or bodily matters are treated and composed in present-day Bosnia. Yet, as much as collective anxieties about poor health and doubts about many forms of (costly) health care sustained my research interests, the sheer effort I was observing, whether enthusiasm about a new remedy on a personal trial or exhaustion, was wearing me down (for who can observe and not be affected?), and I earnestly wished for there to be real cures and genuinely generous practitioners somewhere.

Years after I met Zejneba, her figure and her living and working quarters embody, for me, the full weight of what one seeks in a genuine healer. In the hamlet of Kuge, tucked away from the main road, up on Majevica mountain, she practiced *strava*. This is a common form of traditional therapy across the region that, simply put, treats all sorts of bodily, affective, and behavioral disorders that local etiologies attribute to fear and fright, fretting and stress, traumatic events, or protracted crises, especially if the symptoms nag on and are uncannily resistant to conventional medical or pharmaceutical therapies. Although patients today worry, like late nineteenth-century ethnologists and folklorists used to, that strava is vanishing and that the genuine grandmotherly practitioners, *nene*, are almost impossible to find amid commercially savvy dabblers and imposters, grandmas among them, strava seems to have been never more popular, and never more practiced in towns and villages. Some practitioners' fame attracts health travelers from as far as the Bosnian diaspora spreads. Strava is generally seen as either a supplemental treatment or a more comfortable or more adequate response to complaints that the local clinical and vernacular observers would designate under the rubric of *mental* or *psychological*, though what *psyche* means and entails ends up looking quite different from within the strava practice.

What was plainly *real* about Zejneba was the extravagant, utterly anti-economical care she extended to her patients, whom, it seems, she would rather not see—her daily life would certainly be easier—but could not refuse to treat. If they came, they had to be welcomed, and once welcomed they were guests at her home as much as her patients and she worked on their behalf, beyond all reasonable expectations: feeding them, curing them, hosting them. Her kindness would keep them hostage, actually, for a day-long event. Real was also the elaboration of treatment, which unlike other practices I have seen included a number of devices beyond the strava essentials, which she brought to bear upon the patient in an assemblage particular to each patient's circumstances. More about this later in the chapter, but as a preview: there was no telling how long the treatment would take, no timesaving shortcuts were taken—this was not a kind of strava that professionals underwent during their lunch breaks, as in some practices in Tuzla city—nor were other quotidian events suspended at the expense of therapy. Rather, Zejneba would interrupt strava at the sound of muezzin's *ezan* (from Arabic *adhan*) and would withdraw to pray. She paused to attend to her cow and calf, or to her son's goats, as well as to let the chickens out of the coop. She could walk out to water the vegetables in the garden before the sun rose too high, to feed wood to the stove, where at once she cooked therapeutic implements and our breakfast or lunch, served with a bread she kneaded with her long, gnarled fingers—caramel-crusted, though soft and substantial to the core. If I were to call her treatment a "ritual," the word might trap us in the allure of an extraordinary technique, which primarily strives for effects and meanings that transcend the concreteness and plainness of its tools, whose relevance resides precisely outside their placement in the world.

And yet to speak of Zejneba's craft as "technology" would translate strava too hastily to a more palatable idiom—contemporary and transposable, conveniently bland. Technology, for all the great mileage it gained in social thought since the term's popularization beyond the studies of science and technology would water down the distinctiveness of a curing craft that mobilizes Koranic recitations, and wishful dove (from Arabic *du'a*, supplication). It is more appropriate to describe her strava practice as a curative craft, a technique that is attentive to ingredients as with medicinal cooking, especially if the recipe is secret or committed to memory after numerous trials, and open to improvisations, well attuned to the contingency of this here and now.

Dove were taught to Zejneba by voices she calls friends but otherwise does not name and who too seem to be participant-observers in a way that puts the ethnographer in the room in her relative place of importance: not the only one with notebook in hand, eyes wide open, ears peeled, forever inscribing. The nonhuman scribes, watching over Zejneba's shoulder and from all corners of her home practice, rehearse the grave lessons in acting and record-keeping. What Zejneba remembered (*zikr*, Turkism, from Persian *zikr*, Arabic *dhikr*, remembrance of Allah) and reproduced in a reverent whisper, she drew from revealed knowledge in the local tradition of everyday Islam—as a submission or a receptiveness to the Truth, the Visible and the Invisible, Transcendent and Immanent, Near and Ascendant (Koran, Sura Al-Hadid). But her healing was also framed by a well-practiced wisdom that births bless-ings and responsibilities, that gives insight and presumes inwardness: Zejneba lived in seclusion and can count the number of times she went down the asphalt road into the provincial town, let alone to the iconic site of economic mingling and being social: the marketplace. Yet, in her domestic dwelling and at her preoccupied hands, there issue intense exchanges—transformative and wide-ranging, connecting her, as much as she would like to disconnect, to patients from afar as well as to varied things, fibrous or fine, historical and commercial, vegetal, mineral, and elemental.

Far from the marketplace, strava is inseparable from an economy, which connects singular encounters with a field of expectations, broader than the market and inclusive beyond humans. *Real* was Zejneba's dis-position toward the therapeutic exchange. In the vernacular health refer-ences, women who practice strava are held to especially high standards when it comes to the popular precept that healing has no set price but that gifts are due. As I will show, nene who are actually practicing have adopted a range of tactics to get by or get around this requirement for a generous practice, some of them doing quite well and others barely mak-ing ends meet and complaining bitterly about it. Zejneba refuses gifts with a stubbornness that impresses some patients, endears her to others who search for ways of giving anonymously, sending care packages in parcels with no return address, or caring in turn, including washing dishes or helping around the house. She panics at the sight of a cigarette carton that I bring to her on my second visit—it is customary to bring a little gift when visiting homes in Bosnia—and, since I insist tactlessly, she gives in only to distribute it among her patients before I leave.

"POURING OUT FEARS": A PREVIEW

This chapter circles around the ideal figure of a healer and Zejneba's bony, bent frame that earnestly carried the weight of such expectations. From the premises of her home the chapter ventures a broad exploration of the hugely popular traditional practice of strava that involves patient bodies in contact with the therapist and therapeutic devices, always at a slight distance. Following hectic, circuitous searches for the cure described previously, this chapter arrives at some particular therapeutic encounters to look at how cures and bodies are composed, how they touch, and seeing which tactile economies they affect or suggest. My ambition is to describe the therapeutics of touching while speculating about the metaphysics of contact that underlie it. To get there, however, I will briefly attend to some gritty historical details to show what makes folk commonsense and expertise not only resilient despite many anticipations of strava's vanishing, but also popular and indispensable since the 1990s war and peace. Next, I will shift attention to strava's concrete implements—devices, things, elements—that are integral to the process that translates, literally, to mean an act of "pouring out (*izljevanje, saljevanje, salit'*) of fears (*strava*, a great fear, a fright, a horror)." Thinking of some recent considerations granted to things and nonhumans more generally, I wonder about influences, agencies, and efficacies that make up the therapeutics of touching. However, from the grounds of home practices, I argue that it takes insights of both ontology and of phenomenology to appreciate the sensuousness and effectiveness of the medical touching experience, even when touching primarily lays hands at a distance. Finally, it is a more speculative mood that is in order, I propose after the return visit to Zejneba's, if we want to move from the therapeutics of touching to contemplation about its underlying possibilities. Most importantly, this section shows how irreducibly particular and local (though only provisionally local to the extent that it is also Islamic) the field of metaphysics seems, if we attend to contact from an ethnographer's vantage point at nena Zejneba's veranda.

In short, let me introduce three areas of concern in this chapter: the gritty or historical, the concrete or therapeutic, and the speculative or metaphysical. I will speak to each briefly, before I return to the mode of an ethnographic narrative.

STRAVA: THE GRITTY AND THE HISTORICAL

Three principles of strava are consistently cited in present-day practice as well as in earlier ethnological records: it cures all illnesses (*liječi sve*), it is for everyone (*za svakog*), and it has no price (*nema cijene*).

Strava cures everything—liječi sve: Patients and therapists insist that strava treats all disorders, though they seem to seek a strava therapist for complaints about nerves (*živci*) and nervousness (*nervoza*); excessive or obsessive worry in general or about something in particular (*sikirancija, nasikirati se*); stress, a trauma, or a phobia; great sadness or anger; or apathy. Symptoms include excessive crying—especially for no obvious reason—irritability, restlessness, apprehension, panic, fretting, insomnia, lack of focus, loss of weight and appetite, forgetfulness, and apathy. These symptoms are otherwise managed with various herbal remedies (*odoljen*—valerian root, *majčina dušica*—thyme, *limunček* or *matičnjak*—melissa, as well as with black cumin oil); with home-fermented foods and probiotics; and with pharmaceuticals, anxiolytics, and antidepressants. It is only when the ordinary tactics finally fail or when particular accidents, uncanny events, and life trials make symptoms insufferable or make patients intolerable to family and friends, that one looks for a strava woman who is "for real." As one nena, Fadila, puts it—I will step into her practice, shortly—you turn to strava "when you are worried sick, worried sick, worried sick, today, tomorrow, and then it all kicks in." A few people doubt that anxiolytics help: they are widely prescribed, purchased over the counter, relatively inexpensive, and readily offered by kin, friends, colleagues, or anyone else concerned with one who is upset.[1] Famous brands are iconic for the world gone mad and in need of tranquilization (see chapters 2 and 4). Antidepressants were just gaining wider prescription in 2006–2007, although strava therapists were well-versed in the available brands. But strava points to the limitations of pharmaceutical short-term efficacy and long-lasting side effects, while articulating an alternative therapeutic proposition: a treatment that claims to alter subjects' dispositions, lastingly or through a periodic management plan, without unanticipated side effects. Significantly, many practitioners ask patients to discontinue the use of antidepressants during treatment and proudly cite cases of recovery to the point where drugs were no longer needed. Anxiolytics, by contrast, seem to be irreplaceable even if strava and alternative medicine more generally curbs their consumption to needs-based. Moreover, it is because strava etiology presumes that serious worry or a sudden fright variously affects the entire body, causing lesions and dysfunctions in internal organs as much as a strain in affective relations with the self and others, that this folk practice, and those who subscribe to it, effectively critique the clinical and psycho-pharmaceutical interventions. The following pages will attend to particular treatments to show how strava not only does not differentiate among affective, digestive, and accounting habits, between skin and relational inclinations, but engrosses a singular, biographical person and a "psyche" (*psiha*) in consequential relations to the point where each bodily person is potentially and inconveniently extended into the space of collective affairs.

Furthermore, the claim that strava cures everything, I suggest, is at once a part of its historical legacy and a new concept. Put simply, the objects of strava intervention—contingent bodily lives—have transformed historically and especially so in the brief span of several dramatic decades since the 1990s, and strava has been particularly apt in keeping abreast of the new forms of carnal responsiveness by repurposing the traditional repertoire of treatment techniques and theories about being in illness and health. Late nineteenth-century records associate strava with fright, mostly children's. A Sharia judge from central Bosnia describes visible signs of fright: "[A child] looks like it emerged from the underground, it grows as pale as a piece of white cloth, its body dries up, its eyes fall deep into the sockets, et cetera" (Ugljen 1893:168). Left untreated, strava may cause other illnesses to "latch onto it"; it may come into effect only in the adulthood, and may lead to death, Ugljen writes (ibid). Unlike other contributors to the Bosnian ethnological journals of the time, his article does not assume rationalist or medical-scientific distance from the reported folk beliefs. Rather, strava, in Ugljen's words, is "an excellent remedy" for illness which cannot be cured with the contemporary pharmaceuticals. A few and brief textual references to strava during socialist Yugoslavia assume that it has vanished together with other superstitions of the symbolically rich Slavic peasant past (see Vlahović 1972 and Radenković 1996) while a classic 1980s village ethnography by Tone Bringa (1995) catalogues strava in the rubric of "faith healing" that seems an obvious fit. The rubric, however, seems to overdetermine strava's translation: while her interlocutors speak of using strava for excessive or event-specific worrying (*nasikirati se*), Bringa emphasizes the uncanny causes of fear, such as "spirits" intrusion (177–178; see also Jašarević 2012b). Strava was practiced throughout socialism in relative secrecy though with less frequency, partly because clinical medicine authoritatively defined illness and wellness and denounced folk-healing traditions as backward and embarrassing. When in the 1980s Yugoslav socialist comforts were compromised by recurrent financial crises and IMF-imposed austerities, anxiety was medicated and the popular piece of mind was tended to with a perfectly coincidental launch of a local benzodiazepam, Apaurin, the anti-anxiolytic that reigned supreme in the local psycho-pharmaceutical universe until it was challenged, in the late 1990s, by competitors: Lexaurin and Bosaurin. As I argued in previous chapters, the authority of biomedical and pharmaceutical profession lost the prominence it enjoyed, although medical consultations and the traffic of prescription medicine have never been more lively. Strava therapists have their own theory about this: "Before the war, there weren't these many ailments. It was not like now. People have become too sensitive [*preosjetljivi*]," explains Fadila, and I also heard the point more broadly aired by strava therapists.

Strava is for everyone—za svakog. Patients and therapists often rehearsed this precept for me: strava treats anyone, no matter what their religious disposition or ethnic or class affiliation, and regardless of whether they believe or doubt. Whereas nene begin practicing strava with a Bismillah and recite Koranic suras, at their hands are people of different confessions, with firm or casual ethno-national commitments, as well as people skeptical of religions in general and doubtful about the grandmas' craft but undergoing the treatment anyhow, either under the pressure of concerned familiars or because they were sufficiently frustrated with the condition that they would try anything, just in case it worked. Given how polarized the religious issues and ethno-national identities are in the region, and given the sheer advertisement that various cases of ethnic "mixing," "reconciliation," and "cohabitation" receive from professional as well as academic enthusiasts—the enthusiasm which always also proceeds with a sort of political ambition (to demonstrate age-old interethnic friendships, to find kernels of cosmopolitan secularism, or else to show how the inherent logic of some rational or social instrument or space, such as a market, promotes ex-

changes across and despite the divides) and then invites critical or skeptical reevaluations (to prove age-old hatreds, to find, rather, sectarian
communitarianism)—I am weary of placing too much emphasis on the
open and inviting quality of strava. This is especially because encounters
in strava across embodied, practiced lines of difference take place with
a certain ease that keeps ethnic issues tangential, as people gathered attend to health, broadly speaking. It is important to mention, with equal
light-handedness, that strava, much like other forms of folk medicine,
has a long history of patient pluralism. Contributors to *Bosanska Vila*
(Bosnian fairy), a belle-lettres publication for "entertainment, education, and literature," and *Glasnik* (Herald), the journal of the National
Museum of Bosnia, have described how in the late nineteenth and early
twentieth centuries magic and medicine were shared by or used across
the three confessional communities that the Austro-Hungarian imperial administration inherited from the Ottoman Empire. While strava
was evidently practiced by all three groups (Truhelka 1889; Glück 1890),
one article describes an Eastern Orthodox mother who took her ill son
to an old "Turk"[2] woman with the reputation for the best and cheapest
strava healing (Kovačević 1888:16–7). The author, an Eastern Orthodox priest, makes nothing of the irreverence of the woman who, having
found little relief for her son's condition in a priest's healing prayer, seeks
out a "magical ritual" at the hands of a Muslim woman. The matter-
of-fact tone suggests that irreligious or syncretistic pragmatism was
fairly common, although not everyone approved of the trend. In the
1860s, local Catholic clergy corresponded on the subject of blasphemous
people who not only turned Catholicism into spiritual medicine but
also readily consulted Eastern Orthodox priests and Muslim imams
(see Fabijanić 2004:42–43, 73; Jašarević 2012a). In citing these historical sources briefly, my point is that pragmatism has probably always
accompanied popular medical practice but also that medical concerns
reorder the formal matter of priorities. Everyone quoted the precept not
to showcase ethnic mixing or tolerance—although it may be tempting
to do so at least for the sake of an American-trained ethnographer who
may be taking note—but to advertise the broader claim to efficacy:
strava is oriented to all bodies, bodies that are universally responsive,
rather than essentially defined in ethno-religious terms and beliefs.

Strava has no price—nema cijene. "Everyone knows" that. Ideally, strava is free of charge both because the gift of restored health is priceless and because what nena practices is multiply a gift—she puts to use her skills caringly, empathetically, skills that were not hers proper but bestowed upon her variously, inherited within family, gifted by a strava therapist at deathbed or from beyond death (*ahiret*, Bosnian Arabism), taught on or impressed by presences less than tangible, but perceptible, notable, unforgettable. The expectations guiding a strava encounter are that a patient may give or withhold a gift of money or goods and that the therapist will never ask for it, and, if given money, will either avoid touching it or, as I more often observed, with bills in hand, will interconnect the gift with the patient's body and her own person, with the elements—air and ground, in particular—issuing wishful supplications in the Islamic tradition of dove that emphasizes links between generosity (*sadaka*), a merit-making act or gift (*sevap*), wealth, sustenance or good fortune (*nafaka*), while all along asking for forgiveness (*halali*). Yet, the patient will always ask "how much do I owe" (*kol'ko sam dužan* or *dužna* [feminine, masculine. sg.]), because it is only proper to offer to pay, and because therapeutic efficacy may just hinge on it. You ought to give something, it is said, "for the sake of the hand," as if to further charge its curative potencies by giving money that, significantly, is not a payment (nena asks for none) but a gift. The entire therapeutic economy, the way I see it now, works by constant advancements of gifts, which are also debts, and debts, which are generous and caring and thus gift-like. It is not accidental, I propose, that strava therapeutic give-and-take resonates with the rest of the informal debt economy that I described in the preceding chapters. Later I will discuss how strava presumes and promotes barely a human gift—not least because few people can live up to these expectations and many do not try to—and more than a human accountancy.

TOUCHING: THE CONCRETE AND THE THERAPEUTIC

Strava works with a few basic implements—water, lead, fire, Koranic suras and Islamic wishes, dove—whose effective assemblage hinges on therapists' skilled hands, since, I am told, "not anyone can do strava." The list of items in strava runs beyond the essentials, however, to include, for instance: red cloth (veiling the patient at each lead pouring); Muslim prayer beads (*tespih*, an Arabism); "little towels," controversial inventions of one practicing nena selling for no more than 15 KM (about 9 USD in 2007) to forward strava's remedial action; personal clothing items (and shirts and underwear in particular) of absent patients on whose behalf therapy is sometimes organized; recycled plastic bottles of soft drinks, Coke very often, which bottle up the strava-treated water for use between the subsequent sessions; wood for the stove, sometimes coal; air, which is animate and animated in the course of the treatment that consumes it in fire, transforms it into smoke, and is the medium of breath, which patients are instructed when and how to take, when and where to exhale loudly, and which also escapes in irrepressible sounds of hissing and sighing that molten lead and shaken patents make, almost in tow with each other. In Zejneba's practice, the repertoire is richer still as, depending on the case, it may include iron nails, boiled in an enormous cauldron (such as are used by serious makers of homemade jams and *pekmez*, a medicinal fruit syrup); living water (*živu vodu*) collected from at least three different springs; stems of forest ivy and other herbs.

How do we make sense of these lists as a pharmacopeia of a medical practice rather than simply a strange stock of ritual or symbolic action that aptly expresses or resignifies social conflicts—strife in familiar relations, social disorder, existential precarity—in individual bodily symptoms. The latter was a fashionable analytical gesture in the older anthropology of healing that described in colorful detail native rituals, while avoiding the problems of their truth claims with references to internal logics of concealed meanings, expressive symbols, beliefs, or collective experience (Boddy 1989; Turner 1968; Danforth 1989). Those analytical adventures were written largely prior to the critical examinations of foundational distinctions between knowledge and belief (Good 1994; Lock and Gordon 1988), before anthropologies of medicine and sorcery estranged Western bodies somewhat, from Japan to North America to France (Lock 1993; Favret-Saada 1980), before anthropologists recovered the question of magic in relation to local epistemologies of power and oral archives of colonial history (Wiener 1995), and before inquiries into enigmatic and repressed illnesses and disabilities poked at the confidence about what might be active and how our bodies might register alien animacies, whether or not we can officially diagnose or know them (Chen 2012; Alaimo 2010; Steingraber 2010). Finally, this line of inquiry existed prior to Latour's major campaign to rethink whether we have ever been modern and what the implications are of trying, as well as allied efforts in and outside the social studies of science and technology to reinvestigate what acts and what matters in more generous terms, which is to say with an equal curiosity about all knowledge claims (Latour 1993, 2005; Langwick 2011). In short, to treat all kinds of seemingly strange things as *materia medica*, as active ingredients whose potencies can be neither ruled out by a reference to an external source of authority (say FDA's Orange Book of approved drugs and their therapeutic evaluations) nor known in advance of their coming together in particular encounters, would be to join the good company of contemporary thinkers of things. A growing number of scholars from across disciplines are interested in how thingly and nonhuman doings compose material and political reality, including human bodies and affairs (see Braun and Whatmore 2010; Morton 2013; Daston 1999).

Join I will, except that I do so with a small hesitation about this otherwise inspiring conceptual possibility, which comes from a few of its integral commitments that I will bundle here together, although they come in different analytical intonations and by no means constrain too tightly all the varied scholarly voices speaking of things. First, we have a commitment to "ontological flatness," whereby all action is potentially of equal weight and all agents, big or small, may act with equally weighty consequences. Closely related is the proposal that what power there is, inheres entirely in the things rather than draws from some greater, constitutive forces (say capital, nature, or institution). Second, we have a commitment to either full ontological presence, without a remainder that may be occluded potentially or yet to come, fermenting below the surface, commitment that is most obvious in Latour's writings (see Harman 2009). Or else, a preference for continuous emergence (Connolly 2010), becoming without there ever being a presence (Bennett and Connolly 2012; Pickering 2003). In both cases, the implication is that whatever is and may happen is entirely contingent on the given encounter; no matter the ingredients, the results cannot be ensured or known in advance. Third, is a commitment to a horizontal vision of a human–nonhuman collective, which may not quite allow local knowledges—especially when these travel with strong metaphysics not of the palatable (animist) kind, as I will suggest below—to suggest a thingly order that is otherwise. Finally, we have a commitment to decentering human, which is sometimes achieved by default (once action is democratized, there is no privileged actant with which to enter the story), sometimes pursued with great effort to downplay the relevance of human experience, thought, and intention (Braun and Whatmore 2010; Halberstam and Livingston 1999). This is by now a common set of complaints (see Ihde 2003) and I do not wish to revisit the disputing sides for the sake of the argument but rather to suggest another way—myopically focused on strava—to expand our lexicons of matter and *Materia medica* in particular. To begin with, an adequate understanding of strava, as I see it, must consider how touching, the material act and the experiential fact, arranges, upturns, and stirs up the matters in therapy.

The space of therapy is tight—usually the size of the healer's living room, kitchen, or spare room—and the course of the treatment is shared by those undergoing it, their company, and others patients and their escorts, waiting their turn. Patients' troubles and fears are revealed by and by; everyone observing is taking part by default and so is somewhat exposed. At the very least, each health history offers great opportunity for others to comment, to compare notes, to advance recommendations, or to become more anxious about the general state of health, wealth, and the world. The time it takes for the lead to melt in the fire for the next pouring is also a time to chat. Waiting in strava generates close and concerned, though intermittent, communities: they empathetically share the sense of how a list of common health-related complaints in Bosnia must feel and they rehearse this affective catalogue and leaf through it viscerally, while recharging its historical relevance. Put simply, by sitting tightly next to each other in therapy, people are already touching across the close distance, in so far as touching is moving, pressing, stirring, at least as much as it is about fingers and epidermal follicles crisscrossing skins.

That touching gropes for and inevitably fails to grasp a body, one's own as much as anyone else's, is an insight that I take from Jean-Luc Nancy's post-foundational phenomenology, which I often read across Derrida's shoulder (see the introduction and chapter 3). It is because touching only ever skirts the skin of things, that all touching is superficial, but profoundly so insofar as Nancy doesn't presume that pressing skin-to-skin misses the fleshiness of substantial identity, withdrawn someplace deep below but that with the slightest pressure, the singularity of a composite being spaces out fully: neither here beneath my fingers nor there, in the gut, but is disseminated, inappropriable, most intensely alive, and well in evasions. For the purposes of this chapter, Nancy's most important insight has to do with the proposition that touching always plays up the tangible and the intangible—fingers and sense, the embodied person present but only elusively so (see chapter 3)—and that both are extended into the space. Once we start thinking with Nancy about the extensity of sensing, of feeling, of thinking, wishing, or writing, distance is no longer an obstacle to effective contact. Quite on the contrary. Strava, as I will describe shortly, proceeds with an initial series of contacts between therapist and the patient whereby the therapist connects their bodies to lead, to ground, to water with fingers running along, washing, stroking, knocking, circling, and by finer means of breath, reciting and blowing Koranic suras and *duas.* The rest of the therapy proceeds with the therapist, objects, and elements at a slight distance from the patient body, which comes again in contact with strava-treated water only later, after the treatment.

As I will show in the course of this chapter, Nancy's ideas of inviolable singularities get us only so far, caught up as they are in the fine acts of evading communitarian politics as much as substantial agendas or too clinging attachments. Singularities do not guide us well through the local worlds of intrusive intimacies, pernicious interventions, and etiologies that, for instance, do not keep one man's drinking binges so neatly apart from his wife's intestinal discomforts. Given that therapy is often put to work across still greater distances, on behalf of people who are absent but whose presence is rendered contiguous with the help of things that were or are intended for them, we must stretch Nancy's thought to think uncomfortable, potentially insufferable closeness between bodies and things, and one that is potentially achieved secretly, suspected, partly known. In short, I aim to add some discomfiting considerations to Nancy's thought on touching at a distance.

CONTACT: THE SPECULATIVE AND THE METAPHYSICAL

Nancy, who has been mostly indifferent to things and their ways of touching, has been in the habit of sneaking in metaphysical propositions; long before such speculative ventures turned up in a variety of guises from speculative realisms to vitalisms to new metaphysics (see Niemoczynski 2013; Kohn 2015; Stengers 2011; Bennett and Connolly 2012). His works on touching are related to an ongoing project of deconstructing, and then dis-enclosing Christian metaphysics (see chapter 6), starting with the idea of the Savior's body, resurrected and otherwise curatively and miraculously charged, not least in the host (2008b). Moreover, his pursuits of intangible extension have always been close to what is other to the rational thought: gazes and dreams, psyche and soul (2008a; 2009). Still, Nancy's thought will be at a loss for what to do with particularly local expectations of what passes in touching and what things, agents, and powers are there prior to touching, arranged how and changeable to what extent.

The limitations of Western philosophy have long been obvious to the anthropologists who attended to all sorts of contacts beyond Euro-American, Judeo-Christian commonsense. This started with Mauss's seminal *General Theory of Magic* ([1902] 2001), which rereads older classics while surveying magical propositions worldwide that are "quite outside our adult European understanding" (132). To admit existence to the idea of magic, as a field of experience and a "gigantic variation on the theme of . . . causality" (78), Mauss investigates the "non-intellectualist psychology of a man as a community" (133) and issues a field guide on how to study universal sympathies, which are at once magical and social, experiential and material. Ethnographies have since preferred less universalizing accounts of contact, not as overdetermined or reliably contagious but rather as connections that need be achieved, courted, and cultivated. The questions of underlying sympathies, by contrast, have been rather unpopular. What I shall do in the following pages is explore with strava the possibilities that each of these fields of inquiry and theoretical disposition offers—historical, phenomenological, and speculative—while at the same time arriving at strong, local speculations about prior sympathies and underlying actualities, whose configurations may be below the threshold of experience but may also manifest concretely and sensuously, discerned by expert eyes and hands, and mobilized, supplicated, synthesized, exercised to a point.

FADILA'S STRAVA: THERE ARE ALL KINDS OF US HERE

"Selam." I wish hesitantly at Fadila's door, thinking the greeting will please her. After all, Fadila wears a hijab (or, in the local terms, she is *pokrivena*, "covered," "veiled," or else a *bula*, a Turkism) and is a Hajj pilgrim, so an Islamic greeting is proper, although in 2006 greetings are still so caught-up in the political acts that it is hard to offer the more formal Bosnian transliteration of the greeting in Arabic, *selam alejkum*, or *assalamu alejkum*, without being heard as asserting or recognizing an ethnic identity, especially in the ethnically mixed context of Tuzla where many are proud of the city's stated indifference to the formal differences. *Selam* seems safer and being still fresh in the field, trying hard not to offend, I settle for that greeting. Especially since I only just met Fadila the day before, following a recommendation of her former patient, when I explained myself and asked whether I could observe her practice a form of therapy whose tremendous popularity in northeastern Bosnia I was just beginning to grasp in the spring of 2006. "Selam," Fadila replies, "but not only selam [is due]. There are all kinds of us here," she responds, gesturing across the room. Seated there in the tight quarters of Fadila's living room are two radiant young women, Jasmina and Tanja, friends from the local university, stressed out about exams, which is, partly, why there were here, seeking strava. Seated on the stool closest to the wood-burning stove is a visibly preoccupied middle-aged woman, Ana, whose hands are scrunched up in her lap, her shoulders slumping. She was in the middle of the treatment when I stepped in. The women's names and biographical details, which I will learn in the course of our afternoon at Fadila's, associate each with one of the three dominant religious and ethno-national communities in Bosnia, but I will not employ my index finger in the writerly exercise of pointing out who is who. Writing out the difference bluntly may be too similar to identifying and separating by other means. Besides, fixing the names to ethnic communities would give a false impression that the women's communal affiliations and dispositions are thus made more precise. It could even make some of the strava proceedings that I describe below seem overtly political, whereas everyone in the strava has mostly therapeutic agendas.

Fadila is tiny. Her buoyant, hilarious ways of speaking and moving, however, reverberate about her, all the way to the rippling of the traditional skirt-pants (*dimije*) she wears, whose extensive fabric holds together in restless folds, and in the bobbing of tiny flower bulbs crocheted along the edge of the gauze-thin scarf that frames her face. While Ana is waiting for the medicinal lead—scooped in a soup ladle dipped into flames—to melt, Fadila is preparing Tanja for treatment. Resting a piece of lead in the young woman's lap, she whispers Koranic suras and *ayas* to it, for a while, finishing with a loud blowing. At Fadila's urging, Tanja makes a silent wish and blows three times onto the chunk of lead in the nena's hand. Rising to her feet, Fadila next moves the piece of lead from Tanja's right shoulder to the left, touching each lightly while encircling her head; she swivels it around the young woman's arms extended away from her chest, hands clasping elbows. She does this three times. After each circle she gently taps the lead to the leg of the wooden table. Reciting almost inaudibly, she touches the lead to Tanja's knees, runs it clockwise through the air to Tanja's feet and back, three times, knocking the lead to the ground after each cycle. Lead begins each movement with a light touch of the nena's fingertips to some point on the patient body and travels, swooshing at a slight distance from the person, away to the next point and back to the beginning. Fadila pauses at length at Tanja's toes, whispering, then touches the ground and blows noisily into the chunk of lead cupped in her hand.

Back at Ana's side, Fadila veils the patient's entire figure in red cloth. Ana sighs. "Don't be afraid, Ana, I'm taking a good care of you," Fadila says cheerfully, soothingly. Drawing a bowl of water to a slight distance from Ana's knees, she pours the entire ladle of molten lead into it. When the lead touches the cool water, it sizzles, and sinking to the bottom, it alters its quickened form back into leaden, giving out a trace of squiggly smoke. Ana uncovers herself hastily to listen to the reading which is expected to be at once diagnostic and prognostic, an update on the course of treatment and a statement on the rest of the patient's life: how things are and what might come. Fadila fishes out the lead from the bowl, shiny and still warm, to read the good news: "Here, the whole strava turned up a gain (*dobitak*), an incoming of nafaka (fortune, subsistence, gain). Your wish will come true. The worrying (sikirancija) has left you; a great burden has been lifted. You've been carrying it in you." Dropping the lead back into the soup ladle and back into the fire, Fadila says to the rest of us: "A doctor is an expert, no doubt about that. I believe in doctors. But they can't do what I can do. There is much that they can do—they can perform surgery or such—but for these kinds of troubles, for the stress, disquiet, and restlessness, they can do nothing. They can only issue medicine, Lexaurin, and they are killing you with those, they are only killing the nerves." The speech was not only rehearsed for the sake of the ethnographer, for I have since heard many articulations of it by parties involved with strava, long after my strange presence was domesticated. Nor was Fadila's appreciation of clinical medicine mere lip service. Still recovering from a complicated back injury she sustained during the war when a shell attack from the surrounding hills caught her on the streets of Tuzla and, as of lately, investigating persistent migraines with brain imaging technology and trying to control recurrent urinary infections, she was a frequent visitor to the regional clinic and public health center. She also listed a number of medical professionals among those whom she remembered with gifts from Kaba; these were significant tokens of friendship.

Fadila resumes preparations for Tanja's treatment. Now it's a bowl of water perched on the girl's knees, while Fadila pours over it, reciting quietly from the Koran. Everyone in the room observes silence. Fadila takes her time. Later, I will learn that her recitations of Koranic suras, ayas, and Islamic duas are carefully selected, especially after the first diagnostic pouring. Each curative item is specific to the complaints and causes in strava nosology: for sadness and for worry, for *sihir* and for *urok*. Koran's curative potency is here as taken for granted as it is occluded. It is the medium of Fadila's body that extends it onto the water, her lips moving, her breath rising and falling—and yet her whispering veils the source of power she yields. She blows onto the water, scoops some into an ornate silver cup, and offers it to the girl. Similarly, it is because strava foregrounds as therapeutic implements lead, fire, and the nena's figure, no one regards Tanja's drinking as an act of drinking up a dematerialized Koran: voiced, whispered, breathed, and infused. *Strava is for everyone.*

There is much that is tacit about this claim about strava's indiscriminate accessibility and efficacy, tacit but not secretive. Everyone knows the source of the power that the nena's craft supplicates, but strava proceeds with an ongoing, coordinated understatement, especially compared to other kinds of practitioners of Islamic medicine, and imams in particular, who also heal people across the board. The universal claims about the curative power of Koran and its divine origins are dressed down in the guises of a folk craft but, nonetheless, Koran engenders the effective connections between the therapist's hands and patients' bodies. Thinking agentive capacities horizontally will cause one to miss this prior arrangement of forces and ultimacies that are integral to people's quests for competent therapeutic responses, although the play of contingencies is still possible and expected: patients will tell you that it takes a precise coincidence between the therapist's talents and the ailing body for curing to take place. Nonetheless, it is because the therapy hinges on connections that the therapist works out beyond the patient in question, that potency flows regardless of the humans present or involved: Fadila will later explain to me that strava works because "you bring patients, their names, in connection with the mention of Allah, the Most Merciful, and with Mohammed, peace be upon him." Moreover, the strava therapist uses suras and duas that address *sihr*, the sorcerer who made it (*sihribaz*), the person who has contracted it against the patient, and the nonhumans, jinni, who are carrying out the sihir's design. In Fadila's words: "It helps. It clears out the brain and it cleanses all sorts of stuff in the body. It annuls sihire in the blood, in the organism. You achieve all that, with duas, all down to the roots."

Fadila's hand brushes across Tanja's throat, chest, belly, and knees, and she says: "what beauties came to me today! Thank you for the trust you placed in me, thank you for coming. And someone gave you my phone number?" Tanja explains that the referral came from a fellow student, Fadila's ex-patient. They got lost in Fadila's neighborhood but a man pointed them to her house. Fadila is pleased and boasts, "Yes, people know about me. There isn't a corner of Tuzla city from which people didn't visit. And they didn't come for nothing, I helped them." Fadila now tends to Ana for the seventh and last pouring, at the woman's feet. This time, lead bursts noisily and we hear Ana panic beneath the red cloth. Fadila comforts her: "Uncover yourself, Ana, you ought to sigh out, breathe out, deeply. Look how beautiful your strava is. What weakness you felt! It was there, it no longer is. There are fewer needles." Solidified lead can take many shapes and textures: sometimes it turns green and mossy to the touch, other times it is smooth and flawlessly round, and on occasion bits of it shoot out, thin and elongated like sewing needles. Fadila: "Your strava came out, finally. For days it was terrible to look at. [Addressing us:] This woman is a poor dear, she has been crying her heart out for a long time. Widowed at twenty-eight, she never remarried for the sake of her sons. [Jasmina: "That takes strength!" Tanja: "That takes sacrifice!"] But her sons have not treated her well: they've forgotten her. One son is in America." "My dear woman," she addressees Ana, "you've almost lost your mind. But look, you've thrown it all off. Look at God's gift! It's coming—a great support for you is on its way." Ana: "It's a wonder I stayed alive." Fadila sympathizes, "It is, it is," while bottling the water from Ana's treatment and handing it to her with instructions to add it to her bath but to make sure it does not go down the sewer. Ana knows this; she is nodding, taking her leave, wishing us good luck. Fadila walks her outside.

Back in the room, Fadila seats Tanja on the stool and pours lead near her veiled head. The explosion is modest. Our attention hooks to the strava held in Fadila's hand, as we listen to her reading: "You've gotten yourself worried sick! Here you have some disquiet, restlessness. You have urok [singular, *uroci* in the plural: disorders brought about by too desirous a look, or by active envy], this green stuff, that's what it is. You are full of some fear, nervousness, unrest."

The rest of the session continues in much the same vein as the previous one; while pouring out Tanja's fears, Fadila is preparing the other patient for treatment. Both are instructed to return for two more visits and are sent off with bottled strava water to add to their bath. On the way out, the patients inquire whether they should pay all at once; Fadila replies that "people usually pay little by little, after every treatment. I will not tell you how much, but however much you can, you decide." Each girl gives her 10 KM (around 6 USD in 1997) and Fadila takes the bills, saying "Let my nafaka be good for you." Whispering prayers, she orbits the bill around the giver's head, starting from one shoulder and finishing at the other, circling it around the girl's body, knees, and touching the toes. She thus enacts and vocalizes the expectations in the exchange that ends strava: it is not a payment but a gift that generates income for the therapist and, since the giver is generous and kind, the gift generates in turn an income of sadaka (mercy, merit) for the patient. It takes sadaka for one to recover or to be well, which is why strava nene may ask patients to exercise generosity outside the grounds of the practice: to feed the birds or the fish, to give clothing to orphans, to contribute to local *turbe*.[3]

The friends return the following day and report feeling relief and sleeping better. They are soon joined by a mother and a daughter and the healing sessions draws out, intertwining ritual with casual talk about the women's lives, health problems, and previous treatments. The mother and the daughter, it turns out, have tried another, quite famous therapist, Mevlija, but left her, disappointed. "That one" Fadila says, "is lying." She then proceeds to tell stories about Mevlija: how she employs an assistant who does not know what she is doing, refers patients to a healer imam, her husband ("but he is a fake!" Fadila protests), runs a side-business that includes a restaurant and a bar, keeps a price list of strava services posted at her door, and otherwise is into making money. The mother nods: "Money is a whore."

MEVLIJA'S STRAVA: MOSTLY PSYCHOLOGY

"What is it that you do?" I asked the strava healer Mevlija once. "Mostly psychology," she replied. This confident answer, coming from a grandma who heals by the hearth, some days enveloped in an oversized, stained doctor's white coat, can be seen as amusing: a vernacular joke or a healer's mimetic aspiration for professional authority. But the response could be read more generously, still, especially considering that Mevlija was dead serious and so sure of herself—after all, thousands of people have searched for her to help, have knocked on the doors of the house perched on top of a steep, winding hill in a southern suburb of Tuzla city, among them medical professionals. Like strava healers more gener-ally, Mevlija takes it for granted that she and clinical psychologists and psychiatrists share interest in a host of complaints related to nerves, stress and worry, to fraught perception and poor concentration, and in disorders related to emotional and social relations, mood disorders, and suicidal tendencies, to habits of sleeping, eating, crying. The idea of *psiha* in the Bosnian, Serbian, and Croatian languages has had as promiscuous a popular career outside the professional medical references as the psyche has had in the English-speaking world, except that in Bosnia, psychology and psychiatry are not "stalking" popular imagination nor prescribing psycho-pharmaceuticals nearly as much as in, say, North America (Hacking 1995; Healy 2002; Medawar and Hardon 2004), nor do they exercise as much influence in the shaping of patient subjectivities. The medical rubric of *duševne bolesti*, in particular, carries a surplus of signification that translates the composite psiha (mind, ego, and id/the unconscious, soul) into the language of *duša* (soul): literally, "soul illnesses" (see also chapter 6). Strava intervenes in such a composite, expansive domain of being, relating, ailing, and feeling, showing, in the process, the soul as carnal, thoroughly intertwined with the body, with existential and historical circumstances, while, nonetheless, aspiring to and thriving on finer connections.

Mevlija is the healer who was criticized at Fadila's for treating strava like a business enterprise. A striking presence, at eighty-four Mevlija projects tough, bony vitality. Never ill, never moody, tired, or stressed, she seems to live off coffee and cigarettes and thrives on being involved with people's health needs and living affairs. Her long, clever face bears an expression of amusement, as if suspending a private joke on the tip of her tongue. She wears gorgeous golden hoops, dangling from her soft earlobes. In violet satin dimije, flowering around her, gracefully elastic, she squats by the wood stove chain-smoking, resting a busy cell phone in a nearby bucket of coal. In healing, Mevlija exercises keen interest in the physicality of her patients' disorders, as in this brief exchange with Kata, a woman in her late fifties. Mevlija performs the first pouring of the day with a Bismillah, while Kata takes the cue to cross herself before being veiled by a deep red cloak. It all happens quickly: lead pours out, Kada uncovers her face, Mevlija grasps the chunk of lead to read: "My dear Kata, strava grasped your stomach and your chest." "It's true. I have great discomfort in my stomach. I feel as if someone has been squeezing it like this," Kata responds, making a fist. Mevlija: "And what do you feel in your stomach now? Hunger?" Kata is not hungry, having eaten well, she says, first thing in the morning before taking her medications. "And how's your blood pressure," asks Mevlija, "does it vary?" Kata replies that it used to, but is now steady, "maybe because I used pills for a year, maybe because of something else." She adds: "But my cholesterol is high." A man seated among a few patients waiting their turn speaks his mind: "All of that is related to nerves." Mevlija could not agree more: "All of that is my job."

Nervous disorders are linked to bodily ills as a matter of course. This therapeutic common sense scrutinizes the lead not for its symbolic meanings, not only for existential narratives that it might suggest, but for a quite literal image of the troubled visceral topography. Mevlija is only making this concern more comprehensive by inquiring about Kata's blood pressure, to which Kata adds a report on her cholesterol. The three—blood sugar, blood pressure, and cholesterol—are the usual indices of the condition of "worrying one's self sick" (sikiranje) that so many Bosnians so often discuss. Moreover, Mevlija reads hunger among patients' immediate bodily responses to strava, signs of its therapeutic of action, that may include nausea, lightheadedness, crying, or a sudden urge to urinate.

Furthermore, carnal soul matters are barely separable from one's living circumstances and affective and financial affairs. One day in the spring of 2006, I found a distressed middle-aged woman on a chair by the window, and Mevlija, a cigarette catching the corner of her mouth, whispering prayers, preparing for treatment two pieces of male underwear that belonged to the husband of the crying, sighing woman. Mevlija asks Vahida to make three wishes on behalf of the absent man—the number of wishes in this therapy is inflated, as is the price, since anywhere else you only get to wish once—and the woman throws her hands up in despair: "I no longer know what to wish for! I tried so many things. I no longer know what to do for him." Then quieting down, she complies: "May God give him some common sense. Let dear Allah give him all that's best." Mevlija, drawing the underwear through the prayer beads, comments: "Allah already gave him all that's best: health, which is most important, but he lost it, land, a restaurant. . . ." Vahida interrupts to inform her of the latest fight the husband had with the restaurant staff. He is jeopardizing the family business.

Mevlija's ritual preparations are a fraction of Fadila's—brief prayers over lead, which she circulates either around the patient or on clothing and knocks against the wall before melting ("to shake off all that is bad from the person"), brief whispers over water, a quick run over prayer beads that she draws through either the bowl of water or in cases of remote treatment, the clothes of absent patients. The treatment likewise is significantly shorter, performed at four spots (twice on the head and chest or feet, if necessary).

Setting the bowl of water on top of the underwear tucked in the red sheet, Mevlija pours in the molten lead and concludes a close examination with grave excitement: "Oh, Vahida! It should not surprise you that this man is ripe for a mental hospital, for the psychiatric ward. Before this month is up, he will have to see a psychiatrist. You see, here [pointing to a stick figure protruding from the lead, with a knob for a head], he likes to be alone." Vahida confirms that the man keeps to himself. Mevlija: "His brain is blocked up. Could he have suffered a mild stroke, perhaps while under the influence of alcohol? He will have to see a doctor." While Vahida complains that her husband would not hear of seeking medical help, Mevlija's attention catches another diagnostic sign: "How can he be possessed by such nervousness?" At this, Vahida loses her last bit of self-composure and starts telling how her husband turns red, shakes with rage, and shouts at her and their two daughters who are trying to study for their university exams. Mevlija: "It's a serious depression, believe me. He'll have to be taking [drug] therapy." "He's already taking Lexaurin," Vahida says, but Mevlija shakes her head: "That's nothing compared to what he will have to start taking. But one piece of advice, Vahida. When he falls into this state of great anger, depression, let him be, remain silent." Vahida protests—keeping quiet makes no difference, her husband has become impossible, he suspects her of "having made sihir" (*napravila mu sihir*; sorcery, most simply put; see chapter 4), he mistrusts their daughters. In a different tone, but almost in the same breath, she next gives a careful account of his dietary habits, his stool, his drinking routines, and his bloody underwear. She itemizes all the minute ways in which she cares for him in spite of their strained relationship, while also keeping him under surveillance. In turn, the fact that he seems to rely on her for providing anything from food to clean clothing to monitoring his medical condition, speaks silent volumes about the tacit economies of domestic care that proceed almost under all circumstances. Vahida describes how she secretly, regularly sprinkles his salad, yoghurt, and lemonade with bottled strava water from Mevlija's previous treatments. From nourishing tricks, Vahida's narrative shifts onward along the continuum of matters of concern, that runs from husband's food and stool to her despair and care: her husband was upturning the house last night compiling documents for yet another loan application! The restaurant has been operating at a loss, the house is already mortgaged. He is overextended with bank, micro-credit, and personal loans, while it is she, Vahida complaints, who will be held legally responsible, since she is the principle signee. She chokes up at this point. Mevlija comforts her, encouraging her to endure, to take the business in her own hands, to be patient a bit longer for her troubles will soon end, when the man is forced into therapy. She pours strava once more. "He can no longer count," she says looking at the lead; "he can't tell the difference between 100 KM and 1,000 KM." She concludes the therapy on a solemn note, with the third pouring: "He is like a blind man in a fog. But all of us, you and I and everyone, we have to somehow help this man. I cannot condemn him." Having bottled up the strava water, Mevlija prepares the bowl anew, this time for Vahida, who draws closer to the fire, to be treated herself.

"Everyone scares the life out of me, everything hurts me, my own skin hurts me," Vahida says, seating herself on the floor cushion, now clasping her stomach, now her arms, now her knees. Mevlija asks her to think of three wishes, and shortly after pours out strava, close to her head. Reading the lead: "Exhale deeply, my dear Vahida, unburden yourself. Here he is, alone again. How much does he care for that business of yours?" Vahida: "Not much." Mevlija: "Take everything into your own hands. Don't let him bully the workers so much." Vahida: "I can't, grandma; he shouts at me and I have to go home." Mevlija: "Don't. Try to stay, pretty soon you'll be running things yourself. You will be paying him a visit to Kreka [the regional mental health clinic]. Forgive me, but that's how it is." Vahida: "He's accusing me of having affairs." Mevlija: "Such people are sick." Vahida: "The other day he attacked. . . ." Mevlija interrupts:

"They need a victim." Vahida: "I don't want to go to work again." Mevlija: "You will go!"

After the second pouring of strava, at the level of Vahida's chest, Mevlija touches the woman's back: "You are so tense. Nts, nts, this man will end up in a hospital." Vahida: "If he had a knife, he'd kill someone in a fit of rage." Mevlija: "No doubt, it's a depression." Vahida: "Others think I lead an easy life, a life of luxury, but there isn't anything left in the house." Mevlija: "Just let it be; you'll see, he already suffered a minor stroke. . . . It's just a matter of time. [Looking in my direction] Since this morning I've been seeing the worst cases."

Mevlija is focused on the man's brain, mood, and behavior; she discerns that his brain is "blocked up" after a stroke and makes several predictions: that the man will be forced into clinical treatment and that he will suffer another, more devastating stroke. She diagnoses him with "depression," which may sound surprising to lay ears but is quite in keeping with local psychologists' and psychiatrists' understanding that depression in men often manifests as aggression. The woman's attentiveness to details paints domestic dispute as a matter of health and wealth, and by extension makes both the subject of Mevlija's intervention ("this man can no longer count" and "take everything into your own hands") and of the wife's habitual management: of the husband's diet, with medicinal ingredients snuck in, of faltering business, of accumulating debts.

Vahida's own treatment shows the extent to which her health is involved with her husband's affairs, as his disorders became legible in her lead. Intimacy extends one's presence beyond the immediately sited body, with disordering consequences. But since beings are singular, not interchangeable, the husband here is reached not through his wife's embodied presence but by means of his worn clothes that render him contiguous and legible. Primed for diagnosis and intervention.

WHAT MAKES COKE FLAT, EVERY TIME

Intimacy is powerful but is only one among several vehicles of powerful connections that are being worked out in therapy and that help illustrate the particular economy—of exchange and of influence—at play in strava. I offer three snapshots from the practice to illustrate my point as well as to rehearse an earlier proposition: it may take an ethno-graphic grafting of phenomenological as well as object-oriented atten-tion to grasp adequately some unruly therapeutic proceedings. Still, no prior conceptual commitments can adequately replace local schemes of practical power and action.

One day at Mevlija's, a man in his thirties, accompanied by his moth-er, brings a pair of women's underpants; the undisturbed store tag im-parts to the item the freshness of a recent purchase. A gift meant for his wife, it goes through Mevlija's expert hands, through the hoop of tespih, prayer beads, inspiring a quick cycling of the lead, and rests beneath the red cloth. Mevlija sets a bowl of water on top and pours the lead. The husband came because he was deeply concerned about his wife who, apparently, was much in love—with someone else. The couple's long-planned romantic trip to Morocco ended with a surprising twist when, shortly upon returning, the young woman asked for a divorce and moved back in with her parents. The husband and his mother, however, suspected sihir, which also turns affections around, cools off feelings, and deliberately directs the victim's desires and sexual aptitudes. With a gift of clothing—bought prospectively, a designated gift but yet to be given—the husband is trying to diagnose and treat the distanced wife remotely. Mevlija confirms his suspicions: there is indeed a love sihir on the young woman and she can do her best at a distance, but the removal may require treatment in person.

Another time at Mevlija's, a woman unfolds two pieces of a new cotton undershirt and underpants—mundane gifts intended for her husband. The husband, the woman explains, has been unusually stressed lately, so she thought it was time to intervene, having had her own strava poured out the previous day. A medical doctor employed at the intensive care unit of the regional clinic, she attends strava therapy regularly, every three months, to receive timely relief from existential and professional anxieties. She also regularly and remotely pours out her husband's fears, apparently with his consent; it is not at all unusual for women in Bosnia to assume principal responsibilities for their extended family's medical care: they fill prescriptions on behalf of their husbands, children, elderly parents, and relatives, as well as accompany them on medical quests, whether in or outside the institutional medicine. Mevlija prepares each item, treating water with suras and duas, preparing lead and touching it to the garments, running them through her prayer beads. Next she performs three pourings. Strava lead from the first pouring tells Mevlija that the husband has been suffering the consequences of a major recent fright and the wife relates her account to a barely avoided car accident.

Finally, a brief, noneventful "accident" that I have observed time and again at the tail ends of strava practices at Fadila's and Mevlija's. Nena would reach for a recycled plastic bottle of Coke, or Cokta (a regional brand of soft drinks with a long, socialist history of mimetic difference), that perhaps those people walked in drinking, and would fill it up with strava water to be used, afterwards, in a medicinal bath. When bottles already contained some amount of beverage, they proceeded to add strava to it, telling the anthropologist and sometimes people themselves who reacted, to "never mind it," "it doesn't matter" (*nema veze*), and sometimes "it will only make the water sweeter."

These three examples are telling of hierarchized potencies as well as of actions that, predictably, trump one set of relations with another. In all three cases, there are commodities that enter the therapy, arriving to it following logics and dynamics that make their production, circulation, and consumption possible. Whether we subscribe to critical theories of occulted labor value and the social mediations it affects or we stick to marginalist accounts of market-based relations, it is obvious that the underwear was bought for money, or on credit, and that the relations between the producers, distributors, vendors, buyers, and consumers ought to hinge on its various forms of manipulation and mediation. Distance is abridged, people unknown to each other are brought together—and kept apart—thanks to the convenient medium of universal exchange. However, strava first presumes that a gift can override the plain market relations, subverting them to the point where the intention of a gift, yet to be given, possibly never received (who is to say that the estranged wife can be talked into accepting a suggestive gift from her husband?) turns a commodity into a gift and into a debt: the tangible, consequential extension of the other. Secondly, strava works on the commodity–gift–debt, treating it with the craft's implements in order to achieve diagnostic accuracy and therapeutic efficacy. At a distance, all via extensions made not simply through the fact that people involved are related but through the act of reinvigorating and reconfiguring their relations in the course of buying, intending to gift, gifting in advance of taking, and all its attendant consequences. Moreover, it is because the implements of strava rely on Koranic words and personal wishes and supplications that the things are being rendered medicinally relevant. Equally important here is a nena's presumed obligation toward sound practice and presumed obligations, since doubts may creep in about whether the healer is "for real" or whether his or her talents are reversible, deployed either to heal or harm. The treatment of sihir in particular, the treatment of patients without their consent and knowledge, becomes precariously close to practices of magic themselves, that proceed boldly in disregarding other people's best interests and feelings, on behalf of parties in the business of magic making (pravljene, pravit). Doubts can also open up about whether a nena shortchanges scriptures integral to strava and heals sihir by means of sihir, relying on nonhuman agencies to carry out *her* acts, rather than pleading for Allah's help on behalf of the patients.

As for the Coke, it is the strava water—imbued with suras and duas, with healers' supplicating breath, and with the fears washed off with all sorts of biographical details—that trumps it, all the time, with a potency that a priori overrides its use value, its brand value, its familiar taste, its secret formula, its chemical composition. Combined with strava, Coke remainders remain flat.

SABAHA'S OBJECTION: BARELY A HUMAN GIFT

Strava begins with a gift: a healing gift given to a postmenopausal woman, out of the blue, under grave circumstances. The woman has probably observed the practice in the past, perhaps played as a child at the side of a working strava therapist—as I have seen Mevlija's granddaughters do—but learning the course of the therapy, even learning all the curative suras, ayas, and du'as, alone is not enough. It takes a passing of a special touch from one, whether or not human, to another. Stories of initiation are varied: some received it from a nena before she passed away (or *pre-selila*, literally "moved on"), others from a nena addressing them from beyond, in the intermediary terrain of dreams, between this finite world (*dunjaluk*, from Arabic, *dunya*, "this world" or "that which is close") and the final (or the next): *ahiret*. In some other cases, once strava is given, there is life-long follow-up with instructions and observations by voices without a tangible presence, but voices that can push, stir, point. In any case, the instructions are clear: the woman may never quote a price nor deny treatment. I never heard Mevlija's story of initiation and I often wondered how this clever woman squared her exceptional strava entrepreneurial spirits with the stringent requirement everyone knew about. Mevlija never acted as if she owed anyone an excuse or an apology, even when people were obviously surprised or doubtful about the few other remedies she had up her sleeve, for a price: talismans with Koranic inscriptions (*hamajlije*) and "little towels," which she marketed sometimes as prophylactic and other times as necessary proxies for a person treated. But then again, Mevlija was otherwise uniquely reversible. She regretted the privatization of pharmaceutical and the inflation of drug prescriptions: "Nowadays, medicines are brought in with trailer-trucks," she said disapprovingly. She has turned patients down if they lacked the means to pay, and yet she has donated handsomely to the neighborhood mosque construction project. Each weekend she would take a break from strava, change her dimije for sweatpants, headscarf for a ponytail, and would travel to soccer tournaments to root for her grandson or else would attend dog shows. There was no fitting the many biographical details into a consistent narrative nor a coherent disposition.

Yet, unwavering consistency is what is sought in the healer for real, what seems to be imparted at the heart of the strava gift. It begins with an imposition—one cannot not take it—and an obligation: to practice the gift as a gift. Resistance to marketization and commodification is woven in multiple factors: the circumstances of death or beyond it, thread in the reminder about finitude, which is anyhow readily remembered (see chapter 3 and Jašarević 2012a) and the knowledge itself is a kind that can be neither intentionally taught nor learned, neither standardized nor objectified.[4] As a gift, however, it invites a generous response from patients who have been raised to feel that it is good to give well and only proper to give back. In practices I observed and inquired about across northeastern Bosnia, people mostly tend to give 10 KM per session, which is a rather modest but not an embarrassingly small amount. Everyone tells stories of patients with means who overwhelmed therapists with gratitude of lavish amounts. Returning patients also often bring sweets, coffee, choice foods, or *domaće* products (see chapter 4).[5] Because strava restores health and saves lives, giving in turn does not aim to reciprocate nor commensurate the therapist's gift as much as to give, for what else can one do when gifting is practiced as if it were an irresistible habit, one that aspires to "delight" or "bring joy to" (*obradovat*) as well as meet a need or want.

Irresistible, uncomfortable, unsustainable yet unrestrainable: that seems to be the experience of gift in present-day Bosnia in general, and in strava in particular. Listen to a bit of my conversation with one Tuzla-based strava healer, Sabaha, and her granddaughter, a medical student:

Sabaha: "I do not tell them how much [to give]. I say 'you'll give as much as it is worth to you.'" Her granddaughter adds: "What is it that you usually say, grandma, 'as much as your heart forgives and forgets [halali]'." Sabaha: "I'm not asking you to overextend yourself [*nazor*]. My grandmother had me swear never to say [how much], but to say 'my child, as much as you can.' And no one ever gives me more than 10 [KM] each time. There are some people who never bring [money] or who say 'I don't have it right now, I'll bring it later' and they don't."

The feeling here teeters between forgiving-forgetting, generously, and remembering, begrudgingly a negative balance. Sabaha's standard reply to a patient does put subtle pressure—within an exchange, people read these cues—by speaking of "worth" and valuation. The patient is left to be guided by his or her own sense of plenty, given the circumstances, while the practitioner is expected to forgive and forget, no matter what, even when she gets nothing (but broken promises).

Much has been said about possibility and even more so about impossibility of generosity in anthropology and in philosophy. Skepticism toward gift-giving natives has outlasted initial critical investments in the possibility that there are indeed exceptions to the universal story of *homo economicus,* even if they are confined to islands of ethnographic difference in the sea change of global capital. Bourdieu has accomplished much to at once debunk any romantic ideas about uneconomic, non-Western alterities and to explain the classic, Maussian ambivalence that resides in the gift as at once disinterested and obligatory, but even he reacted strongly to the provocation that was Derrida's (1992) famous

Given Time: I. Counterfeit Money. There, Derrida made the gift impossible by premising it on the forgetting of both the giving and taking, forgetting so radical that not even a trace of the event remains, forgetting, in fact, that is also anticipatory and takes place before "a gift," "a donor," "a taker," "a debt" can take shape. Derrida's contemplation on the gift is powerfully moving and in itself, in many ways, unforgiving and tragic: the doomed subject of his story cannot but be constituted through domination and self-congratulatory self-recognition. He can neither be inclined to selflessly give—without also asserting one's self and appropriating the other in the process—nor to lose one's self in the other, for similar reasons. The bane of giving is time, according to Derrida. There can be no gift insofar as gift presupposes giving time, which is nothing present nor substantial, so can be neither given nor taken but all there ever is, takes place in time. So time, in a sense, is all there is, except that it *isn't* (ever present). Conventionally, time retraces the clock figure of the circle, which is the figure of market exchange (reciprocal, retributional give–take), which is the figure of an ideal Subject constitution, returning to itself, whole. Derrida's story of the gift, fortunately, cannot spell out the terms of "the gift's" impossibility everywhere any more than his idea of a bourgeois subject would find itself at home in many places on earth. If gifts are impossible and unbearable and yet insisted upon and aspired to in strava, they follow a different cultural logic whose pairing of health and wealth, for instance, could not have occurred to our dear continental philosopher. One is supposed to remember to give and forgive as well as to forgive recurrently, whenever remembering anew the given gift or alms. A gift is often given with *halal* or *'alal*, an expression that accompanies ritual or particularly solemn occasions, as well as one solicited to amend an insult, injury, or injustice.[6] More casually, it is given often when one indulges another. Hosts to their guests, in particular, when walking them out, may ask *halali*, on the doorstep, seeking pardon for their excessive care, for the nourishment they pressed upon them, for any unintended slights. Strava women often remember, and remember to forgive their patients' debts. Consider their predicament: they are obliged with a life-long service that consumes time and attention as well as resources—wood and lead—that opens their homes to drop-in visitors, disrupts their routines with appointments, and borrows their sympathetic ears for all sorts of complaints. Among the urban strava healers I worked with were both old-time residents in the suburban Tuzla neighborhoods and refugees who had fled eastern Bosnia. Like most Bosnians since the 1990s, they were caught up in "surviving," tangled up in informal debts and stretching inadequate incomes to maintain a life worth living. Sabaha, quoted above, is a refugee in Tuzla who lives off her late husband's average state pension, which is actually insufficient to meet monthly utility bills and basic costs of living. "My health is poor, the pension being what it is. [This is a life of] worrying-sickness [sikirancija]," she says, and in her words, her poor health has everything to do with the inadequate pension. Strava gifts, therefore, supplement her small income, but the inherited obligation to serve without price prevents her from eagerly anticipating money or withholding treatment from those who cannot pay. She is bound to give. The organ of memory in this practice is the heart, "as much as your heart forgives and forgets," and the heartfelt accounting cannot forget to give and forgive, even begrudgingly, objecting to other people's forgetfulness. Her patients regularly voice their money troubles in treatment, Sabaha says, compelling her further to give: "They are wailing, wailing, wailing that they don't have any [money], and I know why they say it, just so that they don't have to give."[7] Sabaha's patience expires at the sound of popular complaint, even if she knows it only too well and repeats it herself.

Some strava women, however, have done very well in the economy of gifts: Fadila financed a pilgrimage to Mecca (including equally costly gifts that she brought back to her family and friends), repaired a house in Tuzla to live in with her youngest daughter after fleeing eastern Bosnia in the 1990s, and constructed a large family home for her son and daughter-in-law, her youngest daughter and herself, in a new suburban settlement of Tuzla taken up by Podrinje refugees. Fadila was also a constant source of emergency funds for her children until she moved out of Tuzla and the traffic of her patients significantly thinned out.[8] ("This is fine by me," she tells me after the fact; "it means they don't really need me. If they needed me, they'd travel this far.")

And then there is the exceptional figure of Zejneba. Inherited lands, orchards, and a few domestic animals provide her subsistence; she hires help with cultivation and pays for it with surplus produce. She does not depend on her husband, either ("For all these years we've been married, I don't as much as wear his clothes, I don't know where his wallet is, nor do I care"), the husband whom the village has long thought mad and has avoided because of his unpredictable temper. She relies only on Allah, whose Mercy works out her plenty, leaving the means unspecified ("Things come from someplace, I don't know from where"). She refuses gifts. What she is forced to take—insistence on giving is well-drilled (see chapter 2)—she redistributes. "It's not for me, not for me to take. I am obliged to give," she explains, saying literally: "I am indebted to give," or "I owe giving [*dužna sam da dadnem*]." She said these words while nursing a bad shoulder injury—a cow, "a rascal! [*lopov*]" had pinched her—that screwed even further her bent frame, and yet she kept practicing, one hand limp and useless, the other determined, barely allowing me and others to help carry cauldrons to the stove and back. Moreover, her gift of healing keeps no track of clock-time. It is punctured by calls for prayers, themselves ordered according to cosmic agendas and sublunar seasons that cut out the sun's course across the sky; by seasonal and casual tasks (weeding or watering plants); by the habits of the belly and appetites of the soul—for coffee breaks, for instance, at the outdoor veranda.

ZEJNEBA: "UČEVINA, DIJETE, UČEVINA"

Zejneba, I'm told, '*klanja podne*' when I arrive so I wait at the veranda with the other women: her daughter, who is visiting for a day from the capital, Sarajevo; Nena Nesiba, a close friend and formerly a neighbor who came this morning from the nearby municipal town for the sake of a young woman who needs Zejneba's help and who is here with her mother. The old house is tiny, bulging somewhat at the seams, around the architectural waistline in particular the way that traditional houses, made of clay and straw, tend to after a while. The veranda extends far into a garden uncombed and overflowing with flowers, herbs, weeds, and fruit trees. It's a summer day, just about noontime, pleasant in the shade: no one is in a hurry to be anywhere else and we gaze at the garden, waiting. It is *podne namaz*, midday prayer (namaz is a Turkism), that engages Zejneba, though the literal translation of Bosnian seems a more precise description of the embodied disposition presumed by the act—*klanja*: she bows, prostrates herself, submits. Another expression is that someone is '*na sedždi*' or '*na serdžadi*,' which means both seated on the prayer cloth (from Arabic *sajjada*), or on the knees, or more precisely, with forehead pressing onto the ground, whether literally or intentionally, this intent too residing at once in the mind and in the heart

In a while, Zejneba comes out and heads straight to the stove. Pulling a large, square ladle from the fire, hosting a generous amount of molten lead, she pours it out for the girl seated on the floor. She pours gently at a close distance from the water and reads quietly to the girl: "You are nervous, discontent, everything bothers you [*sve ti fali*]." The young woman nods.

The first thing you notice about Zejneba is how she walks: deliberately, head on, slightly hunched as if seeking close audience with what she encounters: from the ladle, to the prayer beads, to the forest ivy string that she will soon be threading into a hoop, on the veranda in preparation for the next round of girls' treatments. This is partly because her vision is terrible—I learn that doctors have recommended surgery to remove her cataracts—and partly because she does not hear very well. I learned to suspect, however, that she doesn't listen much, either, tuned in as she is to more privately sounding worlds. But then, there is also the intensity with which she nears things, with a hushed Bismillah, constantly whispering du'as, deeply personal supplications, many of which she composed over the years and reciting from the Koran. It is as if she is so caught up with a plenitude of things and tasks immediately at hand that the rest of us, a few steps from her, at earshot, blur. Barefoot, very thin, wearing busily patterned dimije, with a scarf, *šamija*, loosely covering her henna-dyed gray hair, she at first strikes me as hostile—displeased that I came to bother her. But she looks me in the eyes, and keeps her gaze fixed for a while—here the world drops off a bit for me, too, and for a second, I think I know what "immediate" means, and then it's gone. She smiles the sweetest smile and I am taken in. Perhaps an ethnography is not supposed to go like this, but it did.

Intensity was the same whenever Zejneba worked: she immersed herself in what she handled, it encircled her in its eventful orbit when she whispered dua's urgently, to the audience of God. Even loud, chattering Nesiba did not come through to her. The girl's mother had to touch

Zejneba's shoulder effectively to ask: which water bottle to prepare for
the next treatment? Later, Zejneba will recite some of the dove for me,
of various lengths, some of which rhymed. She was given them in her
dreams, she says, and gives me instructions on when and how to use
them. But how was I to follow? Let alone write or remember? Her tone is
soft, she speaks fast, often breaking into Arabic, reciting from the Koran,
sometimes translating ayas for my sake. There was no use in asking her to
repeat, and I began to give up the idea of an interview with the grandma.
I just sat there, observing, catching morsels, feeling rather ethnographi-
cally useless, having found the kind of healer everyone is searching for.
Even when she answered my questions, what she said sounded dead-end
straightforward and single-minded. Questions: "What made the water
from three springs 'alive' [*živa*]?" "What about forest ivy acted in strava?"
"Why did she boil rusty nails for the woman's treatment?" Answers:
"God gave it so," "It's God's will," "God's doing and that's that, what to
do about it [*i to je to, šta češ*]?"

Detours, as ever, get me a bit closer to what is meant. Seated on the
veranda, Zejneba is stringing the ivy while the rest of us pick up a favorite
casual topic: garden flower and herbs. Nesiba points out vegetal forms in
front of us and tells how they fare in other gardens—how rare or common they are, are they old, *starinske*, or "bought," *kupovne*, who else has
them, when and how did she get her own bunch, when and why did it
do well or almost perish, and what did she use to save it. At the young
woman's complaint of ovarian inflammation, Nesiba replies: "Ovaries?
I don't even know where they are nor how they look, but I know that this
grass [pointing out one frail, ferny thing] is good for them. And that one
there is *mačkov rep* [literally, a tomcat's tail]"; her listing is unstoppable
as she points next to a startling bush of long stems with furry crowns, "It
is good for women who want to conceive as well as for women's illnesses.
The bush of long ferns is *Čabuša*; it was used as a perfume in olden times.
Girls wore it, you just rub it in and the smell stays. When someone dies,
they carry it into the house and the whole house smells so nice." Next,
Nesiba speaks of *micina* herbal tea as good for ulcers; injections therapy
can break an ulcer "but it forms again, while with tea *od mice*, you remove
it once and for all." Such casual small talk full of rich, prompted, and
randomly recalled details that arises at the sight of grown forms, indexes

history of various uses from medicinal to pleasurable to aesthetic and ritual, and skips from ovaries to a death rite, while all along registering a difference between now and the old times, is the broad field of general reference within which to consider Zejneba's special knowledge. Zejneba joins our conversation to say: "Every herb, Nesiba, is medicine, only it's unknown [*lijek, al se nezna*]," before telling us a story about a man in the village who once happened upon two men in the field, having a drink. They offered him a sip and soon after, all the plants spoke to him, telling him what they were good for. The man could not stand it and walked about frantically, looking for those unknown men until he found them. How he cursed (*opsovo*)! What have you given me, to make me hear all the plants speak! That instant the vegetal voices fell silent, the two men vanished, and soon after, the man died in an accident: a truck rolled over him. There is no joking with God, she says, concluding her story about the responsibilities of a bestowed knowledge.

The ivy that grows up the trees—*bršljen loza*—she says, is medicine, but it is rare and not to be confused with the more common *pandjica loza*. "If there is something on a human [*insanu*—from Arabic *insan*], it takes it off [*svlači*]. When someone has no children, it takes it off." I ask about Čabuša, and Zejneba says that it came from Ka'ba, Mecca, together with squash.

It is not just that Zejneba's attention gravitates to devotional objects and iconic Islamic references—from Koran to Ka'ba; nor is it simply that her insight guides her selectively to the most rare and potent things, deep in the forest, high up in the tree (*bršljen loza*). Rather, her attentiveness dresses the plain with significance, or put another way, her receptiveness undresses common things for their tight connections to the ever-present divine, connections that are always potentially consequential. Speaking of herbs, another time, she remembers encountering a group of herbalists someplace in the southern mountains of Herzegovina, collecting *Trava Iva*, which was new to her. She inquired and they explained its powerful properties (in the marketplace of Tuzla you will hear herbalists promote it with the rhyme "trava Iva, od mrtva pravi živa"; "it turns those once dead, alive") to her, while gifting her with a few sprays. She carried it for a while but then thought to herself, "I dare not keep it. I didn't pay for it, *grehota je* (it's a shame, a harm)." There is no gift innocent enough not to bind, somehow, God knows how, and paying for it is the simplest way of ensuring your entry and exit from the exchange, which may still ripple out in effects long after the original give-and-take, but payment controls the ensuing debts. Importantly, a payment makes you a giver, if like Zejneba you are so inclined to participate in the spiritual economy that starts and ends with a *Bismillahir-rahmanir-rahim*, in the Name of God Most Merciful and Compassionate, where the giving is the divine quality, incessantly recommended throughout the Koran, praised over all other goods collected, coveted, accounted, received, or ensured. She dares not turn people from the door, she says. Once she tried, but then "How did it shake me! I grew too tired [to practice], working on land all day and then strava on top, but when it shook me I was told, 'Accept at least five, even when you are ill.'" She also makes sure, she says, that those who come, eat and drink too. "You know," she says, as if saying the obvious "džumetlija, dženetlija," the generous one is a resident of paradise. The exemplary life of the Prophet of Islam, as collected in Hadith traditions, likewise praises openhandedness, and Zejneba's love for Resulallah is practiced: when she does venture out from the town, she says, she never goes to the market but to *mevlud*, celebrations of the Prophet's birthday or collective zikr that people organize in remembrance of their dear deceased ones.

On the veranda, threading of the dove and Koranic verses into ivy is ongoing. Sometimes her fingers shift from the plant's sharp, deep dark leaves to a long string of prayer beads, lingering at each knob a while or else moving more breezily, in the rhythm of zikr; at other times she intertwines branches and beads. Every now and then Zejneba stirs the cauldron with nails boiling in it, her whispering sustained. When she pauses with ivy she picks up a small bag of wheat seed that the mother and daughter brought along following Nesiba's suggestion, and she sifts through them a handful at a time, applying to them a hum of her pleas and wishes to God. Zejneba's daughter is thinking of their lunch, which has been simmering on the stove inside the house since after breakfast; the bread is already out of the oven, I can smell it. Later, when we step out from lunch, Zejneba will find chickens and a rooster helping themselves to the wheat on the veranda floor and she will scold them: "Aren't you clever? Found wheat, didn't you. But it isn't mine, you cannot be eating it." She takes the seeds inside where they will stay—they need more curing, with water that she breathed Koran into, and with dandelion root—sadly I know neither why nor how nor to what effect—until the women's return visit. Back to the ivy, back to coiling the plant propensities with Koranic Arabic and dove in "our language," but rhymed in the beyond of the waking world. Fingers picking, dropping, fondling, unfurling, lips and breath quickening, relaxing, gathering and releasing, embodying and extending Koran, concentrating it onto a spot, with a blow. Her eyes closed to us whether behind the lids, or slightly upward or to the side, unblinking. At one point she yawns while reciting and keeps reciting throughout the yawning, which Nesiba, our skilled interpreter for the afternoon, explains as a clear sign that the young woman on whose behalf Zejneba worked, suffers from uroci.

Nesiba tells us about the first time she ever came to Zejneba for strava. She was in constant pain following childbirth and there was not a doctor left to visit in the region; no one could help. Later she learned that the illness was caused by sihir she received as a newly arrived bride in her husband's village. She suffered until one night, in a dream, Zejneba's husband showed up to instruct her to seek his wife for help. Of all people, it was a man she had a major fight with and could not stand (Zejneba will tell her later to let the man be; his was a clinically certified madness—*ima potvrdu s klinike*). She swallowed the pride, took the dream's hint, and after some ninety strava pourings, was cured once and for all. She has never been ill since, never been to doctors, and the only complaint she has been developing with age is high blood pressure. Zejneba is sweet to her during the lunch and says: "I rejoice in your visit more than in my sisters." They eat out of the same plate.

After lunch, there is coffee, and then the treatment is resumed. Another pouring of lead—the treatment has been ongoing since 9 AM and it's past 3 PM when we walk out of lunch—and then another. Again, I overhear fragments only: nervoza, and "a burden on your heart [*tegoba na srcu*]." The nails are ready for pouring and Zejneba needs some help. Holding an enormous shallow cauldron by small handles that stick out of its side like the thing's ears, she pours out water with some half kilogram of nails on the bottom. The girl's mother is holding a bowl of water beneath the girl's face, sheltering it from sprinklings but fanning the passage of smoldering smoke toward it, encouraging her to breathe in. She does and begins breathing rapidly and quivering visibly from time to time. "The air must be too hot for her," I say, interpreting the woman's periodic shivers, but Nesiba gives me a disappointed look for misunderstanding the signs: "This pouring, you know, it's not like just anyone can do it, this is *deredže* (a bestowal, recognition, a rank); it comes to someone and she can do it, not everyone can, but only the one to whom it is given [*nemože to svako, to kome se da*]."

Sad to disappoint, eager to show interest, I go back to asking questions: "What is strava?" Zejneba: "When a human [insan] is ill. Učevina, učevina, učevina, my child." *Učevina* sounds folksy and archaic to contemporary ears, a word that references studied knowledge or science. In Zejneba's usage, it principally invokes the Koran, which presumes "učenje"—reciting, reading, or studying the sacred text, not least with medicinal benefits in mind. The imperative form, "*uči!*" begins the first verses revealed to the Prophet, collected in sura el-Alek and translated into Bosnian as: "Uči," or "Čitaj, u Ime Tvog Gospodara" ("Recite [or 'Read']" in the Name of thy Lord). Nesiba wants to clarify, although they were getting up to leave, and offers a list: "Fretting and worrying, and fear and magic and confusion—it expels it all from you. When you happened to *naograjsat*, and when the bad illnesses overcome you so that not even a doctor can help: cancer and diabetes. When there is *ogreb* or *crveni vjetar*." Nesiba takes leave, the other two women are already in the car, and Zejneba carries on with listing: "Nervousness, when you turn aggressive, or become very weak, when you feel slashed right across your chest, Allah gives that this makes it better. This is our weapon, our defense. So is salat and [Koranic] recitation [*klanjanje, učenje.*]" How did she start? God decided so, she says. "When I fell ill, it came to me from God to start working. People started coming from all over and never stopped, from Denmark, from Austria, people dream of me [*usnije narod mene*]; they come from Tuzla, from Lukavac." Her husband would not let her work, she remembers, "but I had to, there was no other way. I was told: 'I gave this to you, I prescribed it to you, the day you were born.' I didn't start this on my own, like some women do." When she fell ill, she went to see an imam, *hodža,* but he sent her to seek direct guidance by means of a dream, *istihara* (from Arabic, *istiqhara*), which is initiated by special *salat* and a dua (see Mittermaier 2011 on istiqhara, and dreams more generally, in an Egyptian context). Then she received directions on how to heal, and her first pouring was for herself. She was told, "Everything will come to you from Allah into your brain." She continues with the list: "From fear. If you fall down, someone attacks you, thieves, a dog startles you. Nervousness comes, all from the heart; this is what your heart does"—her hand tremors at her chest to demonstrate. "Dear God knows how many people I helped, my child, *učevina*; it's all due to *učevina*, there is nothing to strava without it. This girl, she suffers someone's revenge [*osvetio joj se neko*]; it's nothing but blood [showing] in her strava." Strava cures all illnesses, it shows everything: "if you are indebted to someone, if you need to give to a turbe, it all comes out. If [the lead] goes onto the left, that means something too. This girl, she suffers what was 'made to her' [*napravljeno*]."

Sihir, and the intangible agents at work with it, cannot affect her, she says, because she *uči*, and because she keeps her body constantly pure, *pod abdestom*, and her nearness to God and his protection is thus ensured. The protection she works out for others, on behalf of her closeness, are both impressive and limited, always stretched among the cosmological, historical, and biographical. She tells me about her sons. Both were in the trenches, those four long years, and she prayed for them at night. "Allah loves the night salat [*noćne namaze*] the best," she explains, telling me in effect that she practiced submission, remembrance, and intimate supplication outside the time of obligatory salat and in the nighttime that is especially designated as auspicious, when prayers and wishes are kindly received. Islam, as practiced submission, opens up at night, in the hallway of a prostrated heart, into ihsan, "doing what is beautiful," or in Zejneba's words "like a little rose, when it opens up [*ko ružica kad se otvori*]. The tradition of du'a is likewise a part of this inward, intimate practice that recites deeply personal and efficacious prayers passed from the Prophet or from other great Muslims, but also encourages a conversational relationship with the divine. A well-read compilation of dove in Bosnia, Handžić's (2004), describes dova as "a quiet conversation with your Lord. Dova is a mysterious pathway to draw a spiritual strength from the principle source. Dova restores human soul and directs it toward the correct path. Dova is a support, when all other supports weaken, when all hope is lost" (3). Her sons were never wounded, she says, but one of them became ill after he saw his friend blown up by a landmine. He got frightened and has never been the same. He walks between this world and another. He spends time in the forest, alone, with his goats. From a few, he got twenty-seven. Allah gave it to him so. Why doesn't she pour out fears for him? He doesn't want it. He says that: No. He saves money, though, only spends some on cigarettes, but never drinks. He says if I die, all of my belongings will go to the mosque. Since the war, so many people come to Zejneba suffering, so many of them receive the injections. "They have accumulated fears. With lead, you can take them off." She then tells how Prophet Solomon threatened a jinni with lead and she promised to behave. "Imams uče as well, but with Koran and lead, you take it all off."

HAVING FOUND THE HEALER FOR REAL

Having found the healer for real, I never return. Except once more, shortly after, when I came, notebook shoved away, to introduce Zejneba to my mother. What kept me away was not just Zejneba's genuineness that disarmed my ethnographic hand, nor the sheer difficulty of adequately voicing my questions or understanding her answers. Nor was it only a concern that I might be adding to the burden of her daily traffic of visitors. Rather, the field of her practice deterred me for reasons that took years for me to fully understand: my ethnography was not up for the task. Notice that the pages I write on Zejneba's practice are more packed with local terms and codes whose translations are rudimentary; the thickness of the particulars—from gazing at the garden and its medicinal plenty to the merits and perils of gifting and taking—not to mention the particularity of the metaphysical that Zejneba was living, practicing, invoking, left me seriously doubtful, and more precisely put—unwilling—to turn to my rallied conceptual allies to try to study further or properly unpack, let alone to try to grasp the underlying conditions that promise therapeutic success. Visiting with my mother, rather than with a notebook in hand, I cannot quite explain, unless it was an attempt to near Zejneba otherwise, on terms that could have been more sensible to her: as a being related, hence belonging, and, at least through familial ties, knowing something about obligations and responsibilities.

NOTES

1. Bosnia at the time of the fieldwork was among the few places that had not readily followed the global shift in diagnostic practices on anxiety and depression (cf. Applbaum 2006).

2. Turks could have referred either to ethnic Turks who settled in Bosnia since Ottoman times or to Bosnian Muslims.

3. *Turbe* (from turbe in Turkish and turba in Arabic) designates small mausoleums that are sources of blessings and merit. The most obvious translation would be "shrine" or "saint's shrine," which would correctly place these structures within a more global sacred and Sufi geography. Except that *saint* and *shrine* translate too hurriedly and too confidently what is specific about Islamic spiritual tradition in the language of universal mysticism. Turbe might be housing a body of *evlija,* which is Bosnian Arabism for a "friend of God," a person who is holy and imbued with grace, often a *derviš* (a spiritual traveler) or a *šejh* (guide or a teacher) associated with a particular Sufi order, *tarikat* (from Arabic *tarīqah,* "path" or "way"). Many a local turbe across the Bosnian countryside that attracts visitors and supplicants from near and far is not tied to a *tarikat* nor to any known Sufi body but to an anonymous person ("a young woman" or "two brothers") whose stories of life and death are part of the folklore, told often with scarce details. Turbe folklore also testifies to significant historical forgetting and misremembering. For a good overview of the history, ruination, and restoration of turbe across Bosnia see special issues of *Behar,* written by Urjan Kukavica (2010). For a sense of historical forgetting of the role of Sufi orders in Bosnian social history, see Aščerić-Todd (2015).

4. The 1888 article on strava treatment sought out by an Eastern Orthodox Christian woman on behalf of her child reports that the mother gave the healer some Austrian money, one whole cheese, and a large portion of the goat, slaughtered at the healer's recommendation (for it was the goat that gave the child a fright), explaining: "May it be her blessing! I do not regret [giving], since if it weren't for her, my [son], God protect him, would long ago be lying under ground" (1888:16–7). Note the language: she does not speak of payment of a quoted amount, which may or may not seem fair. Instead, her denial of "regret" indexes giving in turn that, upon reflection, could seem extravagant according to the calculus of available means.

5. The offering of a little something, such as coffee, cookies, sugar cubes, or chocolate, sweetens the money and emphasizes its gift quality. The value of these trifles is symbolic only to an extent. These small gifts are currencies in their own right: they can be passed on as tokens in parallel circumstances; they can be shared and consumed at frequent coffee gatherings at work or in the neighborhood that take form of little potlatches. Such little gifts regularly accompany informal payments to the medical staff in the public health system, even when prices for the "free" service have been flatly quoted to the patients' faces.

6. In contemporary Bosnia where language politics fully participate in the making of ethno-nationalist distinctions and claims, *halal* may seem overtly associated with the Bosnian Muslim idiom, but in the vernacular, as heard at the open markets or healing sites, (h)alal is used indiscriminately by all. Janko Balorda, an amateur ethnologist observing the Serb folk in Bosnia between the two world wars, recorded that *sevap* (a

Turkism for good deed and merit) and *halal* are principles surrounding mortuary rites. Balorda writes that those villagers who dress or bathe the deceased, who dig the grave or make the coffin, refuse payment and consider their work "sevap." Furthermore, before the body is lowered into the grave, all the gathered—friends, neighbors and relatives—forgive aloud (*alale*) to the dead all their grievances and claims. Balorda also mentions how visitors brought gifts of food to the dying and their household members, regardless of whether they were rich or poor. After the funeral, mourners are treated to a grand feast (Balorda [1930] 1966). In contemporary context, (h)alal is asked for by the host at parting. The saying goes like this: "eto halali..." or "halali ako je šta..." ("so, forgive... if something has been..."), and is left unfinished, hanging, until the other protests, that nothing "has been" or asks for (h)alal in turn. Such partings are especially practiced by the elderly who worry that there may not be another meeting, and who therefore remind you of that, break your heart at leaving them, every time. (H)alal is asked for after a bargain has been concluded successfully on someone's part. One person asks the other, who suffered monetary loss, to forgive it.

7. The power of compelling here should be considered with due seriousness. Similar sensibility about taking money from someone who does not have it informs personal relations of borrowing and lending so much so that creditors often feel that it is embarrassing or inappropriate to ask for the return of the loan (see Jašarević 2012a).

8. During one of my visits, her married daughter drops by and, in a short while, ends her complaint about a 5,000 KM bill for construction of a water pipeline with: "you will lend to me, won't you." Fadila is quiet and rolls her eyes but ultimately does not resist.

SIX

What If Not for Real?

Troubles with Medical Efficacy

🖋 "How will you describe me?" the queen often asked. Initially, the tone issued clear warnings that my writing would have consequences. Years later, she would repeat the question teasingly, or wondering why my work was taking me so long. At the same time, she would assure me that the time had not yet come, that the world was not quite ready to know her. I kept writing and rewriting and, in the meantime, returned each summer to spend at least one day a week in her clinic, observing and eventually just hanging out. There is, of course, such a thing as too much ethnography, and mine was already much too much, yet I could not resist returning to see her. The queen in 2006 was rather rough— charming and hilariously funny, no doubt—but unpredictable, moody, shifting between high anger and deep laughter between two blinks of an eye. Over the years, she softened, not just toward me, but toward all of us. Returning patients, new ones, would-be-patients' relatives, friends, and parents who intervened or inquired on their behalf found her sweet and comforting. And she was evidently powerful: there were patient stories, records; lives saved and lives conceived; mobilities restored; cancers cured; depressions lifted; suicides prevented; romantic and business relations amended; skin rashes cleared; afflictions caused by *sihir* and jinn-intrusions resolved; chronic conditions managed free of pain and without medications. There were relatively accurate predictions about the lengths of treatments and uncanny precision about internal lesions, percentages of arterial blockages, chemical compositions of urine or blood, and dietary and lifestyle prescriptions that anticipated experiential observations, clinical advice, or simply restored a compromised body over time. There were also silences and secrets, utterances loaded with hints, open-ended suggestions, and the sense of profound misunderstanding, uncertainties, confusion. "Why don't you collect evidence," a man in the queen's office proposed one day, "our names, surnames, and phone numbers, so that people who read your book can call us up to check, if they still doubt? And that would make your research more sound." One after another on a September day in 2007, seven returning patients offered their advice: "Take me as an example." An elegant woman in her late fifties, Šemsa, who travels to the queen's once weekly from Žepče in central Bosnia, extended her manicured hands, adorned with heirloom jewelry, as a proof. The hands showed nothing: no trace of severe rheumatism that, she says, once knotted and disfigured her finger joints. The people gathered around the queen were frustrated, thinking I did not believe them. It did not help when the queen said that she anticipated getting into trouble once my book was published. "Separate the truth from lies; take me for an example," says one of two brothers who used to come together to the queen for treatment, and, getting inspired, he went on to speculate about the possibility of a historically new form of writing that would take note of inconvenient and unbelievable facts. He implicitly designated me as the record keeper and a scientific witness of the new, emergent definitions of reality. The queen liked what he said and raised the wager: "You want material? Here are my records!" pointing to her archive, which I would not take except to look over her shoulder as she leafed through it to tell stories about her patients. My ethnography could not be a scientific trial; it proved nothing. Nothing more nor less than is captured in the photos of some among the reputed seven hundred of her children, those whom she claims to have helped conceive because their parents consulted her for infertility treatments. These were no more obvious than a pair of once-rheumatic hands, nothing more solid than the records of lab exams, x-rays, or clinical diagnoses confirming the queen's insight or efficacy. A patient in a smart suit leans to me on her way out of the office another day to whisper, "That's the queen, the one who's helping [*pomaže*]. She saved my life, she saved my life." For many of her patients, the illness was an experience that radically challenged their sense of the sensible and the real. Among the seven patients who worried about my writing in 2007, one wished that I would fall very ill so that the queen might cure me and thus prove to me the truth of their own experience. The queen's office became a site, perhaps one of many in contemporary Bosnia, where people came face to face with the unknowns of supposedly basic facts: about bodies, about matter, about possible causes and effects. This was also a place where many dealt openly, for a brief time, with radically unsettling possibilities that things were otherwise and where they cultivated livable explanations and arrangements, if not exactly comforts, about the unknown, partly understood, and the uncanny. When they stepped away, they could hesitate to speak of their experiences wherever the official reason—modern, rational, and scientific, if not necessarily secular—seemed securely moored. When an opportunity arose—someone else complained of a health disorder, of ineffective treatment, of a health emergency—they could recommend her warmly. For some patients, the queen offered appropriate responses to the strange new order that succeeded socialism and the war and upturned the normal course of life and death. One day while waiting at the queen's, Šemsa, who is a city clerk in charge of her town's vital statistics, told me, "There were no natural deaths in Žepče the previous week. [Instead] we recorded two heart attacks and eleven cancers of all kinds."

The queen similarly points to the historical urgency of her practice: "I did not want to do this," she often protests, "I was forced [to practice] because of what is happening in the world. There is a mess and much confusion [*zbrka jedna*] out there; there are so many who claim to heal nowadays, who "pour out fears," who write Koranic inscriptions and people keep going to them." She was an alternative, despite herself, she claimed.

People sought her daily, except on Tuesdays and Saturdays. Ever since she started practicing in 1997, the stories of her power have persistently drawn masses to her palatial yellow house out of the way in a village of northeastern Bosnia. Her fame travels without commercial advertisement or media coverage, by word of mouth, with two significant details: no one knows how she treats and she cites no price. This is why the patients wished that I would fall ill, so that I could suspend my urge to know better, that I could write empathetically, that I could better imagine. So let me imagine, but it will only work, dear reader, if

I also do it on your account. Imagine yourself ill. Something happens
that inverts the most ordinary routines: sitting, eating, walking, and
sleeping become ordeals. Your face and body turn into strangers you
scrutinize unhappily and constantly with biometrics or fuzzy records.
Something all of a sudden makes your limbs ill-fitting or your organs ill-
disposed to keeping you well and reasonably happy. Clinical diagnoses
are inconclusive or precise, but medication barely saves you from pain,
therapy takes time and costs money, and something new goes wrong
each time you feel optimistic about the course of treatment. Let's sup-
pose that something transforms the flows into blockages or gluts that
bloat tissues or ooze most embarrassingly, that shorten your breath and
your step, that overtake your mind and feelings. Say you begin to react
to things that ought to yield no such causal power or, at least, they ought
to do it predictably, the way some elusive toxins or triggers do for people
with chemical sensitivities. Or else some ordinary tragedy mutes the
colors, dissolves tastes. Days are bland and living wears you out. Imagine
yourself somewhat shattered, destined as you are to be one day, being a
human like everyone else and so held miraculously together by nothing
more than the good fortune and good state of all the tenuous bits and
pieces that make you up. Perhaps you have been through countless treatments, traveled to public and private clinics, tried alternative, traditional,
and complementary medicines—and now you've exhausted your hope,
patience, and your budget. And then, following an intimate recommendation or a second-hand referral from someone sensible who swears by
this queen, you arrive to see her, fearful, doubtful but also hopeful. So
here you are, waiting.

Until she calls your name and, with the eyes of others glued onto you,
you step into the little room to find the queen walking about, starting and
dropping several separate strands of conversation, pausing to waive her
arms above someone stretched out on the couch, while healing all along,
though doing nothing obvious, the others strewn about, sitting in the few
wicker chairs or standing. She may not look at you for a while or else may
fix you at the doorstep with an inquisitive stare and a mocking remark
about your outfit, your posture, your greeting, or the way you combed
your hair. She may stare at you with her dark eyes, her gaze shaded strik-
ingly by eye-shadow hues—violet, green, sometimes blue—while you

hope that she will let go and smile, that she will approve, or better yet, be inclined to care.

Everyone knows that the queen heals with her hands, without touching, waving her arms at a distance from your body, and some are certain that she works with her eyes alone, at least when she treats people at a distance using their photographs or Facebook profiles. No one knows how. Since the queen is offended by comparisons with "those others" who heal by nonbiomedical means—and there are now very many traditional, alternative, and magical practitioners in the region (since the 1990s peace as the previous chapters explained)—her patients know better than to guess aloud her means or to associate her with any of the three dominant nonbiomedical rubrics: "bioenergy," Koranic medicine, or a variety of folk magic dismissively labeled as *gatanje* ("divining"), *bajanje* ("spell-making"), or *vračanje* ("sorcery"). They also know—or learn when making an appointment—to abstain from any pharmaceutical drugs prior to the visit and not to consume Koranic medicine, specifically those issued by practicing imams. The queen cannot work with these two interfering forces in a patient's body; her reactions to the two, bodily and affective, could be described as "allergic." What is apparent about her practice is that her hands twirl above the patient's head, gesturing downward as if spreading a cover over his or her body, again and again. As her arms rise and fall, their rhythm sways the rest of her body, until the treatment comes to an abrupt stop with her hands chopping the air and producing a peculiar snapping, the source of which I could never locate.

Your turn has come. She motions you to the couch, to which you respond, anxiously, hesitantly, or expectantly, lying down, getting ready for something. Whatever "it" is, the experience that people assembled around the queen have in common is not predictable but varies from body to body. In the queen's own words: "You have to experience that. I can't tell you [about it]. You can't believe it [*nemožeš vjerovat*]. You can ask my patients and they won't be able to explain it. They'll say, I feel something. Someone feels it like electricity, someone like warmth or a chill, someone gets dizzy; others will feel love for me, and they'll say 'you are so beautiful.'" Indeed, patients report feeling flooded with a sense of calm, or else feel the skin of their body intensely, as if it has become too taut or overfilled with jittery vitality; others feel pain in their gut, bones, or chest, while some feel exposed and transparent ("you know, such people see through you, read what you think, . . ." one woman tried to explain). Most patients learn to expect side effects (*reakcije*) that follow the treatment: fatigue, headaches, nausea, bleeding, tingling, numbness, or dizziness.

The queen powerfully intervenes in the lives and bodies of people who have named her so: the Queen of Health. "The queen" for short. A queen (*kraljica*) (or a king—*kralj* or *car*) is a vernacular honorific for someone very cool, effortlessly excellent at what they are doing. She preoccupies the minds and senses of those who have entrusted her with their health problems or with the well-being of their loved ones. She demands no charge. People leave gifts, monetary and otherwise, at the corner of her desk, furtively or conspicuously, such as crinkled local bills or crisp euros, which fail equally to catch her attention except when she refuses to take someone's money or orders her assistant to toss an unopened gift, suspected of sorcery or ill wishes, through the window and into the stream below. She does complain, however, of her expenses, mounting debts, and the fact that people do not sufficiently appreciate her. She can barely make ends meet. The queen's is a peculiar power: it inspires love as often as fear. It found not so much a following—her impulsiveness and professed indifference ("whether you come or not, it's all the same to me," as she often tells people) preclude devotion or any simple affection based on reciprocity—so much as an anarchic gathering, recurrent yet disorganized, and desirous to return to see her, to give something in turn, to earn her affection or friendship. When the crowds disperse, the queen retreats to the upstairs rooms, where she is virtually accompanied by patients throughout the world on whom she works remotely on Facebook. Some among them count her as close friends.

IF NOT FOR REAL: TROUBLE WITH SPECULATING

This chapter describes the queen and the people she assembles, while speculating about the nature of this therapeutic encounter and wondering what it tells us about bodily life and the experience of touching, in Bosnia or perhaps elsewhere as well. More specifically, the chapter is concerned with the queen's practice of reaching and grasping bod-

ies with hands but without touching, and with a vision that sees beyond the phenomenal, outside the usual visual range. With eyes set
on this distance, in this chapter I continue the book's overall project,
which is one of troubling phenomenological and conventional notions
about proximity, and I do so, again, in the good company of Jean-Luc
Nancy and Jacques Derrida, both engaged with the issue of touching.
As the chapter will show, the bodies that enter the queen's treatment
are composed of surfaces, and I will argue that it is a certain form of
"superficiality" that matters and renders the therapeutic and collective
experience around the queen effective. And yet, the bodies in treatment, without depth and without essence, are not crude matter, devoid
of subtle or metaphysical qualities. To the contrary, the queen guesses
that she works with her "psyche" (*psiha*) or, as she puts it at other times,
with her "brain" (*mozak*), and this chapter tries to imagine what putting
the brain and psyche to such work might entail. How does she touch
without a limb, via the unextended or intangible that is the "psyche-
brain"? If contact is always between the fleshly (sensing and sensed) and
the incorporeal (sense sensing), what can the queen's touching without
hands and her grasping vision tell us about touch more generally? How
does contact between bodies work? What sense touches what part of
us? Importantly, the queen's practice strongly suggests that contact is
an exchange, cued by gifting sensibilities and yet deeply steeped in the
broader market. Namely, she often folds both psyche and brain under
the rubric of *self*, an ensouled entity, explaining that she gives herself
to others in order to heal them. What she gives is a gift—priceless,
abundant, and impossible to commensurate—that profoundly indebts
her patients. It is also this gift-debt that I examine more closely in the
following pages.

This chapter, however, has a second project, one that ends the longer
ethnographic journey whose previous five episodes variously picked up a
bundle of the same underlying problems that had to do with visceral and
historical entanglements of the bodily and of the economic, especially
under the conditions of new epistemological uncertainty and medical overabundance of opportunities. Biomedicine may still speak the
comforting idiom of reason and technology, of predictability and pre-
vention, of emergency relief and accurate diagnostics, but the previous

chapters showed many ways in which its competence is effectively and variously challenged by professional practice, private and public, that is compromised by lack of resources, overextended infrastructure, or private interests; by present historical conditions, since the 1990s war and peace, that seem to overwhelm with health risks and threats, that seem to proliferate illnesses, as well as bring about new ones or reinvigorate old ones that exceed biomedical expertise; and by the bodies themselves, which have been historically altered and are far more responsive to influences, therapeutic and pathological, than the clinical practice, formally speaking, finds credible. Hence, people travel far and wide in search of better health, looking for a "real one" (*pravi*), a practitioner who can really cure and who practices medicine as a priceless form of care. The "real one," whether a medical professional or a practitioner by other means, is supposed to be effective and not to charge, but is to receive gifts offered. Previous chapters described such quests, as well as the costs, promises, and disappointments they involved. This chapter, however, returns to the popular quest to further wonder what is at stake in the discernment of the genuine healer. The trouble, I suggest, is not only that those who are less real are fake: charlatans, costing patients dear money, duping them with promises and remedies, harming them in the process, or keeping them away from more proper treatments. Scholars of the region have noted similar preoccupations among patients in post-socialist Euroasia (Lindquist 2006) with the authenticity of medical doctors and they have had good reasons to relate this anxiety to the more general uncertainty about figures of authority in the new and constantly reconfiguring transitional states. In Bosnia, the question of medical authenticity rings a different kind of alarm: if a person is not a "real" healer then what kind? Healers who are less than real can be wonderfully effective, and sometimes this is all that it takes to stop asking further questions. If the healer is "not for real" but still helps, is "not real" but quite obviously yields some form of power to effect a difference, is "not real" but nonetheless demonstrates knowledge of the kind that cannot have been learned nor consistently simulated, then what is he? Who is she? How do they work and know? How can one ever know or tell? Put simply, whether or not the practitioner seems genuinely, more or less selflessly, to care and to be helping the bodies and lives, is he "for real" remains an open question that invites ongoing speculation, generates evaluations and excuses, and produces unsettling doubts.

Popular and private speculations, delivered in confidence and in hushed tones, make a kind of "noise"—an unsteady, ongoing matrix from which redundancy and multiplicity of reality emerge (I lean here lightly on Bennett and Connolly [2012])—that stirs some trouble in the ontological and epistemological "pluriverse" that is Bosnian lived reality. This trouble also contributes a few questions to the anthropology that is (becoming) inclined to speculate about compositions of reality and about theories—and methods—that would be more adequate to the task of grasping it in the field or in the text. Whereas speculative turns in continental philosophy draw sources of inspiration from counterintuitive (re)readings of the classics (as Graham Harman's of Heidegger), from returning to older sources (Spinoza in particular), or from redeeming the once forgotten or unpopular thought (Uexküll or Whitehead), anthropologists have joined speculations with their trademark skills of listening to native, indigenous, and animist philosophies (Ingold 2006; Viveiros de Castro 2009; de la Cadena 2010) or by collaborating with metaphysicians of great philosophical and medical traditions that can barely be called local and only provisionally "traditional" (Farquhar and Zhang 2012), or by hybridizing local insights with canonical theories (Kohn 2013). Bruno Latour (2013) has, not surprisingly, been most methodical about setting out the lines of future research action that begin with an admonition: we can no longer afford to ignore metaphysical questions. Rather, time is ripe "to go back to the old question of 'what is X?'... but in the process" we'll discover "new beings whose properties are different in each case" and gain "power to enter into contact with types of entities that no longer had a place in theory and for which suitable language had to found" (21).

What Latour proposes is compelling: the world of profound ecological crises, ontological uncertainty, and epistemological questions must be thought anew since we can no longer rest confident in the matters of facts; indeed, the institutional sites from which confidence is produced have themselves come under increased scrutiny—from within or without, by rallying activists and dissenters of all stripes. Nonetheless, since the old metaphysics are themselves mired in controversy and traffic in certainties, and since Latour is interested in rethinking the world toward a cosmopolitical democracy, one where symmetry is sacred and uncertainty a cherished condition for the ongoing process of assembling the represented world, he also makes a minimalist metaphysical proposition, one that will not offend, that will clear up and prevent conflict, though it will look at the sites and institutions at odds with each other, productive of differences, such as the familiarly mismatched couple—religion and science. To this effect he proposes inquiry into modes of existence that are parallel and each producing its own conditions for evaluating materiality and relevance of things populating a field of its concern. No mode can be judged in terms of the other. His proposal is no mere matter of description since he urges us to go beyond a language-bound version of inquiry to make these modes of existence more substantial realities (18). What needs to happen "is that language has to be made capable of absorbing the pluralism of values. And this has to be done 'for real,' not merely in words. So there is no use hiding the fact that the question of modes of existence has to do with METAPHYSICS or, better, ONTOLOGY" (19). In effect, Latour asks for representations adequate to ontological pluralism, which would obtain "more diversity in the beings admitted to existence" (21).

I take Latour's admonition seriously, although as compelling as his proposal sounds, I can make little use of it here without mangling it, since I am interested precisely in the moments of profound ontological uncertainty that makes many patients fidget about bottom lines: whether or not a healer is real or rather *what is, who is* the healer who is other than real? Moreover, there is a widely disseminated sense of modes of existence that coexist, overlap, or intersect uncomfortably, and this sense registers as muffled in suspicions and more articulated in expert uses so that I cannot lean on the proposal of ontological pluralism without considering its given metaphysical scaffolding. Here is my major issue with speculating further on a Bosnian context in Latour's company: the metaphysical "noise" referenced here is not minimalist, inoffensive, bound to "clear out" conflict. Quite the contrary, it is the fragments of a strong Islamic metaphysics, partially known, barely believed, and variously conceived and contested among Bosnians, whether practicing Muslim or not, but also loosely familiar but more widely spread among non-Muslims who seek a healer for real, not least those who heal by Koran or specialize in magic-related afflictions (see chapter 4). This chapter then turns to read local and practicing metaphysicians as well as those who are read in translation whose writing professes an urgency—to step into the reigning confusions about healing claims—and proceeds with practical advice: how to tell the difference between healing for real and "curing for the wrong reason" (see chapter 4), how to recognize illnesses that were caused by nonhumans, and how to reconcile these manifestations of an otherwise world with the sense of material, historical, and cosmic reality. I will read selections from three booklets that exemplify a very large and growing field of publications on Islamic literature and medicine in particular. They could be thought of as a genre of Do-It-Yourself manuals, except that the "self" it addresses and encourages is not the ultimate agent of change, whose empowerment aims to bring about more lasting change in consuming, self-cultivating, urban homesteading habits, or wider, communal circumstances. Rather, the reader addressed is reminded of his or her sheer dependence on the divine, urged to remember, taught to read and recite medicinal portions of Koran, invited to contemplate the *ajete* and *sure*,[1] as well as to regard the evidence of their truthfulness in the material, lived worlds. This book has intermittently wondered about the ways in which the magical and the metaphysical seep into the most mundane sites and practices of post-socialist medicine and market; these readings bring the magical and the metaphysical together under the auspices of practical advice.

The chapter proceeds in two parts—Unknowing in Practice, and Reading—and I make no attempt to weave them together, also because this would probably irritate both sources of my inspiration and I have no desire to offend and already worry myself sick (*sikiram se*) about having annoyed those to whom I feel I owe *responsive* writing—one that hears the objections and advice from "the field," writes anticipating them, and attempts tweaking the writing process and prose so that it better resonates, approximates, and responds to what was being forwarded and meant, and how. Rather, in trying to find description proper to each I am hoping, as in Latour's hoping for his modes of existence, that they "allow us to populate the cosmos in a somewhat richer way, and thus to begin to compare the worlds" (2013:21).

For the sake of those to whom two-part writing strategy comes through as too conceptually sloppy or irresponsible, let me reflect briefly on how I see the two theoretical tactics sit side-by-side, the (post-foundational) phenomenological and speculative, or newly metaphysical. The new metaphysics has been also critical of phenomenology (Niemoczynski 2013) although writers are finding various ways in which to square the phenomenological and the speculative (Bogost 2012; Ihde 2003; Bennet 2013; Hawkins 2003). My own sense is that Nancian phenomenology has long been speculative and had always flirted with the metaphysics. There is, for instance, his writing on divine places (1991) or his "Little Dialogues" on heaven and God, addressed to children (2008b). Even without his provocative use of the "soul," his idea of being a body and being together in the proximity that presumes and preserves distance does not separate the material from the intangible. Moreover, his thought on touching and body has been part and parcel of his larger project on the deconstruction of Christianity that contemplated the crucified, resurrected, transubstantiated body of Christ. His recent writing most explicitly sets out with the task of opening the closure of the metaphysical questions, the closure that took place in the West after the death of God, after science and philosophy moved themselves so forcefully and so anxiously away from theology that they closed themselves off to metaphysical questions, confining reason to more pedestrian forms of reasoning. The reason, *logos*, on the other hand, always irreducibly presumes its own other, the *alogon*, what is beyond it, because it cannot resist thinking of what is greater than itself, dreaming of beyond, unearthing all kinds of ways in which sense is non-sense (but not unreason). Nancy, in short, has long been looking for imminence in the world of bodies, exploring how strangeness, space, community, and experience are this excess to which logos–alogon tends. And interestingly, his emphasis on finitude was clearly a commitment to immanence and worldliness, but there was always in his phenomenology space for a kind of transcendence: plurality of being, affinity to others, withness, all prior to every and surviving any being, though a world would close off with each death and open up with each birth. Nancy's phenomenology sets out to explore the alogon, the otherness of language, of adoration, of politics, of dreaming, of somnambulism. The philosopher is clear, however, about the kind of metaphysics he subscribes to: "There is no relation to being that is transcendental, no beyond this world, but this world is beyond the world or beyond the world is here on earth, all the time, sense that exceeds the making sense, the desire to make sense, to ask grand and impossible questions, to speak (in approximation and in inadequacy of language) addressing what sovereignly exceeds it" (Nancy 2008c:10).

UNKNOWING IN PRACTICE

"How can I explain it to you when I don't know it either? If I were making a pie, I'd be able to show you, but for this thing of mine, I don't know how it's done. If I were healing with [Koranic] recitations, I'd tell you [*da učim*]. But I have no time to pray. When I pray, I pray for myself. To me it's nonsense when people say, 'an imam prayed on behalf of someone.' You pray for yourself! It's just that I unburden your psyche. It's the psyche [*psiha*] again and again. It's the brain [*mozak*]. I work with my brain, I guess, I don't know."

In private, the queen openly puzzles about her power and wonders about the limits to her knowing. And yet she practices her "unknowing" confidently and powerfully. When she diagnoses, advises, intervenes, or prepares medicine, she knows what to do without necessarily knowing the content of her knowledge. "Don't ask me what I've put in it," she tells me of the cream she made for a person with a serious skin issue. "I have no idea, all I know is that I was adding in what was needed." The queen regularly demonstrates such insight. Rather than inquire about patients' complaints, for instance, she screens them initially by simply looking or feeling with her hands at a distance before asking them to fill in the gaps with specific details about injuries, surgeries, medications, and symptoms. Her diagnostic language is frequently biomedical (To a man, once: "Your cholesterol is at 7.9. Eat carrots in the morning. Carrots lower cholesterol. And shed some kilograms. Good-bye!").

She would ask patients to confirm her diagnosis with medical technology, but she could also get offended if they were to consult a medical doctor without her prior consent. Yet she keeps some patients in the dark about the nature of their disorder and will not always disclose the expected length of the treatment. Not infrequently, she will claim to have detected health conditions that have eluded clinical attention. Diagnostic images that she draws in her patient's record depict faithful copies of biomedical topography as often as unruly, squiggly anatomies and flows. The queen's idiosyncratic bodily depictions do not present a system that is alternative or complementary to the skeletal–muscular–visceral anatomy of biomedicine. In fact, the queen references, problematizes, and contradicts biomedical facts as well as her own medical inventions. She produces knowledge and undoes it from one moment to the next, affecting powerful experiences but unsettling their interpretation. Without epistemic consistency or unquestioned belief, any certainty collapses around the queen, like a patient's chest, sighing in exasperation at her inventive play. The queen once defiantly laughed at her people: "You believe every [word] I say when you shouldn't!" On the other hand, she will not let others take her lightly, even if it is not always clear when she is joking. A visit to the queen is disquieting precisely because one is in imminent danger of violating codes and transgressing boundaries that are unknown, unpublicized, and constantly shifting. This is why patients earnestly ask for guidance, for some fixed prescriptions and general recommendations to hang onto.

"How do we know in general what is good and not good to wear?" someone once asked the queen, hoping she would develop a theory out of the many prohibitions she regularly issues, alarmingly or impatiently: she criticized one woman for wearing a bracelet that resembled a rosary and had her remove it; she screamed at another for painting her nails black ("Don't you know that black and brown nail polish are bad for you?"); she found fault with the number of beads on a patient's necklace and yanked one trinket off ("The count of eight is proper only for the deceased! The living should use nine or seven or five") and upon closer examination found it dangerous to wear ("Do you know what this is? This is for Buddhists! The Chinese, who have made it, are screwing around with everyone! Whenever you buy something, look carefully. I wouldn't buy it.").

However, when people, the anthropologist included, expect the queen to elaborate her advice on life and health, she only amplifies the confusion. She plays along, issuing generalizations that are inoperable and inconclusive. For instance, the queen once developed a universal, color-coded, weekly dress plan. She, who otherwise insists on the idiosyn-crasies of bodies and illnesses ("no two women are the same"), on par-ticularities of local biologies ("acupuncture is good, but only works for Chinese bodies"), and of fates ("why is it that I drive an Audi and my assistant a Fiat?"), has spelled out a generic theory of life cycles figured in the colors of a rainbow, which translate into dressing tactics: yellow Mondays, blue Tuesdays, green Wednesdays, and red Thursdays.[2] Since Fridays begin the cycle, she says, they should be yellow again. Saturdays should be green like Wednesdays, and Sundays, the week's end, should be met in violet. Black should never be worn and white only to a funeral, explained this same woman wearing a white shirt on a Tuesday and orange pants, a color off the rainbow map.

BODIES OF EVIDENCE

The queen's inconsistencies do not discredit her power as much as baffle her patients and discourage any attempts at systematization. She exag-gerates, muddles, and retracts claims, making any simple "belief" or knowledge likewise impossible. Her impulsiveness invites scrutiny, and while she seems to enjoy the unsettling, she also demands her patients' loyalty and trust, without producing conventional conditions for it: she does not explain her therapeutic proceedings, illness categories, or the logic and length of the treatment. Even questioning her about symptoms and side effects can get one into trouble or yield unhelpful answers.

All this uncertainty and epistemological fluidity notwithstanding, both the queen and her patients are deeply invested in material and ex-periential evidence. They point to the queen's diagnostic insight, her ability to register subtle discomforts that evade biometrics as well as read disorders in the idiom of medical technology: "65, 45, and 75 per-cent—that's how much your main heart arteries are blocked. Go to a doctor for an ECG [electrocardiogram] to confirm it," she told a man in his late fifties, who had traveled from the Serb Republic to see her. To a first-time visitor, a silent young woman, she said, "you are feeling pain in your stomach, you have frequent [vaginal] discharge and migraines." To a father who accompanied his daughter with undisclosed mental-health issues she stated, after a brief examination, that the girl "gets possessed with uncanny strength, becomes violent, and starts swearing" (as the man nodded silently in agreement). The queen regularly performed, and patients reverently recounted, her ability to affect palpable bodily transformations and to sense other people's sensations or cravings ("be patient now, this will make you lightheaded," she often warns patients in her office or tells them, "endure, this will hurt" or "thinking coffee, aren't you? I'll order some to be brought for you"). Most of all, the queen and her people stressed the importance of biographical evidence of her therapeutic success. She opens a record for each patient and updates it periodically with notes on their recovery. Notebooks filled with patients' histories occupy an entire bookshelf in her office and while the data is not catalogued in any obvious way she navigates the archive with ease.

IN THE QUEEN'S HANDS

It is Monday, August 6, 2006. The traffic of visitors is heavy, typically so for the summer when the queen's regular patients are joined by seasonal ones on a break from life and work abroad in Europe, North America, or Australia. As people move in and out of treatment, four people remain in the queen's office, receiving her protracted therapeutic attention. One has accompanied her daughter, a pharmacy student in her early twenties, whom the queen has directed on and off the couch for the forty minutes since I have been here. This is the young woman's first visit. She turned to the queen after a year of suffering a range of symptoms, including nervousness and limb numbness, that medical practitioners whom she consulted could neither define nor treat adequately. A neuropsychiatrist whom she saw last in a public health clinic diagnosed her with a panic disorder and prescribed antidepressants. Three months into the drug therapy, she felt no difference. All the tests that she took, including an EEG and a CT, showed nothing abnormal. Beneath the queen's hands, the student reports feeling nausea and a burning sensation in her stomach. Her mother also looks nervous and discomfited. In the course of the treatment, the queen attends to both women, explaining that the mother is implicated in her daughter's illness and that the daughter's recovery depends on her mother's health. The queen's practice more generally reiterates the point that there exists an effective contiguity between near family members, whose ailments are not discrete affairs but somehow etiologically interrelated. As the young woman's mother is getting up from the couch, looking somewhat unstable, the queen tells her: "Your blood pressure is high, 195 over 125. For two and a half years now, you've been having fainting spells. That's because you get your organism so upset. So, eat onion and *ciao*, for now. But go easy or you'll fall down."

Among the lingering patients is a beautiful young woman who lives in Germany, shadowing a child unsure on his legs and walking in jerky steps backwards and forwards. Queen: "Watch the child, he'll fall down! If he falls down.... Watch his back!... He's getting weak now because I'm working him, watch him, watch him closely. The queen sums up the woman's previous visits on behalf of the child: "First she was saying [feigns whimpering] 'will he walk?' and now he walks and she's asking 'will he talk?'" The child's mother tells us how her husband thought her mad for bringing the child to the queen, while she was confident that she had arrived at the right place, finally, to someone real, having already "taken him everywhere" to no avail. "To take someone everywhere" registers an urgent quest for a medical cure that expands one's search inside and outside the biomedical establishment (see chapter 4). Given that this family has lived in Germany since the 1990s, this health pursuit started in German clinical centers and extended across Bosnia in search of conventional, traditional, alternative, and magical treatments. "I only doubted a little," says the woman, but the queen fires back, though in good humor: "Why are you lying? You didn't believe me! I wouldn't have believed me either. The child was completely immobile; how could you have expected him to start walking.... He was a plant, a plant! Only Allah can do that. You should thank him every hour."

If it were not for the queen, the child's mother tells me, her hands still outreached toward the boy's back, she would have gone crazy. Soon after birth, her son was diagnosed with CHARGE syndrome and the German doctors she consulted suggested drug therapies and physical exercise while making it clear that these could only ameliorate a life-long condition of mental and physical disability. When they brought the boy to the queen, the mother says, he was "like a doll," barely moving except for his head, bobbing uncontrollably back and forth. He was constantly crying, which, the queen explained, was due to the pain between his shoulder blades. "But I worked on that child out of spite," the queen says, "to prove to his father how wrong he was [to doubt me]. I made progress in just ninety days! According to the medicine and everything else he should have started walking when he was nine, but I worked on him fast."

The first signs of improvement, the boy's mother says, occurred two to three months after the first treatment. She noticed that he was holding his head better. That winter they came back to the queen for four consecutive treatments: "When he started walking, it was a miracle. When the doctors saw him back in Germany they said, 'It's a miracle,' they couldn't believe it. And they didn't like it when they heard that we took him to Bosnia for therapy. The doctors also proposed a hearing-aid implant, but the queen told us that he doesn't need it, he hears already, and she's still working on his hearing. The queen told us that he'll go to school, like a normal kid." The queen here, typically, begins joking, toning down the emotion rising in the woman's voice, making the whole scene more comfortable though no less moving for that: the story is perfectly compelling, the child obviously walking, the promises hang in the air that he will walk to school, the mother's disbelief and adoring gratitude against the biomedical professional skepticism, invoked in the exemplary figures of German, quintessentially "Western" doctors. All together, the scene is full of invitations to ponder the strangeness of what may be believable, curable, and real.

TOUCHING WITHOUT TOUCHING

The queen touches patients without touching with her hands. In her office, beneath her dancing hands or merely in her presence, patients report various sensations: swaying and dizziness, trickles of warmth or prickly currents of needles and pins down their limbs, release of pain, muscle relaxation, calming or energetic joy. Still further, at a distance of thousands of miles, in different time zones and on different continents, the queen's patients feel her powerful intervention, before finding Facebook messages alerting them to her planned treatment. Her therapeutic power puts into an ethnographic play questions that Jean-Luc Nancy—and Jacques Derrida writing on Nancy in *On Touching* (2005)—raise about the phenomenology and the common sense of contact. I mention Nancy throughout this text, but here I want him to take us to the far limits of his imagination, where the intangibility of tactile sense delivers a soul. In short, with Nancy, Derrida, and the queen I want to ask what does any touching touch and how? Together they make us wonder whether touching is even possible between fleshy surfaces pressing into one another, and whether it grasps anything beyond the presumed presence of the other. Can anyone be properly accessible and readily held? And if the surfaces are not exactly tangible and the other's presence does not easily fill up one's eager hands, then what is touchable and how *does* one touch without touching in any ordinary sense? Finally, what is it that senses the senses touching? I want to bring together Nancy's and Derrida's philosophical investigation with the ethnographic insights of the queen's practice. The post-structural philosophers proceed with precepts about the mind and the body, although doubting their universal explanatory power, and so presuming some radical alterity, some alien, non-Western bodies and psyches that would be subject to other rules of contact. As Nancy puts it: "not a single one of *their* words tells us anything about *our* body." (2008a:7) and Derrida similarly writes that we do not know what touching or kissing means outside home, the "West." The queen rejects universalizing theoretical attempts but exercises power that claims to intervene indiscriminately and universally: nothing is foreign to it, no one could resist its appeal, it requires neither epistemological consent nor a heartfelt belief. The queen's power works at a distance while her theory regularly upsets Western as well as local expectations of the real. If the two philosophers are daring, the queen's over the top, but the philosophical and therapeutic imagination curiously converge around the idea of bodies in surfaces and extensions, and of touching as always presuming a distance.

Nancy seeks to upset foundational ideas of "primal interiority" and of the plenitude of presence that has defined phenomenological and lay thought on touching. In other words, he reacts against the assumption that touch is the most literal of the senses, grasping the other, undeniably, physically here, in one's hand, the iconic limb of touching. Skin is usually seen as the prime surface of the encounter between the self, hidden inside and others, outside. Skin-to-skin contact is presumed to bring most fully together the touching subjects, to abolish distance and realize an intimate closeness in an amicable, coital, marital, or communal union. Skin is thought to be the proverbial surface, the opposite of profundity, a site ruled by social conventions and aesthetic norms, the reverse of an authentic inside. Emerging with a historically cultivated distinction between public and private, skin is evidently the modern man's obsession; as James Joyce quipped, "Modern man has an epidermis rather than a soul" (quoted in Connor 2004:9). A number of contemporary social thinkers on skin seem to agree that skin has never been more visible, never more anxiety-inducing, never so enticing to think or tinker with (see Jablonski 2006; Benthien and Dunlop 2002; Connor 2004). These recent texts are valuable explorations of evolutionary and cultural history of the tactile sense, cultural sensibilities that envelop it, politics of difference that surround it, as well as of the psychology and psychoanalysis of subject formation.

Nancy, however, thinks touch differently. He begins by thinking bodies in terms of spatial extension. Nancy's body is all on the surface, feeling itself on the outside, handling the skin, which is at once a point of encounter and a limit to appropriation. "I" am no more fixed here beneath my fingertips than you are fully, firmly fixed with my poking finger. My sense of self is disseminated in thinking and feeling, already removed from the proclaimed "I" the moment I opened my mouth. As Nancy puts it in *Corpus*: "Bodies are first and always other—just as others are first and always bodies" (2008a:29). In other words, body is the central medium of contact since subjects are embodied by default, but bodies are contiguous, not identical with selves, and are also foreign and distant, even if our physical presence in the world hinges on them. It follows that contact is also an experience of distance and displacement of both self and the other, neither of which are fully here and now as much as also elsewhere. Touching feels that there is no immediate nor interior presence, finds the distance that always remains in contact.

Nancy rereads Aristotle's treatise *On Soul*, which deals with the problem of touching. For Aristotle, all living bodies have souls, which is to say that they have particular forms of life. Living bodies have tangible properties that are extended in space as well as intangible ones, extended inward. Body and soul are in union to the point that soul (a life form) is inseparable from material form, which it animates and defines. Nevertheless, Aristotle distinguishes the nonbodily parts or potencies of soul (such as thinking, contemplating, or sensing) that are in the body but not of the body, and as such are unextended and untouchable. Touching in particular shows the curious ways in which the Aristotelian body–soul union is at once touchable and intangible, extended and withdrawn, bodily and not. Touching prods the sensible faculty that senses the other senses sensing (and senses itself) but it itself cannot touch, cannot be touched except indirectly via the body, and cannot affect itself without external stimuli. What we grope for in touching, then, following Aristotle, is the soul, this untouchable faculty, sensing the world, sensing the body sensing, and self-sensing. And it is the soul, the sensible untouchable, that eludes the grasp. In short, in Aristotle's understanding of touching, senses participate in the perception of the external world, and flesh is the medium of touch, but an inner organ or faculty of perception provides a coherence to all sensing, discriminates among the sensory materials, and feels the senses sense.

Nancy picks up the contradiction of touchable and untouchable at the point of contact but he dislodges Aristotle's "untouchable" inner sensitivity from the depths of the body onto the surface, into the open. At the same time, Nancy opens up the body, extends it across space, surface next to surface. Body and soul are all exposed. This openness, extension, and exposition, which make a body, are precisely the body's other, which is the soul,[3] whose form is extended along the body's extensions. Soul, for Nancy, is body's idea of itself as being all on the outside, and not only in the sense that my face is always facing another but also in that I am touching myself from the outside and on the surface, fingertips pressed to the skin or tending to the finer surfaces of the body gaping open in a wound (2006:25, 128). Because psyche or soul is spatially extended along the body, it too is a body of sorts.

However, the superficiality and exposition of bodily being does not render it more properly touchable. On the contrary, touching only skims the surface, the skin, which is the limit at which a groping hand can handle the other. No matter how close two or more beings are, no matter how much caressing, consuming, or sharing takes place between them, they are spaced apart. But for Nancy, this spacing is not a gap that precludes intimacy. On the contrary, the other and the self are most effectively "there" in the evasion, on the verge of departure (ibid., 33). The apart-ness is the conduit for closeness, achieved through affect or exchange. Without the space between, two would be self-same, would consume each other to the point of nondistinction, their mutual annihilation. Touching does not intervene, Nancy suggests, does not tamper or tear; in touching "nothing gets through" (2008a:11). Because tangible and intangible equally elude touching and are accessible only at a distance, every body, therefore, is untouchable.

Distance is integral to Nancy's thought as much as it is to the queen's healing. The queen's touch, however, indeed "goes through" and effec-tively reaches across space to grasp all kinds of "insides" usually thought of as untouchable: gut, blood pressure, heart arteries, spinal vertebrae, moods, or nerves. Her hands count on a certain superficiality of the bod-ies, extended at the level with the skin, remotely accessible. The queen profoundly alters the body and being of her patients. If the law of her therapeutic touch is distance, the condition of the bodies she treats—and as we shall see, of her own body—is a risky extensity and permeability.

FACTS AT HER FINGERTIPS; GRASPING

The queen not only touches without touching, but also "sees" remotely. Her vision, however, regularly confuses the senses. Just as in her office she often demonstrates that her hands "see" disorders and "read" them in precise metrics, so does her vision grope for the absent bodies and touches them. Or is it her eyes that extend the grasp of her hands to peel the bodily surfaces and watch-touch closely at the living organs maintaining life? Her insight is not only anatomical: she also sees the biographical and existential circumstances of the body in examination, and feels convoluted histories and pathways of pain.

It is in the queen's living quarters, after hours, that I hear the most about her distended vision. After a long day in her office, in May 2007, the queen invites me upstairs to talk. A butterfly printed across her shirt sheds sequins all over her neck and arms. The queen glitters in the sub-dued light of her little bedroom. I am listening:

"You see, my gaze always stands out. 'The gaze of her eyes' people say about me. No one can understand my eyes. I'll show it to you; maybe it will be easier to explain." In excitement, the queen runs off barefoot to get a book from another room and is back with a fat volume of illustrated anatomy. "You see," she says, "I study all of this. I know it already by looking alone, without the book, but I like to confirm that I'm right." She flips pages impatiently to effect a blur of images: bones, muscles, organs, tissues, veins, and nerves, before singling out an image of the spine: "Imagine that you are piercing this, and then [the cerebral fluid] goes out, drip by drip. The person is finished. His backbone starts drying up. And doctors do it all the time. You see, all these [illustrations] are from dead bodies, but can you imagine that I see all of this? I see it alive. Every nerve is connected, you can touch organs by touching these," she says, tapping her finger at an illustration of nerves that innervate the thighs. "You can do it yourself." The queen thus gives an anatomy lesson not intended by the medical textbook in her lap: body exposed and accessible in surfaces, each of which effectively leads to another: skin to nerves to viscera.

I ask how she sees multiple patients at the same time or at a distance. "Just like I'm looking through the window now and seeing seven kinds of trees," the queen replies. "Do you see that I see them? But I see them faster than you do. Because I have a gaze more powerful than anyone else's. For me, it's all within a matter of seconds. I experience every human [*doživljavam svakog insana*]. I experience, feel, and see every pore in every moment. . . . When I look at you I see circumstances at your home, I see who is having a good life, who's tranquil, who's nervous. I see their brains. The brain is water, all of that is liquid, little tubes, . . . it's not flesh, not a solid matter which it becomes in touch with air. I see where the ailments are coming from. Someone may complain of pain here [pointing to her stomach], but I see that the pain comes from here, from the spine. I sense who did what [treatment] before because you can feel everything. I have a stronger field of vision than anyone else in the world. The strongest. But it can disappear in one second. I used to ask myself, did I make this up?"

Her vision splinters, too. Another afternoon in the same room, we are having coffee. I am looking at the queen, seated cross-legged across from me, while the queen is looking at her reflection in a round table mirror. In fact, she tells me, she is looking beyond the mirror image, at two young women at the same time, one in the nearby city of Tuzla and the other in Denmark. Both women, the queen explains, are suicidal, consuming antidepressants, and as of recently, receiving her care at a distance. Looking at her eyes thus reflected, the queen explains, doubles her vision and her power. Sometimes the queen reaches her patients via photographs, especially if she never met them in person but has agreed to treat them at a distance at the urging of their spouses, friends, and relatives. She treats a privileged few via Facebook, looking at their profiles. Of course, I wonder what her eyes—if indeed her eyes—are seeing, if indeed seeing, beyond the visible, and how. And why is it that our conventions of spatial distance scramble under her gaze?

For Nancy, in fact, a scrambling of senses is a given. He thinks of touch as a haptic ambition of all senses as well as of the sense that "makes sense" of sensations, that ponders. To perceive is to grasp and in grasping vision sees "with *touches* from other senses, smells, tastes, timbres, or even, with sounds, from the senses of words" (2008a:47). In short, Nancy proposes a vision that coincides with its objects, sees not what is visible "Because we would see nothing of this body here if we only saw it in the pure visibility of its presentation" (45) nor what is hidden beneath the appearances but sees all the many fragments that gather and disperse to make up a living being. It is a peculiar vision of "an eye planted in the swerve of being" (45), appropriate to the busyness of constant expositions of existence and departures and displacement of the being groped for.

Nancy's mysticism is partly a provocation: the philosopher says as much in his discussion on the soul (2008a:122), a certain "interruption" of the discourses on the body with an incorporeality. He is reacting against the long-standing Cartesianism in biomedical and much of folk understandings of body and health; he does so by deliberately avoiding the term *mind* that calls to mind the binary division between mind and body. Nancy's soul is neither Freud's psyche, inwardly extended into the unconscious, nor Descartes's mind, severed from the body, nor is it a theological, transcendental category. Rather, Nancy turns to Aristotle's idea of the soul as an articulated form of existence, particular to the given body, which renders the soul material, "but a different matter, without place, size, or weight" (151). But Nancy goes further still to depict the soul as a bodily matter. According to him, forms of embodied life are so many different souls: "Body's simply a soul. A soul, wrinkled, fat or dry, hairy or callous, rough, supple, cracking, gracious . . ." (152). So body, for Nancy, already tangles up the material and the metaphysical, while perception, visual as much as tactile, entails a further meeting between tangible and intangible that takes place in the open: "When I look at extension and the extension is extended to my eyes, then an emotion and an extension touch one another. . . . The mind is then moved . . . even into extension and [the extension] is extended all the way to the mind. . . . The soul is then touched" (144).[4] This is how the incorporeal spatializes and gains tangibility, but also how a body (perceived and perceiving) interrupts the sense/soul. Touching is the exposition of the soul, of the sense of sensing and of thought, making sense, in such a way that the incorporeal fully participates in the material and meddles with it, to the point that both are extended in touching the world.

Furthermore—and this is where Nancy gets us even closer to imagining Queen's touch—while body is limited in space to a place, the incorporeal extension is potentially infinite, can stretch as far and as long as does the thinking. But because the soul/thought/psyche is inseparable from the physical body, it is the body that is extended infinitely in this motion of experiencing.

GIVING: PSYCHE, BRAIN, SELF

The queen's is obviously a curious vision, one that mixes up the sense of sight with other senses and potencies. Like "the eye planted in the swerve of being," the queen's seeing, in her own words, "experiences every patient down to the every pore of their body." Hers is a "sight" that "experiences" (*doživljava*), undergoes a close and empathetic encounter with another, while at the same time fragmenting him, zooming in too closely, down to "every pore in every moment," without losing the grasp on the whole. "Did I make this up?" she wonders aloud.

The queen herself often attributes her haptic vision to another faculty of sensation. She speculates that her therapy works by the means of "psyche" (psiha) or at times she simply names the anatomical point: the brain (mozak). This vagueness is typical for the queen. But if we allow the possibility that she is speaking from the standpoint where distinctions among matter, brain, and psyche/mind make no practical difference, we are left to imagine just how physical and intangible, biological and mental cooperate in contact.

Furthermore, the queen folds both brain and psyche under the concept of the self when she says "it is myself that I give." Her gaze thus implanted in others, she gives. Of course, *psyche* in the psychoanalytic and philosophical tradition is also a conception of *self*, but for the queen *self* is thingly, alienable, and bodily, extended and divisible so it can be given and received. While Nancy dreams of contact that respects and preserves the distance, the queen relies on the touch that touches the entire other's being, in its minute details and fragments—pores, blood cell counts, enzymes, heart rates—interfering, coinciding to the point where she feels what her patients feel. "Every illness you've got, I too go through," she says; "I wouldn't be able to help you otherwise." Searching, groping, feeling, the queen recruits a radical form of empathy to work on others. This affective contiguity must be managed at times. She asks her patients to abstain from pharmaceuticals prior to her visit because drugs in their bodies interfere with her work and "poison" her. She refuses to treat alcoholics because, she says, their intoxication intoxicates her. In summer 2012, she attributes the redness on the skin of her arms to traces of psoriasis on a ten-year-old patient whom she treated earlier that day. And after a day of work she typically points to her abdominal swelling that persists for hours: she says that her stomach receives her patients' ailments.

Nancy thinks of contact as sharing, a relationship that is uneconomic and symmetrical, between equals who preserve their differences. The queen's empathic contact, however, persuasively reminds us of the power inherent in a bodily encounter and paints contact as a contagious, yet unequal exchange. It is the queen who gives overwhelmingly, though she is not immune to the patient's influences. And yet she is drawn into the exchange, and she too is subject to it—obliged to give as well as to receive, and regularly giving too much: "I give too much of myself to others," the queen often complains. Or as she sometimes puts it: "I spend myself too much [*previše se trošim*]." How does one give oneself, though? And how does one give self excessively, and in the excess of what? I want to listen the queen's words, issued at this significant and exceptional site of healing for clues they broadcast about popular economy more generally.

WE ARE ALL CAPITALISTS: SURVIVING

In the course of the working day, money piles up in the corner of the queen's table, although she quotes no price for treatment and ignores the giving hands. Some patients leave nothing, others furtively drop scrunched, threadbare local konvertible marks or else deliberately spread out crisp euros; no gesture draws the queen's attention. The queen is known to refuse the money offered to her: she stops the bills in mid-air or returns them from the pile (she gives a bill back to one grandma, shouting: "Screw the Mark!"). On her terrace, one summer day in 2007, she explains: "I don't ask [for money]. People just give me what they want. I ask for nothing. There are times when I see that they've borrowed money to pay me and I tell them, no, don't be mad, take that back to your neighbor [who lent it]. Why do you give it to me? I tell them, look, you paid money already [for transportation] to come and see me, 10 KM here and 10 KM back; you're spending money, why don't you help yourself instead? Sometimes I give them [money] for food, when I see that they don't have. But all of this, all of this is built by the people. They built it for me."

The queen herself seems to spend very little and then mostly on inexpensive clothes available at the open-air markets. She dresses carefully and flamboyantly, often in fashions gifted to her by returning patients who know her sizes as well as the colors she favors at the moment.

Whatever it is that the queen gives, her giving is in excess of calculation, of computing that minds the incomes and outcomes, concerns itself with the balance of positive numbers that promise security and futurity: a stash to count on in case of trouble, a firm foundation from which to plan the use and disposal of resources. The queen receives and passes money with no regard for its potential to accumulate, appreciate, or transform into capital or a hoard. She does not save. She spends and gives with a marked indifference toward property. She takes things lightly, showing comfort with the impermanence that trails all human effort at having, keeping, and enjoying: "All this might disappear," she says motioning around her room, one day: "I'm just afraid of being hungry." She prudently arranges a planting and harvesting of her own wheat, just in case.

And yet, the queen does not downplay the importance of money. On the contrary. She often comments on the economy of the new historical present, regretting that "everything now has come down to the market [*sve se svelo na tržište*]." She troubles this new market logic by refusing to profit from her practice, but her gift-minded routine also demonstrates the fact that "market" in Bosnia nowadays presumes traffic of money, commodities, as well as gifts. She finds these broadly economic affairs inseparable from the state of one's health. In her own words: "A Bosnian needs money and he'll be healthy. The fact that there is no money, that he owes all over the place, that he has not [money] is ruining his health." Other times she makes it clear that the connectedness of health and wealth is universally valid: "The people of Bosnia live in a cramp. They have stomach cramps, which they have caused themselves.... And people are concerned with surviving not only in Bosnia, but everywhere on the planet: in Germany, in America, in Australia." She concludes that "Everything always comes down to finances. . . . We are all capitalists. From me to you."

I TOO AM HUMAN: INDEBTED

Whether the queen refuses or takes the offerings, she indebts her patients infinitely. No gift can be taken lightly, as ethnographers of giving–taking around the world have argued since Marcel Mauss. Taking on debts obliges the receiving party to reciprocate, to give back and to give better. In the meantime, the unreciprocated gift burdens the recipient with a felt obligation. Taking the queen's gift of self is particularly burdensome considering that she gives what cannot be paid nor properly returned. As she often reminds her patients: "I give myself for you; it is my self I'm giving." Or another way she puts it: "I'm giving myself so that someone else survives." I asked her once if there is anything that people can do in return for what she does for them, whether they can *odužit se,* settle their debt. The expression *odužit se* signals returning gifts that exceed monetary calculation, which is to say returning splendidly in a way that corresponds to the gesture of giving and obliges in turn. "No, there is no such money," the queen simply says, denying the adequacy of money and, at the same time, rejecting the possibility that any other act or thing could potentially compare with or approximate her gift.

It is obvious to her patients that the queen cannot be given anything that she needs, craves, or cares to have. Her gift always exceeds yours and the indifference with which she takes, your gratitude or your money, is such that you might get in trouble with her whether you give or withhold, when you calculate how much is reasonable to give ("I hear them thinking, should I give 20 or 30 or 10?") or you give unreasonably much, running into debts to pay her, with the fact that she finds out and refuses ("You should only give within limits," I listened to her explain. "You give as much as you have; not more than what you have," the queen tells me; "most people give 10 or 20 [Marks]"). In the culture that is marked by a certain tendency toward inordinate generosity (see chapter 2), perhaps the only adequate response to the queen's overexpenditure of self is to give excessively, above one's means, overextending oneself until it troubles or hurts, or in other words compromises the subject. But the queen prevents such acts, recommending prudence, and so remains the supreme giver in her domain.

And yet, "I too am indebted [*i ja sam dužna*], like everyone else," the queen told us once in her office, "I too am human." Indebtedness, as the queen describes it, is the human condition in contemporary Bosnia. Thus the queen, whose extraordinary gifts of touch, vision, and excessive generosity make her a people's queen, nevertheless stakes her membership too in the human community, divulging her debts. She too is in need of scarce money, available mostly through informal borrowing or personally negotiated deferred payments and promises: to the construction company, electricians, plumbers, painters, to the home improvement dealers, and such. For even the queen who is otherwise so strangely carefree about money and property, and is so unencumbered by worldly ambitions to possess, who proclaims that she is "ready to die," and who predicates her healing and living on this disowning of attachments to things and people; even she is caught up in market debt. Nonetheless, her professed money debts inadvertently remind patients further that she may not care for money but that she could use some.

HAVING STUMBLED UPON FATE

I searched for the queen following stories and footsteps of so many health travelers to and from her village, proverbially far away. When I faced a woman on a terrace of a yellow house (then under construction), in tight white clothes and red rubber boots with yellow duck images printed on them, hosing carpets, I did not yet know I had found the Queen of Health. Only when she grew tired of teasing me, and agreed to talk—for no obvious reason, since my research description failed to impress her—I learned that our appointment had already been made: "It was fate that we should meet," the queen explained. Apparently, I arrived right where I was supposed to, next to the queen, listening, licking an ice cream that her young assistant brought for us. Over the course of my weekly visits in 2007, the queen would repeat to the audience of her patients: "I looked into her future and allowed her to write," sometimes adding a reason: "So that the world knows that there once existed such a woman. Because that book will remain." If fate has kindly made arrangements for me to write, the process of visiting and observing the queen practice, and the trials of writing in the years since, did not guarantee that I would get this far: it was rough. I too was the subject of her fickle, tactless power, an object of ridicule and criticism. It took years for me to feel the queen's more tender attention, and when I did I almost regretted it. This may sound perverse, but it was easier to bear her abuses than her infinitely obliging generosity, her sweetness, her undeniable, irrepressible closeness. Then there was the feeling of indebtedness—under what conditions could an anthropologist escape it? Transantlantic distance ensured no forgetting, years passing depreciated no negative balances in my favor. There was nothing I could properly give in turn, and the text I was long producing promised to disappoint her; at best it failed properly to describe her and at worst it offended the queen, and her patients, by running off on apparently irrelevant tangents of interest to academic readers only. Let alone the detour to the forms of Koranic curing that she found so vehemently irritating.

Her patients worried whether I was up to the task, and they offered leads: beginnings, conclusions, as well as evidence. "You should begin your book like this," said a man who survived liver cancer "thanks to the queen and the queen alone," "like this: 'In a place where there are many [healers], there is only one person with a real gift to do good.'" The queen, too, planned "my book" from the opening lines to the cover design. "Your book is good for nothing if no one reads it. You need to think about the book covers, how to draw people to it. Do not have it in black nor in gray; those are too dark and too depressing. People will pick it up and drop it down," she said on the first day we met. Thinking, smoking, in silence she got an idea: "The best would be to have your book in the colors of a rainbow. There's not a single book in the world with the colors of the rainbow. It says light will come after dark. That way both believers and nonbelievers will read it. It will be a book not for just some nationalities but for all the people. Also, you should write directly, without an introduction. You have to attract people; I know this, believe me. Now, don't talk about darkness of life right away. You have to introduce it a bit." The queen laughs: "I end up being your consultant. Because people always have to be attracted somehow. I know because I can penetrate into people's brains. Then you have to think of the colors in which you will paint all of us who are [medically] working. Warm words are made of warm colors. You too, when you are writing, do not give people a puzzle but the truth. You will be world-famous with your book. With my knowledge, you will succeed."

In the summer of 2012, the queen gave me a gift: she pulled out of the closet a well-loved dress she had worn as a young woman in the 1980s. A little black dress with large prints of crimson hibiscus flowers and green leaves, that almost fit me. She insisted that I try it on and, confused and much moved, I kept it on while resuming our interview and recording, diligently, our conversation in a field notebook. Later, I often tried to write this chapter in her dress: the lengths I would take to write "responsively," not just responsibly (see the introduction), could seem playful rather than very productive or could be read more generously as mimetically powerful exercises that could achieve the embodiment of all kinds of sympathetic ties, that could achieve a thoroughly empathetic sense of the obligations I felt I owed to the queen and her following. I wanted my textual production to press against the fabric, the hems of the gift, to keep my skin as a background reminder of discomfiting ways in which the ethnographic and the writing subject-project sit with its powerful, irresistible, object-subject. Yet, as skilled readers of mimesis, the likes of Michael Taussig (1993) would point out, mimetic rituals of first and second contact between the object of power and conditions of its reproductions should not be meddled with—even experts have a hard time managing the course of possible efficacies and consequences. There is such a thing as too much ethnography and too much closeness, especially when the field, as research fields tend to be, holds such potential exuberance that no one involved quite knows its sources nor its limits. George Bataille, very much interested in pervasive and perverse expenditures that bind earthly economics with cosmic principles of supply and demand, thought about it in *The Accursed Share*. He writes: "Certainly, it is dangerous, in extending the frigid research of the sciences, to come to a point where one's object no longer leaves one unaffected, where, on the contrary, it is what inflames" (1998:10). Bataille thus introduces a general economy modeled on the sun's exuberance, whose giving he could no more escape than he could reciprocate. The rest of the quotation reads: "Indeed, the ebullition that animates the globe is also my ebullition. Thus, the object of my research cannot be distinguished from the subject at its boiling point. I could not personally resist effervescence" (ibid.). This irresistible contact, the messy coincidence, and contagious contiguity were the conditions of my ethnographic and quotidian being in the field and of my writing this text. It is with relief, though thoroughly affected and richer in debts that I am inching, desirously, toward the end. Dreaming of exits and closures, as if they spelled a better life.

READING

Bookstores and bookstands, whether explicitly Islamic or not, near a mosque or by a madrasa, carry a rich and growing selection of books on Islamic medicine, of all kinds: from herbal and api-therapy to Prophetic medicine to the prophylactic properties of ablutions (*abdest, ghusl*). Very many among them, however, address the problem of a cluster of illnesses that sit in the domains between the magical and the metaphysical and that are caused by *sihr*, a deliberate manipulation of nonhuman potencies with the aim of harming or helping; by various forms of accidental interferences by nonhumans, jinn in particular (*ograma, mess, nagaz*); by ill effects of desirous or covetous gaze (*urok*) as well as actively envious ill-wishing (*zavist*). Collectively, the books introduce the subjects, which they expect to strike the readers as less than credible, as confusing, daunting, and unfamiliar, perhaps fascinating or experientially only too familiar. The authors count on the latter group of readers who might be suspecting the case of such disorder, whether for themselves or for the near and dear, weathering or recovering from such ailments. There is a redundancy here that seems not to bother the publishers nor the readers, judging by the reported sales in a place where books are no longer among the hot staples of market exchange, although some authors are precisely reacting to such overabundance, worrying that it may be obscuring and further confusing.

What one picks up from these books is a short introduction to Islamic metaphysics and a brief, instructional history of universal magic and magic in Islam, but the brunt of the texts are practically oriented: how to tell symptoms, how to find properly Islamic cures and, importantly, how to discriminate between efficacies: permissible, questionable, and forbidden.

It would not help, I think, to simply catalogue this reference literature under the heading of spiritual medicine. First because what these readings do, effectively, is to broaden the regional category of *duševne bolesti* (see chapter 5), which is the older but still current rubric that keeps together the ontological ambiguity of domains of *duh* (spirit), *duša* (soul), and *duševni* (of soul, of spirit) in the way that *psihička oboljenja*, maladies of the psyche, or *mentalne bolesti*, mental illnesses, resolve in favor of cleaner concepts, more legible in the global diagnostic and prescription technologies. Second, they do not simply elaborate on the precepts of Islamic faith in relation to pious body, ritual practice, and the world of purity and danger, but venture very particular, more or less elaborate, anatomies of human bodies composed of physical and intangible elements, of spirit and soul, mind, heart, and viscera, of earthly elements and elements that are transcendent. It is such a body, intricately related to all other existents and to the plural worlds—18,000 according to the Koran—that suffers and heals in ways that require medicinal attention to the composite at hand: flesh and skin, secretions and desires that manifest the reality of affliction and efficacy of cure. Third, the books themselves sport a number of genres but typically mix the educational with cautionary, advisory, and instructional, devotional with pragmatic: how to prepare herbal medicine, how to tell pure honey, how to recite particular Koranic *ayas* and suras in order to heal which host of symptoms, how to recruit the help of friends and family during illness and recovery, how to exercise a healthy suspicion toward advertised curers. Some of these books, by design or inadvertently, uncover the secrets of the sihir trade only too well, undressing the veiled contents of curative or harmful talismans and consumable inscriptions, to the point where they may offer instructions for reverse engineering to those so inclined. Others worry about being misconstrued as doing precisely that, and so start with a *dova* (from Arabic *dua*, supplication, see chapter 5) or on a personal note, explaining themselves.

U Ime Allaha Milostivog, Samilosnog (In the Name of Allah, Most Merciful and Compassionate), is how Vehid Pekarić begins his book, addressing first of all God, stating his good intentions (*ispravan nijet*) to help people follow the correct path and to write a book that will offer protection. The address itself may be flagged as a reminder to those of us sympathetic to Latour's quest for a language more "capable of absorbing the pluralism of values," an idiom that would "obtain more diversity in the beings admitted to existence" (2013:21). The gravity of the first address, the dutiful granting of the first address to the Divine in the audience, as well as the remainder of the contents of the manual that relies on the Koran, God's speech, to cure, suggests that we, scholars, twirling our fingers at new objects and new routes of inquiry into ontologies are not alone capable of such a capacious imagination, nor are we, perhaps, most adept, or perhaps entirely free, to proceed inventing from scratch a more elastic and receptive language. Isabelle Stengers, whom this book has recognized as exceptionally attuned to the opportunities and inconveniences of the new materialisms and cosmopolitical imaginations (see chapter 4), writes in response to the ready and easy academic citational fashions suggesting that we may also have to invoke other, more compromising voices. "It is academically fashionable to quote Spinoza today, but less so to recall that both religion and the craft of magic implied some knowledge of what language can do—of the power of words crafted to bless or kill, or save, or curse—of ritual or ancestral words" (2011:369).

That what is "more compromising" may be more globally recognizable as such, whether in North America or Bosnia, or may need some explaining—this much is obvious from the preface, preparing the reader for what is to come in the pages of Pekarić's book, published in 1998 by a small local press in northeastern Bosnian town of Gračanica. "This text is a bit unusual [*pomalo neobičan*], forwarding a theme that remained unknown to our wider public," writes a fellow imam in a foreword, adding that, nonetheless, the text has great practical value. "It points to the fact of existence of invisible, spiritual [*duhovnog*] world that is beyond the grasp of human senses." The preface presumes an incredulous public and reflects on the modern conditions of being a human that are at once bringing about a crisis in experience and in health and are sending people in search of alternative and traditional forms of knowledge. For his part, Pekarić proceeds with two precepts very popular in Bosnia (see chapter 4): that one has a duty to take care of one's health and that every illness has a cure but it must be searched for. He makes it clear that health presumes both body and soul, and raises the question that those of his readers most in need of practical advice are probably eagerly expecting "how to treat illnesses, how to find a cure, to whom to turn for help?" He then writes an apology on behalf of imams who have always been practicing forms of healing but whose skills have been prosecuted by the communists (who, nonetheless, have sought their help furtively, he adds), and are greatly misunderstood by the wider publics who have suspected imams *hodže*, of healing entrepreneurialism. In short, Pekarić gives four classes of medicines: herbal medicine, Koranic medicine, dhikr (remembrance of Allah), and duas (dove).

A book by Muharem Štulanović also starts by acknowledging the world of strangeness that the topic introduces, sited at the intersection between superstitions and religious truths; but really, he says, sihir happens. On a personal note, he narrates two key moments of his introduction into Koranic healing—one was an official discrediting of the theme itself he proposed for a thesis at the Faculty of Islamic Sciences and the other was his shock at the sheer mass of Bosnian patients who sought and responded to the medicinal recitations of selections of Koran by the Cairo professors of Koranic commentaries at the visiting Bosnian Islamic center in Vienna, where the imam Štulanović acted as a translator. It was the second experience, followed by the sheer pressure of the masses of Bosnians who sought Islamic curing, that convinced him to carry on with the practice and, eventually, to take it back to Sandžak in southwestern Serbia and elsewhere in the region. Štulanović, importantly, explains that the mass incidence of Bosnian illness complaints is logically related to the war circumstances that render a human particularly unstable—profoundly sad, angry, frightened, witnessing violence and suffering—and thus vulnerable to nonhuman infection. Eventually, it was the popular misunderstanding of the Koranic medicine, various superstitions, and the mass rise in all forms of professed healing, professional practitioners, and authoritative texts that convinced Štulanović, in his own words, to offer an explication of forms of healing that are in accordance with *shariat* (*šerijatski dozvoljeno*) as well as those that are suspicious and better avoided. Štulanović offers a sober, understated critique of contemporary forms of Koranic healing that are conducted professionally and commercially or that invest too much personal power in the figure of the healer. He is particularly keen on listing the ways to tell authentic Koranic healers from those who are not, whose powers are suspicious, and who themselves may be curing sihir by the same means—in association with occult powers, powers other than God's, and thus into poison. He references Hadith traditions to recommend the form of healing he clearly prefers: patients take up the task of themselves reciting medicinal Koran according to the three-stage healing process he describes, or, if they are unable, to turn to someone trained in Islamic sciences.

A book by Rijad Muhamed Semaha, translated as *Koranic Healing* from Arabic and published by the same small publisher in Gračanica, also in 1998, gives a few special insights, though it proceeds in a similar vein. Speaking from the grounds of another local milieu—contemporary Egypt—it observes the alarming rise in illnesses and the popular quests for cures everywhere, many of them futile. This is just one obvious reminder of the fact that the literature on Islamic medicine is only "tentatively" local: rather, they are pan-Islamic in their reading and referencing habits, transnational in their learning and expertise, and universalist in their metaphysical ambitions and knowledge claims. Semaha's book also gives a comprehensive, if brief, overview of the anatomy of physical and spiritual being, which is human: the anatomical lesson is also cosmological, connecting the constitutive elements of human to the elements found in nonhumans, including the planet earth. The book, like Štulanović's, recommends that the patient treats himself or herself or entrusts treatment to those who are loyal and dear. Finally, Semaha offers a classification of illnesses that helps clear "a great deal of possible confusion about what is Koranic medicine for: *duševne bolesti* or physical ones?" In a word, both, he says. His scheme resonates with the symptoms and diagnostic strategies that one finds disseminated elsewhere, including in Pekarić's and Štulanović's books, while trying to make explicit the logic that seems to be mixing physical symptoms, sensations of pain, and visible bodily manifestations (from pimples to impotence to cancer) with affective disorders, changes in personal habits and dispositions toward others, with illnesses that seem to have clear pathogens or lesions at work. In his three-partite etiology, illnesses can be purely physical, purely spiritual, or spiritual-physical where nonhuman interferences, through healing or curing or accident, can take any form.

Like most healing practices I described here, the manuals on Koranic healing and practical guides to recognizing illnesses caused by a host of uncanny causes and searching for the right cures are not exclusively bought nor read by practicing Bosnian Muslims. Rather, they are consulted by all those who might be concerned, having traveled widely across the medical terrain to find no cure, and having been convinced, or at least been ready to consider the possibility that their bodily beings might be stranger than they imagined. The major difference among the reading publics is that only Muslims well-grounded in the practice are likely to undergo treatment on their own: others, Muslim or not, use the books as reference while seeking expert help from imams or from otherwise established Koranic healers or healers whose wide therapeutic portfolio also incorporates select recitations from Koran (*ruk'ja,* Bosnian Arabicism). Moreover, imams' and Koranic healers' expertise attracts visitors from across ex-Yugoslavia and in their offices one finds patients from everywhere, from Slovenia to Montenegro. Signed impressions from one imam's guest book read as postcards from the region on tour. Nonetheless, established popularity and efficacy do not end the trouble with speculating that the three manuals I read here attempt to avoid: the question remains about who is the healer for real and what if he is not real? Those who pick up the manuals with the intention of cross-referencing bodily symptoms or personal or firsthand experience with authoritative descriptions of ontological possibilities may be profoundly unsettled. What flies off these open pages is not a picture of ontological plurality of the most ordinary world that is politically promising, composing a more inclusive collective and an agentive plenty, but, in principle, already assembled, stakes already divided, lines between harming and hurting, good and evil drawn out. What may sink in, turning these pages, is the sense that the reader, presumably new to the topic, is bumbling into a unfamiliar zone where very little, including one's body, can be taken for granted and where therapeutic efficacies may be both more accessible (best if you do it yourself, writes Štulanović) and more beyond the reach, obscured.

NOTES

1. Plural forms of Bosnian Arabicism for *ayat,* meaning "sign" as well as the smallest section of the Koran and *sura,* literally "form," designating a chapter of the Koran.

2. It goes like this: yellow is rebirth; blue is becoming, childhood, and self-awareness; green is youth and marriage; red is maturity, crisis in love life; violet is old age, financial crisis, death, the end of life and the fulfillment of life.

3. Nancy distinguishes between soul, as the form of body, mind as the force producing soul, and body which expresses the mind, "meaning that it makes it spurt outside . . . tosses it all outside" (2008a:157).

4. In one of Nancy's many unprofessed Bergsonisms, perception takes place in the world where the extensions of retina, optical sense (memory) of the object, and the object sensed meet.

REFERENCES

Alaimo, Stacy. 2010. *Bodily Natures: Science, Environment, and the Bodily Self.* Blooming-ton: Indiana University Press.

Applbaum, Kalman. 2006. "Educating for Global Mental Health: The Adoption of SSRIs in Japan." In *Global Pharmaceuticals: Ethics, Markets, and Practices*, edited by Adriana Petryna, Andrew Lakoff, and Arthur Kleinman, 85–110. Durham, NC: Duke University Press.

Aščerić-Todd, Ines. 2015. *Dervishes and Islam in Bosnia: Sufi Dimensions to the Formation of Bosnian Muslim Society.* Leiden: Brill.

Balorda, Janko. (1930) 1966. "Običaji Oko Smrti i Pogreba u Okolini Visokog." *Etnološka Gradja*, 391–396. Zagreb: Akademija Nauka i Umjetnosti Bosne i Herzegovine.

Bataille, George. (1954) 1998. *Consumption.* Vol. 1, *The Accursed Share.* Translated by Robert Hurley. New York: Zone Books.

———. 1988. *Inner Experience.* Translated by Leslie A. Boldt. New York: SUNY Press.

Bennett, Jane. 2013. "Thing-Power." In *Political Matter: Technoscience, Democracy, and Public Life*, edited by Bruce Braun and Sarah J. Whatmore, 35–63. Minneapolis: University of Minnesota Press.

Bennet, Jane, and William Connolly. 2012. "The Crumpled Handkerchief." In *Time and History in Deleuze and Serres*, edited by Bernd Herzogenrath, 153–171. London: Continuum.

Benthien, Claudia. 2002. *Skin. On the Cultural Border Between Self and World.* New York: Columbia University Press.

Berlant, Lauren. 2007. "Nearly Utopian, Nearly Normal: Post-Fordist Affect in *La Promesse* and *Rosetta*." *Public Culture* 19 (2): 272–301.

Bockman, Johanna. 2011. *Markets in the Name of Socialism: The Left-Wing Origins of Neo-liberalism.* Stanford, CA: Stanford University Press.

Boddy, Janice. 1989. *Wombs and Alien Spirits: Women, Men, and the Zar Cult in Northern Sudan.* Madison: University of Wisconsin Press.

Bogost, Ian. 2012. *Alien Phenomenology, or What It's Like To Be a Thing.* Minneapolis: University of Minnesota Press.

Bokovoy, Melissa K., Jill A. Irvine, and Carol S. Lilly, eds. 1997. *State–Society Relations in Yugoslavia, 1945–1992.* New York: St. Martin's.

Bourdieu, Pierre. 1984. *Distinction: A Social Critique of the Judgment of Taste*. London: Routledge.

———. 1990. *The Logic of Practice*. Stanford, CA: Stanford University Press.

———. 1997. "Marginalia—Some Additional Notes on the Gift." In *The Logic of the Gift: Toward an Ethic of Generosity*, edited by Alan Schrift, 231–241. London: Routledge.

Braun, Bruce, and Sarah J. Whatmore, eds. 2010. *Political Matter: Technoscience, Democracy, and Public Life*. Minneapolis: University of Minnesota Press.

Bridger, Sue, and Frances Pine. 1998. *Surviving Post-Socialism: Local Strategies and Regional Responses in Eastern Europe and the Former Soviet Union*. London: Routledge.

Bringa, Tone. 1995. *Being Muslim the Bosnian Way: Identity and Community in a Central Bosnian Village*. Princeton, NJ: Princeton University Press.

Burawoy, Michael. 1979. *Manufacturing Consent: Changes in the Labor Process Under Monopoly Capitalism*. Chicago: University of Chicago Press.

Burawoy, Michael, and Katherine Verdery, eds. 1999. *Uncertain Transitions: Ethnographies of Change in the Postsocialist World*. Lanham, MD: Rowman & Littlefield Publishers.

Cadena, Marisol de la. 2010. "Indigenous Cosmopolitics in the Andes: Conceptual Reflections beyond 'Politics.'" *Cultural Anthropology* 25 (2): 334–370.

Cain, Jennifer, Antonio Duran, Amya Fortis, and Elke Jakubowski. 2002. "Health Care Systems in Transition: Bosnia and Herzegovina." European Observatory on Health Care Systems. http://www.euro.who.int/__data/assets/pdf_file/0018/75132/E78673.pdf.

Chen, Mel. 2012. *Animacies: Biopolitics, Racial Mattering, and Queer Affect*. Durham, NC: Duke University Press.

Chu, Julie. 2010. *Cosmologies of Credit: Transnational Mobility and the Politics of Destination in China*. Durham, NC: Duke University Press.

Ćimić, Esad. 1970. *Socijalističko Društvo i Religija. Ispitivanje Odnosa Izmedju Samoupravljanja I Procesa Prevladavanja Tradicionalne Religije*. Sarajevo: Svjetlost.

Cohen, Ed. 2011. "The Paradoxical Politics of Viral Containment; or, How Scale Undoes Us One and All." *Social Text* 29, 1 (106): 15–35.

Comaroff, Jean. 1980. "Healing and the Cultural Order: The Case of the Barolong boo Ratshidi of Southern Africa." *American Ethnologist* 7 (4): 637–657.

Comaroff, Jean, and John Comaroff. 1999. "Occult Economies and the Violence of Abstraction: Notes from the South African Postcolony." *American Ethnologist* 26 (2): 279–303.

———. 2000. "Millennial Capitalism: First Thoughts on a Second Coming." *Public Culture* 12 (2): 291–343.

Connolly, William. "Materiality, Experience, and Surveillance." In *Political Matter: Technoscience, Democracy, and Public Life*, edited by Bruce Braun and Sarah J. Whatmore, 63–86. Minneapolis: University of Minnesota Press.

Connor, Steven. 2003. *The Book of Skin*. Ithaca, NY: Cornell University Press.

Cooper, Melinda. 2008. *Life as Surplus. Biotechnology and Capitalism in the Neoliberal Era*. Seattle: University of Washington Press.

Csordas, Thomas. 1994. *Embodiment and Experience: The Existential Ground of Culture and Self*. Cambridge: Cambridge University Press.

Danforth, Loring. 1989. *Firewalking and Religious Healing: The Anastenaria of Greece and the American Firewalking Movement*. Princeton, NJ: Princeton University Press.

Daston, Lorraine, ed. 1999. *Biographies of Scientific Objects*. Chicago: University of Chicago Press.

Daston, Lorraine, and Katherine Parker. 2001. *Wonders and the Order of Nature, 1150–1750*. New York: Zone Books.

Derrida, Jacques. 1967. *Of Grammatology*. Baltimore, MD: Johns Hopkins University Press.

———. 1992. *Given Time: I. Counterfeit Money*. Chicago: University of Chicago Press.

———. 1995. *The Gift of Death*. Chicago: University of Chicago Press.

———. 2005. *On Touching—Jean-Luc Nancy*. Stanford, CA: Stanford University Press.

Evans-Pritchard, E. E. 1976. *Witchcraft, Oracles, and Magic among the Azande*. Oxford: Oxford University Press.

Fabijanić, Radmila. 2004. "Zapisi, Hamajlije, i Moći od Pomoći. Odjeljenja za Etnologiju Zemaljskog Muzeja u Sarajevu." *Glasnik Zemaljskog Muzeja Bosne i Herzegovine* 46: 37–88.

Farquhar, Judith. 1996. "Market Magic: Getting Rich and Getting Personal in Medicine after Mao." *American Ethnologist* 23 (2): 239–257.

———. 2002. *Appetites: Food and Sex in Postsocialist China*. Durham, NC: Duke University Press.

Farquhar, Judith, and Qicheng Zhang. 2005. "Biopolitical Beijing: Pleasure, Sovereignty, and Self-Cultivation in China's Capital." *Cultural Anthropology* 20 (3): 303–327.

———. 2012. *Ten Thousand Things. Nurturing Life in Contemporary Beijing*. New York: Zone Books.

Favret-Saada, Jeanne. 1980. *Deadly Words: Witchcraft in the Bocage*. Cambridge: Cambridge University Press.

Filipović, Milenko. 1982. *Among the People: Native Yugoslav Ethnography—Selected Writings of Milenko S. Filipović*. Edited by E. A. Hammel, Robert S. Ehrich, Radmila Fabijanić-Filipović, Joel M. Halpern, and Albert B. Lord. Ann Arbor: University of Michigan Press.

Foucault, Michel. 1994. *Power*. Edited by James D. Faubion. New York: New Press.

Galbraith, John Kenneth. 1958. *Journey to Poland and Yugoslavia*. Cambridge, MA: Harvard University Press.

Geschiere, Peter. 1997. *The Modernity of Witchcraft: Politics and the Occult in Postcolonial Africa*. Translated by Janet Roitman and Peter Geschiere. Charlottesville: University of Virginia Press.

Gilbert, Drew. 2008. "Foreign Authority and the Politics of Impartiality in Postwar Bosnia-Herzegovina." PhD diss., University of Chicago.

Glück, Leopold. 1890. "Hamajlije i Zapisi u Narodnjem Ljekarstvu Bosne i Herzegovine." *Glasnik Zemaljskog Muzeja* 2: 49–53.

Godelier, Maurice. 1999. *The Enigma of the Gift*. Chicago: University of Chicago Press.

Good, Byron. 1994. *Medicine, Rationality, and Experience: An Anthropological Perspective*. Cambridge: Cambridge University Press.

Graeber, David. 2011. *Debt: The First 5,000 Years*. New York: Melville House.

Hacking, Ian. 1995. *Rewriting the Soul: Multiple Personality and the Sciences of Memory.* Princeton, NJ: Princeton University Press.

Halberstam, Judith, and Ira Livingston, eds. 1999. *Posthuman Bodies.* Bloomington: Indiana University Press.

Han, Clara. 2011. "Symptoms of Another Life: Time, Possibility, and Domestic Relations in Chile's Credit Economy." *Cultural Anthropology* 26 (1): 7–32.

———. 2012. *Life in Debt: Times of Care and Violence in Neoliberal Chile.* Berkeley: University of California Press.

Handžić, Mehmed. 2004. *Zbirka Izabranih Dova (Iz Kur'ana i Hadisa).* Sarajevo: El-Kalem.

Hann, Chris M., ed. 2002. *Postsocialism: Ideals, Ideologies, and Practices in Eurasia.* London: Routledge.

Haraway, Donna. 2008. *When Species Meet.* Minneapolis: University of Minnesota Press.

Harman, Graham. 2005. *Guerrilla Metaphysics: Phenomenology and the Carpentry of Things.* Chicago: Open Court Publishing.

———. 2009. *Prince of Networks: Bruno Latour and Metaphysics.* Melbourne: re.press.

Harrington, Anne, ed. 1997. *The Placebo Effect: An Interdisciplinary Exploration.* Cambridge, MA: Harvard University Press.

———. 2007. *The Cure Within: History of Mind–Body Medicine.* New York: W.W. Norton & Company.

Hart, Keith. 2001. *Money in an Unequal World: Keith Hart and His Memory Bank.* New York: Texere.

Harvey, David. 1989. *The Condition of Postmodernity: An Enquiry into the Origins of Cultural Change.* Oxford: Blackwell Publishing.

———. 1991. *The Limits to Capital.* New York: Verso.

———. 2003. *The New Imperialism.* Oxford: Oxford University Press.

———. 2010. *The Enigma of Capital and the Crises of Capitalism.* Oxford: Oxford University Press.

Hawkins, Gay. 2010. "Plastic Materialities." In *Political Matter: Technoscience, Democracy, and Public Life,* edited by Bruce Braun and Sarah J. Whatmore, 119–139. Minneapolis: University of Minnesota Press.

Hayden, Robert. 1999. *Blueprints for a House Divided: The Constitutional Logic of the Yugoslav Conflicts.* Ann Arbor: University of Michigan Press.

Healy, David. 2002. *The Creation of Psychopharmacology.* Cambridge, MA: Harvard University Press.

Hedges, Ellie, and James Beckfort. 2000. "Holism, Healing and the New Age." In *Beyond New Age: Exploring Alternative Spirituality,* edited by Steven Sutcliffe and Marion Bowman, 169–87. Edinburgh: Edinburgh University Press.

Heelas, Peter. 1993. "The New Age in Cultural Context: The Premodern, the Modern and the Postmodern." *Religion* 23 (2): 103–116.

———. 1996. *The New Age Movement.* Oxford: Blackwell Publishers.

———. 1999. "Prosperity and the New Age Movement: The Efficacy of Spiritual Economics." In *New Religious Movements: Challenge and Response,* edited by Bryan Wilson and Jamie Cresswell, 51–78. London: Routledge.

Highmore, Ben. 2001. *The Everyday Life Reader.* New York: Routledge.

Hill, Michael. 1992. "New Zealand's Cultic Milieu: Individualism and the Logic of Consumerism." In *Religion: Contemporary Issues. The All Souls Seminars in the Sociology of Religion,* edited by Bryan Wilson, 216–236. London: Bellow Publishing.

Horvat, Branko. 1969. *Ogled o Jugoslovenskom Društvu.* Zagreb: Mladost.

———. 1970. *Privredni Sistem i Ekonomska Politika Jugoslavije. Problemi, Teorije, Ostvarenja, Propusti.* Belgrade: Institut Ekonomskih Nauka.

Hromadžic, Azra. 2015. *Citizens of an Empty Nation: Youth and State-Making in Postwar Bosnia-Herzegovina.* Philadelphia: University of Pennsylvania Press.

Ihde, Don. 2003. "If Phenomenology Is an Albatross, Is *Post-phenomenology* Possible?" In *Chasing Technoscience: Matrix for Materiality,* edited by Don Ihde and Evan Selinger, 147–166. Bloomington: Indiana University Press.

Ingold, Tim. 2006. "Re-Thinking the Animate, Re-animating Thought." *Ethnos* 71 (1): 9–20.

International Monetary Fund. 2004. IMF Country Report No. 04/67, March 2004. Available at https://www.imf.org/external/pubs/ft/scr/2004/cr0467.pdf.

Jablonski, Nina. 2006. *Skin: A Natural History.* Berkeley: University of California Press.

James, William. 1976. *Essays in Radical Empiricism.* Edited by Fredson Bowers and Ignas K. Skrupskelis. Cambridge, MA: Harvard University Press.

———. 1977. *A Pluralistic Universe.* Edited by Fredson Bowers and Ignas K. Skrupskelis. Cambridge, MA: Harvard University Press.

Jansen, Stef, Čarna Brković, and Vanja Čelebčić, eds. 2016. *Negotiating Social Relations in Bosnia and Herzegovina: Semiperipheral Entanglements.* Aldershot, UK: Ashgate.

Jašarević, Larisa. 2005. "Everyday Work: Subsistence Economy, Social Belonging, and Moralities of Exchange at a Bosnian (Black) Market." In *The New Bosnian Mosaic: Identities, Memories, and Moral Claims in a Post-War Society,* edited by Xavier Bougarel, Elissa Helms, and Ger Duijzings, 273–294. Aldershot, UK: Ashgate.

———. 2012a. "Pouring Out Postsocialist Fears: Practical Metaphysics of a Therapy at a Distance." *Comparative Studies in Society and History* 54 (4): 1–28.

———. 2012b. "Grave Matters and the Good Life: On a Finite Economy in Bosnia." *Cambridge Anthropology* 30 (1): 25–39.

———. 2014a. "Speculative Technologies: Debt, Love, and Divination in a Transnationalizing Market." *Debt: Women Studies Quarterly* 42 (1–2): 261–277.

———. 2014b. "Interplanetary Present: On a Public Spectacle of Healing and Gifting." In *The 21st Century Gift.* Special Issue of the *Anthropology Forum.* 24 (4): 427–439.

———. 2015. "The Thing in a Jar: Mushrooms and Ontological Speculations in Post-Yugoslavia." *Cultural Anthropology* 30 (1): 36–64.

Jay, Martin. 1995. "The Limits of Limit Experience: Bataille and Foucault." *Constellations* 2 (2): 154–174. Oxford: Blackwell Publishing.

———. 2005. *Songs of Experience: Modern American and European Variations on a Universal Theme.* Berkeley: University of California Press.

Kardelj, Edvard. 1954. *Problemi naše Socijalističke Izgradnje.* Belgrade: Kultura.

———. 1978. *Pravci Razvoja Političkog Sistema Socijalističkog Samoupravljanja.* Belgrade: Komunista.

Kleinman, Arthur. 1980. *Patients and Healers in the Context of Culture: An Exploration of the Borderland between Anthropology, Medicine, and Psychiatry*. Berkeley: University of California Press.

Klima, Alan. 2002. *The Funeral Casino: Meditation, Massacre and Exchange with the Dead in Thailand*. Princeton, NJ: Princeton University Press.

———. 2006. "Spirits of 'Dark Finance' in Thailand: A Local Hazard for the International Moral Fund." *Cultural Dynamics* 18 (1): 33–60.

———. 2008. "Thai Love Thai: Financing Emotion in Post-Crash Thailand." In *The Anthropology of Globalization: A Reader*, edited by Jonathan Xavier Inda and Renato Rosaldo, 121–137. Oxford: Blackwell Publishing.

Kohn, Eduardo. 2013. *How Forests Think: Toward an Anthropology beyond the Human*. Berkeley: University of California Press.

———. 2015. "Anthropology of Ontologies." *Annual Review of Anthropology* 44: 311–327.

Kovačević, Kosta. 1888. "Kako se Liječi od Strave?" *Bosanska Vila*, September 1.

Kukavica, Urjan. 2010. "Sveta Povijest i Duhovno Viteštvo u Bosni i Herzegovini (tekije, elvije, sufije, ratnici, pjesnici)." *Behar* 95: 3–74.

Kurtovic, Larisa. 2012. "Politics of Impasse: Specters of Socialism and the Struggles for the Future in Postwar Bosnia-Hercegovina." PhD diss., University of California, Berkeley.

Lampe, John, Russell Prickett, and Ljubiša Adamović. 1990. *Yugoslav-American Economic Relations Since World War II*. Durham, NC: Duke University Press

Langwick, Stacey. 2007. "Devils, Parasites and Fierce Needles: Healing and the Politics of Translation in Southeastern Tanzania." *Science, Technology, and Human Values* 32 (1): 88–117.

——— 2011. *Bodies, Politics, and African Healing: The Matter of Maladies in Tanzania*. Bloomington: Indiana University Press.

Latour, Bruno. 1993. *We Have Never Been Modern*. Cambridge, MA: Harvard University Press.

———. 2005. *Reassembling the Social: An Introduction to Actor-Network-Theory*. Oxford: Oxford University Press.

———. 2010. *On the Modern Cult of the Factish Gods*. Durham, NC: Duke University Press.

———. 2013. *An Inquiry into Modes of Existence: An Anthropology of the Moderns*. Translated by Catherine Porter. Cambridge, MA: Harvard University Press.

Levi-Strauss, Claude. 1962. *The Savage Mind*. Chicago: University of Chicago Press.

———. 1969. *The Elementary Structures of Kinship*. Boston: Beacon Press.

———. 1976. "The Sorcerer and His Magic." In *Structural Anthropology*, 167–185. Chicago: University of Chicago Press.

Lindh de Montoya, Monica, and James Kent McNeil. 2003. "Microcredit Organizations and Savings Mobilizations in Bosnia and Herzegovina. An Assessment for USAID." USAID Financial Center for Advocacy and Training.

Lindquist, Gallina. 2006. *Conjuring Hope: Healing and Magic in Contemporary Russia*. New York: Berghahn Books.

Lock, Margaret. 1993. *Encounters with Aging: Mythologies of Menopause in Japan and North America*. Berkeley: University of California Press.

————. 2001. *Twice Dead: Organ Transplants and the Reinvention of Death*. Berkeley: University of California Press.

————. 2008. "Living with Uncertainty: The Genetics of Late Onset Alzheimer's Disease." *General Anthropology* 13 (2): 1–9.

Lock, Margaret, and Judith Farquhar, eds. 2007. *Beyond the Body Proper: Reading the Anthropology of Material Life*. Durham, NC: Duke University Press.

Lock, Margaret, and Deborah Gordon. 1988. *Biomedicine Examined*. New York: Springer Science & Business.

Lock, Margaret, and Vinh-Kim Nguyen. 2010. *An Anthropology of Biomedicine*. Oxford: Wiley-Blackwell.

Lockwood, William. 1975. *European Moslems: Economy and Ethnicity in Western Bosnia*. New York: Academic Press.

Low, Setha, and Sally Engle Merry. 2010. "Engaged Anthropology: Diversity and Dilemmas. Introduction to Supplement 2." *Current Anthropology* 51 (S2): S203-S226.

Lūse, Agita, and Imre Lázár. 2007. *Cosmologies of Suffering, Post-Communist Transformation, Sacral Communication, and Healing*. New Castle, UK: Cambridge Scholars Publishing.

Luthar, Breda, and Maruša Pušnik. 2010. *Remembering Utopia: The Culture of Everyday Life in Socialist Yugoslavia*. Washington, DC: New Academia Publishing.

Malinowski, Bronislaw. (1922) 1984. *Argonauts of the Western Pacific: An Account of Native Enterprise and Adventure in the Archipelagos of Melanesian New Guinea*. Long Grove, IL: Waveland Press.

Manning, Robert. 2000. *Credit Card Nation: The Consequences of America's Addiction to Credit*. New York: Basic Books.

Marchart, Oliver. 2007. *Post-Foundational Political Thought: Political Difference in Nancy, Lefort, Badiou, and Laclau*. Edinburgh: Edinburgh University Press.

Marx, Karl. (1867) 1967. *Capital: A Critique of Political Economy Volume 1*. London: Lawrence & Wishart.

Masquelier, Adeline. 2001. *Prayer Has Spoiled Everything: Possession, Power, and Identity in an Islamic Town of Niger*. Durham, NC: Duke University Press.

Matić, Milan, Stanislav Stojanović, and Čedomir štrbac. 1972. *Tito o Radničkoj Klasi*. Radnička štampa: Belgrad.

Mauss, Marcel. (1902) 2001. *A General Theory of Magic*. London: Routledge.

————. (1954) 1990. *The Gift: Forms and Functions of Exchange in Archaic Societies*. New York: W.W. Norton.

Mazzarella, William. 2003. *Shoveling Smoke: Advertising and Globalization in Contemporary India*. Durham, NC: Duke University Press.

McIntosh, Janet. 2009. *The Edge of Islam: Power, Personhood, and Ethnoreligious Boundaries on the Kenya Coast*. Durham, NC: Duke University Press.

Medawar, Charles, and Anita Hardon. 2004. *Medicines Out of Control? Antidepressants and the Conspiracy of Goodwill*. Amsterdam: Aksant Academic Publishers.

Merleau-Ponty, Maurice. (1945) 1958. *The Phenomenology of Perception*. Translated by Colin Smith. London: Routledge.

Meyer, Birgit, and Peter Pels, eds. 2003. *Magic and Modernity: Interfaces of Revelation and Concealment*. Stanford, CA: Stanford University Press.

Mijatović, Jova. 1982. *Travar. Trave i Melemi.* Belgrade: Porodica i Domaćinstvo.

Miles, Anne, and Leatherman, Thomas. 2003. "Perspectives on Medical Anthropology in the Andes." In *Medical Pluralism in the Andes,* edited by Joan D. Koss-Chioino, Thomas Leatherman, and Christine Greenway, 3–15. London: Routledge.

Mittermaier, Amira. 2011. *Dreams that Matter: Egyptian Landscapes of the Imagination* Berkeley: University of California Press.

Miyazaki, Hirokazu. 2009. "The Temporality of No Hope." In *Ethnographies of Neoliberalism*, edited by Carol Greenhouse, 238–251. Philadelphia: University of Pennsylvania Press.

Morton, Timothy. 2013. *Hyperobjects: Philosophy and Ecology after the End of the World.* Minneapolis: University of Minnesota Press.

Munk, Kristine. 2004. "Medicine-Men, Modernity and Magic: Syncretism as an Explanatory Category to Recent Religious Responses and Magical Practices among Urban Blacks in Contemporary South Africa." In *Syncretism in Religion: A Reader,* edited by Anita Maria Leopold and Jeppe Sinding Jensen, 362-75. New York: Routledge, 2004.

Munn, Nancy. 1986. *The Fame of Gawa: A Symbolic Study of Value Transformation in a Massim (Papua New Guinea) Society.* Cambridge: Cambridge University Press.

Nancy, Jean-Luc. 1991. *The Inoperative Community.* Translated by Peter Connor. Edited by Peter Connor, Lisa Garbus, Michael Holland, and Simona Sawhney. Minneapolis: University of Minnesota Press.

———. 2000. *Being Singular Plural.* Translated by Robert Richardson and Anne O'Byrne. Stanford, CA: Stanford University Press.

———. 2008a. *Corpus.* Translated by Richard A. Rand. New York: Fordham University Press.

———. 2008b. *Noli me tangere. On the Rising of the Body.* Translated by Sarah Clift, Pascale-Anne Brault, and Michael Naas. New York: Fordham University Press.

———. 2008c. *Dis-Enclosure. The Deconstruction of Christianity.* Translated by Bettina Bergo, Gabriel Malenfant, and Michael B. Smith. New York: Fordham University Press.

———. 2009. *The Fall of Sleep.* Translated by Charlotte Mandell. New York: Fordham University Press.

Neumann Fridman, Eva Jane. 2004. "Ways of Knowing and Healing; Shamanism in the Republics of Tuva and Buryatia in Post-Soviet Russia." In *Divination and Healing; Potent Vision,* edited by Michael Winkelman and Philip Peek, 139–165. Tucson: University of Arizona Press.

Nichter, Mark, and Lock, Margaret, eds. 2002. *New Horizons in Medical Anthropology: Essays in Honor of Charles Leslie.* London: Routledge.

Niemoczynski, Leon. 2013. "21st Century Speculative Philosophy: Reflections on the 'New Metaphysics' and Its Realism and Materialism." *Cosmos and History: The Journal of Natural and Social Philosophy* 9 (2): 13–31.

Panagio, Davide. 2009. *The Political Life of Sensation.* Durham, NC: Duke University Press.

Pedersen, Morten Axel. 2011. *Not Quite Shamans: Spirit Worlds and Political Lives in Northern Mongolia.* Ithaca, NY: Cornell University Press.

Pekarić, Vehid. 1998. *Spoznaja Duhovnog Svijeta i Liječenje Duševnih Bolesti.* Gračanica: Grin.

Pelagić, Vasa. (1888) 2008. *Narodni Učitelj.* Belgrade: Beoknjiga.

Pickering, Andrew. 2003. "On Becoming: Imagination, Metaphysics, and the Mangle." In *Chasing Technoscience: Matrix for Materiality,* edited by Don Ihde and Evan Selinger, 96–116. Bloomington: Indiana University Press.

Pine, Frances, and João de Pina-Cabral, eds. 2008. *On the Margins of Religion.* New York: Berghahn Books.

Plestina, Dijana. 1992. *Regional Development in Communist Yugoslavia: Success, Failure, and Consequences.* Boulder, CO: Westview Press.

Portata, Barbara. 2007. "Regressing into the Past: Past Lives and Collective Memory in Post-socialist Slovenia." In *Cosmologies of Suffering, Post-communist Transformation, Sacral Communication, and Healing,* edited by Agita Lūse and Imre Lázár, 107–128. Cambridge: Cambridge University Press.

Possamai, Adam 2005. *In Search of New Age Spiritualities.* London: Ashgate.

Principe, Lawrence. 2013. *The Secrets of Alchemy.* Chicago: Chicago University Press.

Pugh, Michael. 2005. "Transformation in the Bosnian Political Economy since Dayton." *International Peacekeeping* 12 (3): 448–462.

Radenković, Ljubinko. 1996. *Simbolika Sveta u Narodnoj Magiji Južnih Slovena.* Niš: Prosveta.

Rajan, Kaushik Sunder. 2006. *Biocapital: The Constitution of Postgenomic Life.* Durham, NC: Duke University Press.

Rajan, Kaushik Sunder, ed. 2012. *Lively Capital: Biotechnologies, Ethics, and Governance in Global Markets.* Durham, NC: Duke University Press.

Rihtman-Auguštin, Dunja. 1988. *Etnologija Naše Svakodnevnice.* Zagreb: Školska Knjiga.

Rivkin-Fish, Michele. 2005. "Bribes, Gifts, and Unofficial Payments: Rethinking Corruption in Post-Soviet Russian Health Care." In *Corruption: Anthropological Perspectives,* edited by Dieter Haller and Chris Shore, 47–64. London: Pluto Press.

Sadiković, Sadik. 1988. *Narodno Zdravlje.* Sarajevo: Svjetlost.

Schatz, Edward. 2009. *Political Ethnography: What Immersion Contributes to the Study of Politics.* Chicago: Chicago University Press.

Schrift, Alan. 1997. *The Logic of the Gift: Toward an Ethic of Generosity.* London: Routledge.

Scott, Joan. 1991. "The Evidence of Experience." In *Questions of Evidence: Proof, Practice and Persuasion across the Disciplines,* edited by James K. Chandler, Arnold I. Davidson, and Harry D. Harootunian, 363–388. Chicago: University of Chicago Press.

Šefer, Berislav.1965. *Životni Standard i Privredni Razvoj Jugoslavije.* Zabreb: Informator.

Shevchenko, Olga. 2008. *Crisis and the Everyday in Postsocialist Moscow.* Bloomington: Indiana University Press.

Smith, James Howard. 2008. *Bewitching Development: Witchcraft and the Reinvention of Development in Neoliberal Kenya.* Chicago: University of Chicago Press.

Štahan, Josip. 1974. *Životni Standard u Jugoslaviji.* Zagreb: Globus.

Steingraber, Sandra. 2010. *Living Downstream: An Ecologist's Personal Investigation of Cancer and the Environment.* Philadelphia, PA: Da Capo Press.

Stengers, Isabelle. 2000. *The Invention of Modern Science*. Translated by Daniel W. Smith. Minneapolis: University of Minnesota Press.

———. 2003. "The Doctor and the Charlatan." *Cultural Studies Review* 9 (2): 11–36.

———. 2010. "Including Nonhumans in Political Theory: Opening Pandora's Box?" In *Political Matter: Technoscience, Democracy, and Public Life*, edited by Bruce Braun and Sarah J. Whatmore, 3–35. Minneapolis: University of Minnesota Press.

———. 2011. "Wondering about Materialism." In *The Speculative Turn: Continental Materialism and Realism*, edited by Levi Bryant, Nick Srnicek, and Graham Harman, 368–380. Melbourne: re.press.

———. 2012. "Reclaiming Animism." *e-flux journal*, July (36): 1–10.

Stewart, Kathleen. 2001. "Real American Dreams Can Be Nightmares." In *Cultural Studies and Political Theory*, edited by Jodi Dean, 243–257. Ithaca, NY: Cornell University Press.

Stites, Elizabeth, Sue Lautze, Dyan Mazurana, and Alma Anic. 2005. "Coping with War, Coping with Peace: Livelihood Adaptation in Bosnia-Herzegovina, 1989–2004." Feinstein International Famine Center (FIFC), Friedman School of Nutrition Policy and Science, Tufts University, and Mercy Corps International. http://reliefweb.int /sites/reliefweb.int/files/resources/98E8BFFC00C9FB83C1257019003774D3-FIFC %20MCI%20Bosnia%20Livelihoods%20Study.pdf.

Stitziel, Judd. 2005. *Fashioning Socialism: Clothing, Politics, and Consumer Culture in East Germany*. Oxford: Berg.

Strange, Susan. 1986. *Casino Capitalism*. Oxford: Blackwell.

Štulanović, Muharem. 2007. *Liječenje Kur'anom Od Ograisanja, Sihira, i Uroka*. Novi Pazar: El-Kalimeh.

Subotica, Andreja, and David Wildman. 2003. "Health Profile—Bosnia and Herzegovina." DFID Health Systems Resource Center with the London School of Hygiene and Tropical Medicine (LSHTM). http://www.lshtm.ac.uk/ecohost/see.

Sutcliffe, Steven. 2003. *Children of the New Age: A History of Spiritual Practices*. London: Routledge.

Taussig, Michael. 1987. *Shamanism, Colonialism, and the Wild Man: A Study in Terror and Healing*. Chicago: University of Chicago Press.

———. 1993. *Mimesis and Alterity: A Particular History of the Senses*. New York: Routledge.

———. 1995. "The Sun Gives without Receiving: An Old Story. *Comparative Studies in Society and History* 37 (3): 368–398.

———. 2003. "Viscerality, Faith, and Skepticism: Another Theory of Magic," In *Magic and Modernity: Interfaces of Revelation and Concealment*, edited by Birgit Meyer and Peter Pels, 272–306. Stanford, CA: Stanford University Press.

Truhelka, Ćiro. 1889. "Bosanci Žive u Vjeri o Dobrim Dusima i o Zlodusima." *Gradja Zemaljskog Muzeja*, 1 (IV): 237–239.

Turner, Victor. 1968. *Drums of Affliction: A Study of Religious Process among the Ndembu of Zambia*. Oxford: Clarendon Press.

Turner, Victor, and Edward Bruner, eds. 1986. *The Anthropology of Experience*. Urbana: University of Illinois Press.

Ugljen, Sadik. 1893. "Olovo kao Narodni Lijek." *Glasnik Zemaljskog Muzeja*, 5: 168–170.

Velimirović, Danijela. 2006. "Odjevanje Jovanke Broz." *Anthropologija* 1: 50–60.

Viveiros de Castro, Eduardo. 2009. "Intensive filiation and demonic alliance." In *Deleuzian Intersections: Science, Technology, Anthropology*, edited by Carl Bruun Jensen and Kjetil Rödje, 219–253. New York: Bergahn Books.

Vlahović, Petar. 1972. *Običaji, Verovanja, i Praznoverice Naroda Jugoslavije*. Belgrade: Beogradski izdavačko-grafički zavod.

Wagner, Sarah. 2008. *To Know Where He Lies. DNA Technology and the Search for Srebrenica's Missing*. Berkeley: University of California Press.

Whyte, Susan Reynolds, Sjaak Van der Gist, and Anita Hardon. 2000. *Social Lives of Medicines*. Cambridge: Cambridge University Press.

Wiener, Margaret. 1995. *Visible and Invisible Realms: Power, Magic, and Colonial Conquest in Bali*. Chicago: University of Chicago Press.

Williams, Brett. 2004. *Debt for Sale: A Social History of the Credit Trap*. Philadelphia: University of Pennsylvania Press.

Williams, Raymond. 1981. *Politics and Letters: Interviews with New Left Review*. London: Verso.

Winkelman, Michael, and Philip Peek. 2004. *Divination and Healing: Potent Vision*. Tucson: University of Arizona Press.

Woodward, Susan L. 1995. *Socialist Unemployment: The Political Economy of Yugoslavia, 1945–1990*. Princeton, NJ: Princeton University Press.

———. 1996. "The West and the International Organisations." In *Yugoslavia and After: A Study in Fragmentation, Despair, and Rebirth*, edited by David Dyker and Ivan Vejvoda, 155–176. New York: Longman.

Zupčević, Merima, and Fikret Čaušević. 2009. Case Study: Bosnia and Herzegovina. Sarajevo: Center for Developing Area Studies—McGill University and the World Bank.

INDEX

LARISA JAŠAREVIĆ is Senior Lecturer in the Global and International Studies Program at the University of Chicago. An anthropologist, she is interested in health, bodies, and natures as well as medicine and popular knowledges in contemporary Bosnia.

Printed and bound by CPI Group (UK) Ltd, Croydon, CR0 4YY

27/10/2024

14580187-0001